Harm Reduction

Pragmatic Strategies for Managing High-Risk Behaviors

Edited by

G. ALAN MARLATT

Foreword by David B. Abrams
and David C. Lewis

THE GUILFORD PRESS
New York London

© 1998 The Guilford Press
A Division of Guilford Publications, Inc.
72 Spring Street, New York, NY 10012
www.guilford.com

Printed in the United States of America

This book is printed on acid-free paper.

Last digit is print number: 9 8 7 6 5 4

Library of Congress Cataloging-in-Publication Data

Harm reduction : pragmatic strategies for managing high-risk behaviors
  / edited by G. Alan Marlatt.
      p.   cm.
    Includes bibliographical references and index.
    ISBN 1-57230-397-2 (hc.)   ISBN 1-57230-825-7 (pbk.)
    1. Substance abuse—Complications—Prevention.   2. Substance
abuse—Treatment.   3. Health behavior—Social aspects.   I. Marlatt,
G. Alan.
RC564.H364   1998
616.86—dc21   98-37938
                                                                   CIP

*To my mother, Vera, and her mother, Winnifred,
who set the tone for this book*

Contributors

John S. Baer, PhD, VA Medical Center, Seattle; Addictive Behaviors Research Center, Department of Psychology, University of Washington, Seattle, WA

Arthur W. Blume, MA, Addictive Behaviors Research Center, Department of Psychology, University of Washington, Seattle, WA

Fransing Daisy, PhD, HIVNET Project, School of Medicine, University of Washington, Seattle, WA

Linda A. Dimeff, PhD, Addictive Behaviors Research Center, Department of Psychology, University of Washington, Seattle, WA

E. Mike Gorman, PhD, MPH, MSW, Alcohol and Drug Abuse Institute, University of Washington, Seattle, WA

Elizabeth H. Hawkins, MS, Addictive Behaviors Research Center, Department of Psychology, University of Washington, Seattle, WA

Jason Kilmer, PhD, Addictive Behaviors Research Center, Department of Psychology, University of Washington, Seattle, WA

Mary Larimer, PhD, Addictive Behaviors Research Center, Department of Psychology, University of Washington, Seattle, WA

G. Alan Marlatt, PhD, Addictive Behaviors Research Center, Department of Psychology, University of Washington, Seattle, WA

Elizabeth Miller, MS, Addictive Behaviors Research Center, Department of Psychology, University of Washington, Seattle, WA

Heather Brady Murch, MA, Addictive Behaviors Research Center, Department of Psychology, University of Washington, Seattle, WA

Peggy L. Peterson, PhD, MPH, Alcohol and Drug Abuse Institute, University of Washington, Seattle, WA

Lori A. Duthie Quigley, PhD, Department of Psychiatry, University of California, San Francisco, San Francisco, CA

Lisa J. Roberts, MA, Addictive Behaviors Research Center, Department of Psychology, University of Washington, Seattle, WA

Martin J. Stern, PhD, Psychology Services, Santa Clara Valley Medical Center, San Jose, CA

Susan Tapert, PhD, Psychiatry Service, San Diego VA Healthcare System, San Diego, CA

Lisa R. Thomas, BA, Addictive Behaviors Research Center, Department of Psychology, University of Washington, Seattle, WA

Kenneth R. Weingardt, PhD, Alcohol and Drug Abuse Institute, University of Washington, Seattle, WA

Imani Woods, Center for Health Education and Research, University of Washington, Seattle, WA

Charlene Worley, ScM, North American Indian Center of Boston, Inc., Boston, MA

Foreword

Hippocrates, writing in the 5th century B.C., advised people coming to a new city to assess whether it was likely to be a healthy or an unhealthy place to live. He suggested that they evaluate its geography and water supply—was it "soft, hard, or salty?" He advised them to observe the behavior of its inhabitants—"whether they are fond of excessive drinking and eating, and prone to indolence, or else fond of exercise and hard work." These recommendations were an early articulation of a harm reduction approach, an approach we can reemphasize now, at the dawn of the 21st century.

Viewing individuals as responsible for their own choices and as both agents and recipients of environmental influence is central to the harm reduction paradigm. Individuals must be engaged "where they are" and moved from there in small manageable steps to increasing levels of improved self-care, health, and well-being.

The modern harm reduction movement effectively deals with already afflicted individuals and high-risk groups because it is a pragmatic, nonjudgmental, and humane philosophy. It chooses health and personal responsibility over punishment for behavioral misadventures. It chooses treatment of all varieties, including abstinence-based approaches, over incarceration of the addicted. Moreover, it is less costly. On the average, treatment of addiction to illegal drugs costs $1,800 to $6,800 annually compared with $25,900 on the average for incarceration. Treating tobacco addiction costs $500 to $6,000 per quality adjusted life year saved (QUALY) compared with from $30,000 to over $150,000 per QUALY for treatment of tobacco-related cancers and heart disease.

But harm reduction is much more than a humane approach to those at highest risk and already suffering the consequences of their behaviors, it can apply to the whole population, stretching along a continuum of risk from high to low. The broadest way that harm reduction can be conceptualized is in relation to prevention in populations who are not yet afflicted by the problem in question. A great number of individuals in a society fall into these low- and moderate-risk groups, making the potential benefit of harm reduction large.

It is now well accepted that lifestyle factors such as tobacco, diet, alcohol abuse, and sedentary lifestyle are the leading causes of disease burden in developed countries. Moreover, socioeconomic factors, especially poverty, result in the clustering of lifestyle and environmental risk factors, further contributing to the absolute disease burden in populations. In impoverished communities, individuals are at greatest risk and face enormous barriers to becoming healthier. Behavioral choices have been documented as the source of over half of all preventable deaths and disabilities in the United States, raising convincing humanitarian and socioeconomic imperatives to intervene.

The situation in the developed nations will be dramatically repeated for the developing world by the year 2020 as estimated by the World Health organization's Report on the Global Burden of Disease, 1996. The next two decades will see huge changes in the health needs of the world's population. The traditional enemies—infectious diseases and malnutrition—will be replaced as the leading causes of disability and premature death by behavioral factors. In fact, by 2020 tobacco product use will be the leading cause of preventable disability in the world. These trends will overwhelm smaller scale solutions such as acute care medicine or rationing care. Every developed country now faces the increasing social and financial burden of preventable disease. The very large numbers involved impose serious challenges to health care systems and force difficult decisions about the allocation of limited resources.

In light of these trends in developed and developing nations, health delivery systems will have to change. Up to now, the industrial nations have focused on the prevailing medical model by placing the overwhelming majority of their resources into acute care interventions. If our mandate is to prevent or lessen the negative impact of lifestyle behaviors, we will need a prevention strategy and newly energized delivery system. As foreseen by George Pickering in 1954, the idea of a sharp distinction between health and disease is a medical artifact for which nature, if consulted, provides no support. The delivery systems must shift to population-based health planning and the management of chronic disease. Fortunately, medicine and public health, insulated from one another for most of the 20th century, are now beginning to explore the advantages of interdisciplinary collaboration.

In his book *The Structure of Scientific Revolutions*, Thomas Kuhn defines a paradigm shift as occurring through crossdisciplinary collaboration in which there is a loosening of old paradigms. New syntheses are born as simplistic dichotomies, break down, and give way to a deeper understanding of complex interactions between genes and environment, nature and nurture, individual and community, health and disease, mind and body. At every level of society, we possess greater knowledge that can be applied both individually and collectively to improve our well-being.

Traditional disciplinary boundaries are dissolving, creating unprecedented opportunity for new solutions to old problems. There is growing transnational interdependence with new cultures being shaped by global social and economic forces. Burgeoning information facilitates policy and public health planning within and across nations. Breakthroughs in biology, behavioral and social sciences, and epidemiology are facilitating understanding of the complex molecular, genetic, and psychosocial interactions underlying addictive and other risky behaviors. New ideas can be disseminated with amazing speed. Harm reduction strategies are gaining momentum all over the world.

In the United States, there are calls to create a new agenda for health care for the next century, one that effectively addresses behaviors. Inevitably, the sharp distinctions between the medical/disease model and harm reduction will begin to be altered as their principles and practices draw more closely together. This shift has already begun. Primary care physicians who embrace the disease model of addiction are also often active practitioners of harm reduction. For example, there is an increasing willingness to ask all patients those uncomfortable questions about alcohol, tobacco, other drugs, and sexual practices, and then provide brief interventions to prevent harm.

Harm reduction is a good model for helping to loosen old boundaries and for bridging the gaps between medicine and public health. In fact, the history of public health practice centers on harm reduction strategies, from cleaning up the water supply to tracking infectious disease. Preventive and harm reduction measures go hand in hand. Measures such as discouraging youth from tobacco addiction, slowing or reversing progression to hard drug use, encouraging sexual abstinence and "safe sex," and fostering the maintenance of normal body weight, a healthy diet, and regular physical activity, will have to be applied as early in the human lifespan as possible to help prevent cancers, heart disease, addictions, and communicable and infectious diseases later on.

Harm reduction is not new to medicine. After all, it is not so far from the Hippocratic advice to young physicians *primum non nocere*—first, do no harm. In its modern dress, harm reduction takes on special meanings which make it an attractive and fundamentally sound approach. In particular, it helps challenge basic dogma and unproved emotional assumptions on either side of the medical–public health divide. The current movement encourages a critical reappraisal, a common-sense, pragmatic integration of the best each has to offer. Avoiding the traps of abstract theory or moral philosophy, a balanced rational collaboration between medical and public health paradigms may help achieve what neither can do on its own and encourage not only synergism but new creative solutions to age-old problems.

What is true in our general approach to health care is equally true when considering addictions. It is no longer possible to simplify concepts of addiction into physiological versus psychological versus sociocultural or to draw a clear line between the gradations of addiction liability from mild to moderate to severe. There is growing recognition that addictive and other risky behaviors result from complex interactions among biopsychosocial factors with exquisite individual variations in choice of behavior or drug, pattern of use, and reasons for use.

We envision a prevention strategy that can be built by matching interventions to levels of risk, focusing on policies and communities as well as on individuals, and applying a spectrum of approaches—some preventing the problem from getting started, others preventing progression once the problem has occurred. The emerging harm reduction strategy can provide new energy for a revamping of the delivery system. Harm reduction is a new synthesis, a paradigm to guide action—in the Kuhnian sense, a scientific revolution.

Fundamentally and perhaps above all, the harm reduction strategy is a movement intended to empower the patient and the consumer of health services. It seeks to blunt the power differential between those who administer and deliver health services and those who receive them, to give a voice in the decisions of how, where, and in what manner people are to be treated.

The breaking down of old rules and the formation of new movements is always filled with strong emotion, deep fear, and great hope. Policies and other cultural "rules" designed to balance community and individual needs generally exist in a tension between extremes. Education can become brainwashing, police protection can become oppression, and public leadership can become monomania. Similarly, harm reduction can be oversimplified and then demonized as an extremist movement. Alternatively, it can be viewed as a new overarching conceptual blueprint for integrating the best of medicine, public health, and prevention policy. Harm reduction can address the emergent needs of societies in a rapidly changing 21st century.

This book by G. Alan Marlatt and colleagues is timely, searching for common ground to provide a step-by-step pathway toward practical solutions that lead to new public policies. Not only do the first three chapters (Part I) place the extremist views in perspective, they dispel the myths about harm reduction, zero tolerance, and the medical model. The next four chapters (Part II) are the heart and soul of this remarkable book, and present evidence supporting the basic tenets and strategies of harm reduction. The diversity of strategies are placed firmly within the framework of the real world—what any worker in the front lines can do to help empower people, improve their well-being, and reduce their burden on society. Part III examines population groups at disproportionate risk and most in need. Part IV explores policy and organizational issues. Marlatt and his colleagues have done an enormous service to humankind by documenting the potential for harm reduction in a straightforward manner.

Within the context of the wrenching and rapid social changes that today's societies are undergoing, can the voices of reason and maturity prevail against the extreme oversimplification and polarization that have characterized so many of the largely ineffectual approaches for treating drug problems and other risky behaviors? Is our society secure and mature enough to allow for the shades of gray that reflect the reality of how to approach individual, collective, and policy recommendations for the 21st century and beyond? Can society embrace the best ideas from harm reduction paradigms and can the harm reduction movement avoid being labeled extremist? The authors of this excellent book think that it is possible. We hope so.

DAVID B. ABRAMS, PhD
Center for Behavioral and Preventive Medicine
Brown University, Providence, Rhode Island

DAVID C. LEWIS, MD
Center for Alcohol and Addiction Studies
Brown University, Providence, Rhode Island

Preface

People often ask me how I first became interested in harm reduction. In 1990, I had the good fortune to spend two months working and living in Amsterdam at the invitation of Jan A. Walburg, general director of the Jellinek (named after E. M. Jellinek, an American expert on alcoholism), an internationally recognized center for the prevention and treatment of substance dependence and addiction problems in the Netherlands. In return for my teaching clinical courses in relapse prevention, I was taught the basics of the Dutch model of harm reduction (described in detail in Chapter 2).

During the months I spent at the Jellinek, I had the privilege of joining staff members on several occasions as they drove the "Methadone van" to meet addicts "where they were"—often in neighborhoods lacking adequate housing or other basic services. The nurses and other staff members on the van provided their clients (who often waited in long lines for the van to arrive in the morning) with basic outreach services, such as methadone maintenance, needle exchange, condoms, first-aid kits, medical referrals, and information on drug treatment programs. But far more than just providing medical and health services, staffers offered something else of great value: They showed deep compassion and acceptance for their clients.

The members of the Jellinek did not talk down to their clients and did not tell them what to do. They talked with their clients, not at them. They worked together to help their clients help themselves. They did not demand that their clients relinquish their existing coping strategies, including drug use, before more adaptive coping resources were set in place. The care and help offered by these dedicated staff members exemplified for me the essence of harm reduction. As the summer of 1990 continued, I began to view harm reduction as a humane and compassionate alternative to what I was familiar with back in the United States—namely, the "war on drugs" and its punitive "zero-tolerance" approach to drug users. I began to realize that zero tolerance + zero compassion = zero.

Now, close to a decade later, the basic gap between the Dutch harm reduction approach and the U.S. drug war policy continues to widen.

Advances in the Dutch model were reviewed in the December 1997 issue of the *Jellinek Quarterly*, a news bulletin of the Jellinek Institute and the Amsterdam Institute for Addiction Research. In the following excerpt from an editorial in this issue, the humane care and tolerance of the Dutch approach come across clearly:

> In 1998 the Netherlands will be witnessing the start of medical supply of heroin to a group of addicts that do not seem to have a perspective of abstinence. The number of potential participants exceeds the space available in the experiment. There will be enough addicts left who will have to score their heroin on the streets, who will be homeless, and therefore, not be in a position to use drugs in a quiet and familiar environment. Within the framework of harm reduction the city of Amsterdam has put forward a solution in behalf of the Amsterdam street users. So-called "tolerance rooms" are due to be created, in which participating users will be able to use their street heroin while being supervised. Furthermore, in shelters for the homeless space will be made available for street users. . . . The city of Amsterdam also take[s] care of other addicts. In the care circuit, people with alcohol problems can turn to the same shelters that will open their doors for drug users. Alcohol users wanting to kick or reduce the habit of drinking will find help and guidance with the health centres subsidised by the city government. (Hurkmans, 1997, p. 3)

The other critical lesson that I learned during my visit to Amsterdam is that the harm reduction approach applies to a variety of high-risk or potentially harmful behaviors other than alcohol or drug use. Visitors to the "red-light" district of Amsterdam soon become aware that sex workers provide legal, safe sex activities under the supervision of local police and health administrators. As a result, the potential harm associated with unprotected sex (especially the risk of contracting HIV) is minimized.

During one tour of Amsterdam and the surrounding countryside, my guide from the Jellinek pointed out the intricate system of highways and paths employed by the Dutch to manage traffic and pedestrian risks. In addition to the main highways, where traffic is restricted to motor vehicles, there are usually two additional pathways that parallel the main road—one for bicycles, and another for pedestrians. Each is clearly marked with traffic signals and other safety features. Remarking on this system of traffic management, my guide told me, "You see, we even apply harm reduction principles to manage the risks of travel. Since this separate traffic routing system has been introduced, the harm associated with traffic accidents and pedestrian injuries has been dramatically reduced."

My guide pointed out to me that harm reduction principles can be applied on three key levels: first, working with individuals to reduce harmful behaviors (e.g., teaching individuals safe driving skills); second, modifying the environment to enhance safety and reduce risk (e.g., establishing separate traffic lanes for motor vehicles, bicycles, and pedestrians);

and third, changing policies, laws, and regulations so as to reduce harm to both individuals and the larger society (e.g., arranging for stiffer penalties for driving under the influence of alcohol). He concluded that the harm reduction approach can also be applied to a wide variety of other high-risk or harmful behaviors, including violence and the use of firearms, excessive eating, and compulsive gambling.

Toward the end of my stay in Amsterdam, it began to dawn on me that harm reduction is much more than just an alternative to abstinence in the treatment of addiction and the prevention of HIV/AIDS. Harm reduction is about safely managing a wide range of high-risk behaviors and the harms associated with them. The focus is not on whether the specific behavior is good or bad, right or wrong; in harm reduction, the emphasis is on whether the behavior is safe or unsafe, helpful or harmful. Harm reduction is about what works (pragmatism) and what helps (compassion).

Meanwhile, back in the United States at the time of this writing (summer, 1998), several significant developments regarding the plight of harm reduction efforts in this country have occurred. Perhaps the greatest setback was the U.S. government's refusal to lift the ban on federal funding for needle exchange programs for injection drug users. As reported in the *New York Times,*

> After a bitter internal debate, the Clinton Administration today [April 20, 1998] declined to lift a nine-year-old ban on Federal financing for programs to distribute clean needles to drug addicts, even as the Government's top scientists certified that such programs did not encourage drug abuse and could save lives by reducing the spread of AIDS. The decision, announced by Donna E. Shalala, the Secretary of Health and Human Services, was immediately denounced by public health experts and advocates for people with AIDS, who had been told in recent days that the ban was about to be lifted. . . . "At best this is hypocrisy," said Dr. R. Scott Hitt, chairman of the President's Advisory Council on HIV and AIDS, which last month issued a vote of "no confidence" in the Administration. "At worst, it's a lie. And no matter what, it's immoral." Many Administration officials strongly supported lifting the ban and were disappointed with the final decision. But the position taken by Gen. Barry R. McCaffrey, the Administration's director of national drug policy, was that lifting the ban would send the wrong message to the nation's children. (Stolberg, 1998, p. A1)

In a second development, the U.S. government is now seeking to expand the "war on drugs" approach to a global level. In June 1998, President Clinton addressed a special summit-level session of the U.N. General Assembly, which was convened to discuss ways to counter drug use and trafficking in all countries (Wren, 1998a). Clinton called for both drug-producing and drug-consuming countries to stanch the supply and demand for illegal drugs. Although reducing the demand for drugs was addressed briefly, the primary emphasis was placed on reducing the world's supply of drugs (supply reduction). The director of the U.N. International Drug Control Program, Under-Secretary General Pino Arlacchi, promised to eliminate all coca leaf and opium poppy plants (the sources of cocaine and heroin, respectively) throughout the planet within the next 10 years.

The U.N. meeting to enhance the global "war on drugs" faced considerable criticism in the mass media. An editorial in *The New York Times* lamented the absence of any discussion of alternative perspectives to supply reduction solutions:

> The U.N. kept off the program virtually all the citizens' groups and experts who wanted to speak. There is no discussion of some interesting new ideas such as harm reduction, which focuses on programs like needle exchanges and methadone that cut the damage drugs do. Like previous U.N. drug conferences, this one seems designed to primarily recycle unrealistic pledges and celebrate dubious programs. ("Cheerleaders against drugs," 1998, p. A20).

The U.N. conference was also criticized in a public letter published in *The New York Times* on the first day of the conference. An article about this protest letter was published on June 9 (Wren, 1998b):

> A drug reform institute financed by the billionaire George Soros has amassed signatures of hundreds of prominent people around the world on a letter asserting that the global war on drugs is causing more harm than drug use itself. The signers include the former United Nations Secretary General Javier Perez de Cuellar, the former American Secretary of State George P. Shultz, the Nobel Peace Laureate Oscar Arias of Costa Rica, the former CBS television anchorman Walter Cronkite, two former United States Senators, Alan Cranston and Claiborne Pell, and the South African human rights activist Helen Suzman. (p. A3)

The purpose of the present book is to provide an alternative to the "war on drugs," that is, a framework for a new approach to working with people who use drugs or who engage in other high-risk behaviors. Harm reduction provides such an alternative, and I highly recommend it as a safer and saner approach for dealing with these problems in the new millenium. It's time to relegate the "war on drugs" to the historic list of failed wars in the 20th century, as we have tried to do with the Vietnam War.

The book is intended for a wide audience, including students, professionals, researchers, policy makers, and others who might be interested in harm reduction (including active drug users and others engaging in risky practices). The descriptions of theory and research in the text constitute a selective rather than a comprehensive review of the vastly expanding literature on harm reduction. This selectivity has led to an emphasis on empirical research findings, along with a focus on emerging theoretical models that may guide future work in the harm reduction field.

This book is divided into four parts. Part I consists of three chapters that provide an overview of the harm reduction field as it was represented at a recent conference (Chapter 1); a history of how harm reduction has been developed in Europe, Australia, and Canada (Chapter 2); and a description of harm reduction's basic assumptions and principles (Chapter 3). Part II provides a comprehensive review of the harm reduction literature as it applies to various addictive behaviors, including drinking problems (Chapter 4), smoking (Chapter 5), and illicit substance use (Chapter 6); Chapter 7 is devoted to harm reduction programs for HIV/AIDS prevention. Part III consists of two chapters describing the application of harm reduction principles within two ethnic minority populations: African Americans (Chapter 8) and Native Americans (Chapter 9). Finally, Part IV contains a single chapter on the implications of harm reduction for drug policy (Chapter 10).

Many people have helped in the preparation of this book over the past several years. I have had the honor and pleasure of inviting my students and colleagues (both past and current) at the Addictive Behaviors Research Center here at the University of Washington to share in the writing of this book. Almost all of the chapter authors have worked with me as students (both graduate and postdoctoral) or as faculty colleagues in recent years. Each has contributed tremendously in summarizing the harm reduction literature as it applies to various problems and populations, and I would like to take this opportunity to thank them all for their persistence and for the quality of their work (their names are all in the list of contributors). The preparation of this book has truly been a team effort.

In addition, I wish to thank Judith Gordon and Chris Owen, both of whom provided extensive and valuable editorial feedback on earlier drafts of the book. Thanks also to Rebekka Palmer, who was responsible for much editorial work and the final preparation of the text. And I would like to thank once again my friend from the Netherlands, Jan Walburg, who was the first to bring the topic of harm reduction to my attention.

G. Alan Marlatt
Addictive Behaviors Research Center,
Department of Psychology, University of Washington
Seattle, Washington

REFERENCES

Cheerleaders against drugs [Editorial]. (1998, June 9). *The New York Times*, p. A20

Hurkmans, I. (1997). Care clients [Editorial]. *Jellinek Quarterly*, 4(4), 3.

Stolberg, S. G. (1998, April 21). President decides against financing needle programs. *The New York Times*, p. A1.

Wren, C. S. (1998a, June 9). At drug summit, Clinton asks nations to set aside blame. *The New York Times*, p. A3.
Wren, C. S. (1998b, June 9). Anti-drug effort criticized as more harm than help. *The New York Times*, p. A3.

Contents

II. APPLICATIONS TO ADDICTIVE BEHAVIORS AND HIGH-RISK SEXUAL BEHAVIORS

III. MATCHING STRATEGIES TO DIVERSE ETHNIC COMMUNITIES

IV. CAN HARM REDUCTION PLAY A ROLE IN U.S. DRUG POLICY?

PART ONE
OVERVIEW OF HARM REDUCTION

CHAPTER ONE

Highlights of Harm Reduction

A Personal Report from the First National Harm Reduction Conference in the United States

G. ALAN MARLATT

Harm reduction has finally arrived in the United States. Broadly conceived, harm reduction is founded on a set of pragmatic principles and compassionate strategies designed to minimize the harmful consequences of personal drug use and associated high-risk behaviors. Although, as we shall see in Chapter 2, harm reduction has its historical origins outside North America, the movement is quickly taking hold as a public health alternative to both the moral model (as exemplified by the ongoing "war on drugs") and the medical model (addiction defined as disease). These two traditional approaches have long dominated U.S. drug policy and addiction treatment philosophy (Bertram, Blachman, Sharpe, & Andreas, 1996).

Advocates of harm reduction see it as a grassroots movement that has emerged as a middle path between the polarized opposites of the moral and medical models—a path that promises to provide humane and practical help for drug users, their families, and our communities. Active drug users themselves have provided much of the impetus for the development of harm reduction, including their advocacy in the Netherlands to establish "needle exchange" programs, designed to reduce the risk of HIV infection among injection drug users who would otherwise be forced to share potentially infected syringes. Critics of harm reduction reject it as being overly permissive in its rejection of strict "zero-tolerance" policies and its promotion of alternatives to abstinence. Some critics have gone so far as to label the entire harm reduction movement a "front" for drug legalization.

The purpose of this book as a whole is to provide an introductory guide through the terrain of harm reduction, so that readers can make up their own minds about what harm reduction is, how it has been applied, and whether or not it is a viable approach. To many in the field, harm reduction offers new and exciting ways of assisting people to help themselves by reducing the harm and suffering associated with licit and illicit drug use and associated high-risk sexual activities. To others, the area of harm reduction, with its advocacy of such formerly taboo concepts as needle exchange programs and medical marijuana, is a potentially damaging crack in the zero-tolerance armor of contemporary U.S. drug policy.

In this chapter, readers are provided with a "grand tour" of harm reduction, based on highlights of the First National Harm Reduction Conference held in Oakland, California, in September 1996. Sponsored by the Harm Reduction Coalition (HRC), the conference was heralded as marking the national birth of a U.S. harm reduction movement.[1]

Like the evolving field of harm reduction itself, this chapter consists of a broad sweep of ideas and issues, which have been selected to provide a representative sampling of the wide range of material presented at the conference. (I personally attended many of the conference sessions, and subsequently reviewed the audiotapes of other conference meetings and panels.) I feel that this diverse sampling of topics subsumed under the general rubric of "harm reduction" is important for readers to digest before any specific definitions of the term are offered. I hope that readers will inductively generate their own working definitions of "harm reduction" as they read through the examples. Although space does not permit a complete listing and description of all presentations at the conference (a total of eight plenary sessions and 63 workshops or symposia were presented), the ones described here exemplify the offerings presented.

MY ARRIVAL: LESSONS FROM A T-SHIRT

The 4-day conference attracted over 700 registrants. The meeting was held in a large chain hotel located in downtown Oakland. After arriving at the airport only to find that my checked baggage had been misplaced (my luggage remained missing for another day), I took a taxi to the hotel and registered for the conference. Near the registration desk, a table was set up to sell T-shirts designed especially for the conference by the Chicago Recovery Alliance. Needing a change of clothes, I purchased a black T-shirt; imprinted on the front was this slogan: "The Power of Any Positive Change!"

Wearing the shirt on the elevator on the way up to my hotel room, I became aware that several businessmen dressed in suits and standing behind me (apparently at the hotel to attend a different meeting) were whispering to each other in a disparaging tone while one of them pointed at my back. When I got to my room, I took off the T-shirt and read a list of "positive changes" printed on the back, which I had not noticed earlier. The list is given in Table 1.1; it appears to me to provide an operational definition of the many facets of harm reduction. The recommended changes range from tips on how to use drugs more safely ("Prepare a clean shot," "Inject where it isn't red or swollen") to suggestions for decreasing drug use ("Reduce frequency of use," "Reduce amount of drug used") and even messages consistent with a goal of abstinence ("Choose not to use drugs," "Have sober sex"). Additional tips recommend improved general health habits ("Eat well," "Sleep well"), safer sexual behavior ("Make condom use fun"), and a more positive self-image ("Respect yourself," "Overcome shame and resentments"). The changes vary from benign suggestions ("Work for peace," "Have fun") to radical drug management recommendations ("Use clean, purified drugs," "Enjoy your high in a safe place"). No wonder the businessmen were talking behind my back!

TABLE 1.1. The Power of Any Positive Change

• Talk safety with your partner	• Choose your time to use
• Use a sterile syringe for each shot	• Cop safer
• Drive sober	• Choose not to use drugs
• Wipe with an alcohol pad before injecting	• Keep Narcan around
• Prepare a clean shot	• Cultivate good veins
• Build strong relationships	• Learn to inject yourself
• Rotate injection sites	• Enjoy your high in a safe place
• Inject where it isn't red or swollen	• Have fun
• Use clean, purified drugs	• Use less harmful drugs
• Work for peace	• Know the law
• Use the smallest needle possible	• Use a kind tourniquet
• Apply pressure to site after injection	• Reduce frequency of use
• Use your own cooker, cotton, and water	• Use one drug at a time
• Develop safer ways to split drugs	• Open your senses naturally
• Dispose of syringes safely	• Learn to detox safely
• Take thiamine if you drink heavily	• Overcome shame and resentments
• Reduce amount of drug used	• Know CPR and first aid
• Eat well	• Help others to make their own positive changes
• Have sober sex	• Know your drugs
• Sleep well	• Know where you can get help and what it offers
• Respect yourself	• . . . And other positive changes as you define them for yourself
• Make condom use fun	
• Use lube to excite	

Note. From the back of a T-shirt designed by the Chicago Recovery Alliance, 1996. Reprinted by permission of the Alliance.

OPENING ADDRESSES

The welcoming address in the opening plenary session was delivered by Allan Clear, executive director of the HRC, who noted the diversity of the audience, including drug policy makers, academics, researchers, law enforcement representatives, alcohol and drug treatment counselors, addiction outreach and front-line workers, peer educators, and drug user activists. The atmosphere was casual, with most conference attendees dressed informally. Many in the audience were young, and many different ethnic minority groups were represented.

In his talk, Clear described the three main goals of the HRC and the conference itself: (1) to develop resources for drug users; (2) to provide training in harm reduction; and (3) to facilitate community organization efforts to promote harm reduction. Reluctant to provide a fixed and firm definition of "harm reduction," Clear noted that the movement was in a state of "perpetual revolution" and that different people defined the term in different ways. The HRC brochure distributed with the conference registration materials included the "principles of harm reduction" listed in Table 1.2.

In the published version of his introductory remarks, Clear stressed the point that the harm reduction movement in the United States has largely sprung from the grassroots level, particularly in response to political opposition at the national level:

> Let me make it clear that we don't believe change comes from the top. . . . We cannot even get equal access, democratic access, to HIV prevention materials for all people in this country. So, we're not going to get it given to us, and what we have to do is work from the ground, from the grass-roots. . . . (Clear, 1997, p. 11)

Next to speak was David Purchase, director of the North American Syringe Exchange Network, known for his work in establishing the first U.S. syringe exchange program—the Point Defiance AIDS Project in Tacoma, Washington, in 1988. During his talk, Purchase noted that harm reduction is more "an attitude" than a fixed set of rules or regulations. He described this attitude as a humanitarian stance that accepts the inherent dignity of life and facilitates the ability to "see oneself in the eyes of others" instead of judging or condemning them. He denied that harm reduction is a front for any political agenda (i.e., drug legalization), describing it instead as a "living thing" not to be found in the field of dogma. Purchase emphasized that the essence of harm reduction is an individualized approach to positive changes in behavior:

> Harm reduction is against harm, neutral on the use of drugs *per se*, and in favor of any positive change, as defined by the person making the change.

TABLE 1.2. Principles of Harm Reduction

Harm reduction is a set of practical strategies with the goal of meeting drug users "where they're at" to help them reduce any harms associated with their drug use. Because harm reduction demands that interventions and policies designed to serve drug users reflect specific individual and community needs, there is no universal definition of or formula for implementing harm reduction. However, HRC considers the following principles central to harm reduction practice. Harm reduction:

- Accepts, for better and for worse, that licit and illicit drug use is part of our world and chooses to work to minimize its harmful effects rather than simply ignore or condemn them.
- Ensures that drug users and those with a history of drug use routinely have a real voice in the creation of programs and policies designed to serve them, and both affirms and seeks to strengthen the capacity of people who use drugs to reduce the various harms associated with their drug use.
- Understands drug use as a complex, multi-faceted phenomenon that encompasses a continuum of behaviors from severe abuse to total abstinence, and acknowledges that some ways of using drugs are clearly safer than others.
- Establishes quality of individual and community life and well-being—not necessarily cessation of all drug use—as the criteria for successful interventions and policies.
- Calls for the non-judgmental, non-coercive provision of services and resources to people who use drugs and the communities in which they live in order to assist them in reducing attendant harms.
- Recognizes that the realities of poverty, class, racism, social isolation, past trauma, sex-based discrimination and other social inequalities affect both people's vulnerability to and capacity for effectively dealing with drug-related harms.
- Does not attempt to minimize or ignore the many real and tragic harms and dangers associated with licit and illicit drug use.

Note. From HRC (1996, pp. 3–5). Copyright 1996 by the Harm Reduction Coalition. Reprinted by permission.

> That's ANY positive change. We all set our own rate of change. . . . We change at the pace that is possible for each of us. (Purchase, 1997, p. 22)

Edith Springer, clinical director of the New York Peer AIDS Education Coalition and a pioneer in introducing harm reduction to U.S. drug workers (Springer, 1991), also gave a talk on the opening morning of the conference. She introduced a "spectrum of harm reduction," an overview of a variety of methods and approaches that can be subsumed under the four general categories of harm reduction presented in Table 1.3 (Springer, 1996). Springer noted that in contrast with fixed drug policies that promote a black-and-white, dichotomous stance (e.g., a zero-tolerance policy), harm reductionists adopt a value system that accepts many "shades of gray"— one that promotes an individualized approach, and that recognizes and responds to unique differences among individual drug users. In harm reduction programs, consumers (clients) are treated with dignity and respect

TABLE 1.3. Spectrum of Harm Reduction

1. HIV/AIDS-related interventions, including both direct services (e.g., syringe exchange and bleaching equipment for injection drug users, promotion of safer sex, referrals to HIV testing and medical care) and ancillary interventions (referrals for primary health care, psychotherapy, and alternative treatments such as massage, acupuncture, yoga, and meditation; providing access to housing and entitlements).
2. More compassionate drug treatment, for both abstinence-oriented treatment (e.g., using moderation goals as a "recovery readiness" strategy to get to abstinence) and drug substitution treatments such as methadone maintenance (e.g., making methadone available upon prescription by primary care physicians). The goal of abstinence is freely chosen by the consumer, who sets the time frame for change.
3. Drug use management, "for those who want to continue using drugs," including safer drug use (e.g., proper injection techniques, changing route of drug administration, substitution of less harmful drugs, advice regarding drug combinations) and more responsible drug use (e.g., "more control over when, how, and with whom one uses; taking care of business first: maintaining entitlements and housing, keep[ing] medical appointments, respecting the rules of agencies regarding drug use on the premises, buy[ing] the Pampers first!")
4. Advocating for change in drug policy, including making treatment more readily available (as opposed to incarceration), changing drug paraphernalia laws (e.g., legalizing syringe purchase), reducing penalties for drug-related offenses, and providing rehabilitation and vocational training in prison.

and are free to choose their own goals, including goals of abstinence or moderation, instead of being forced to accept goals set by treatment providers. Workers adopt a client-centered approach in helping consumers set their goals. One such goal is long-term drug maintenance (e.g., methadone maintenance), to stabilize drug consumers and reduce the harm associated with illegal activities that users might otherwise engage in to obtain money to support their drug habit. Springer's talk reinforced a position she first set forth in a 1991 publication:

> In psychotherapeutic training, we are taught never to remove a defense mechanism until there is another in its place; we run the risk of causing a person to decompensate and become worse off than when he or she was before they used the regressive or harmful defense. This is no different for drug users. It is important for workers to understand that when a person has multiple problems, one of which is drug use, ripping that defense from them as the first step is inappropriate and countertherapeutic. (Springer, 1991, p. 144)

One of Springer's former students, Imani Woods, presented the next talk. During her inspiring and humorous presentation, she talked about her gradual transition from her original adherence to a strict abstinence-only approach to one of accepting harm reduction alternatives:

I'm here to represent all of us who believe in abstinence. That's where I come from: abstinence. Years ago, when I would come into a room and hear somebody say "harm reduction," I said, "You must be crazy." . . . I didn't come to harm reduction saying "Yippee!" I was like, "Uh-uh, that ain't gonna work." But I'm telling you, I tried these different things and tried to develop my own things in different cases and it worked. I began to think about drug users in a different way. Drug users have families. Drug users are employers. Drug users have jobs. Drug users want to stay healthy, and the access to services we offer should not be regulated by whether or not you're using. That was something that even way back, I couldn't agree with. For a lot of services, users can't even get in. Drug users pay taxes, and therefore drug users should have the same quality of services as everyone else. (Woods, 1997, pp. 4–6)

Because of her expertise in harm reduction programs for the African American community, I have asked Imani Woods (who has since moved from New York to Seattle) to outline her ideas more fully in Chapter 8 of this book.

Ricky Bluthenthal, a researcher with the Alameda County Exchange Program (Oakland is situated in Alameda County), presented the next talk. He gave a summary of the legal difficulties experienced by the 24 existing syringe exchange programs in California. Many people working in needle exchange programs have been arrested because of the illegality of their actions under current California state law.

In sharp contrast with the situation as described in California, Washington State has provided a warm welcome to supporters of harm reduction. As noted by the next speaker—Patrick Vanzo, division manager and county coordinator of the King County (Seattle) Division of Alcohol and Substance Abuse Services—Washington was the first state in the country to have a needle exchange program (the one started in Tacoma by David Purchase, as noted above),[2] and Seattle was the host city of the first of a series of regional conferences (held in January 1995) sponsored in the United States by the HRC. Among Vanzo's official duties is the coordination of public health funding for drug and alcohol treatment programs in Seattle and King County. He noted that if harm reduction is to make an impact with city and county representatives of both drug treatment providers and elected public officials, supporters of this approach must learn to communicate and collaborate with members of these community-based groups. Vanzo has found the following five principles of harm reduction (drawn in part from Springer's work) to be both useful and pragmatic in his efforts:

1. Abstinence should not be the only objective of services to drug users, because it excludes a large proportion of people who are committed to long-term drug use.

2. Abstinence from drug use should be the final goal in a series of harm reduction objectives designed to reduce harmful consequences.

3. Harm reduction programs should offer user-friendly services to attract and make contact with drug users, and to empower them to change their behavior and develop suitable intermediate objectives for change.

4. Harm reduction should be multidisciplinary and should include health care providers, police, drug treatment and prevention workers, and others who work with drug users.

5. Harm reduction should include four areas of service: treatment, care, control, and education.

Vanzo further observed that in his official position, he could back a "consumers' union" (e.g., to help consumers of treatment services by providing programs such as needle exchange), but was less likely to get community backing for a "users' union" (e.g., providing "clean crack pipes" to cocaine users). To gain community support for harm reduction, Vanzo recommended five arenas of collaboration with treatment providers: collaborative data collection, planning services, training, seamless service delivery, and accountability for program outcomes (measured in terms of quality, quantity, cost, and time). He concluded his talk with a plea for increased partnership and alliance between the domains of public health and harm reduction.[3]

THE POLITICS OF HARM REDUCTION

The plenary session on the first afternoon of the Oakland conference was devoted to a discussion of the political environment within and surrounding harm reduction. The panel was moderated by Cheryl Epps of the Drug Policy Foundation, a national organization formed for the study and reform of U.S. drug policy. She introduced the first speaker, Ethan Nadelmann, director of the Lindesmith Center, a drug policy "think tank" located in New York City.

Nadelmann noted some historical antecedents and parallels with current drug policy reform efforts. In particular, he drew attention to alcohol prohibition—a policy that was eventually rescinded in the United States as it became increasingly clear that the problems and harms brought about by this policy (e.g., the development of organized crime) outweighed those caused by the use of alcohol itself. In this context, he described two main goals of harm reduction: to reduce the negative consequences of both drug use and harmful drug policy (e.g., less incarceration). Although most harm reductionists agree on the first goal, disagreement exists with regard to the second. Some advocate free-market legalization as a solution to the problems caused by prohibition, whereas others focus primarily on reducing the harm caused in part by current drug policy. Nadelmann urged reform of harmful drug policies by the development of alternative policies based on a combination of "common sense, science, public health, and human rights."

Nadelmann also described harm reduction as constituting a "wide swath" of divergent topics; the movement includes individuals who agree on some points and disagree on others. Opinions vary on such topics as decriminalization of marijuana, provision of marijuana as medicine, access to psychedelic drugs for psychotherapy or for religious ceremonies, and harm reduction as a general approach to risk management (e.g., safe sex, safe driving, safe sport, etc.). Points on which most movement members agree include acknowledgment of the harmful consequences of drug prohibition and the domination of drug users by the criminal justice system. Nadelmann also observed that harm reductionists do not reject abstinence as an ideal goal. Rather, they reject an abstinence-only approach that withholds help from drug users unless they adhere to abstinence.

Next to speak on the panel was Nick Pastore, then chief of the Department of Police Service in New Haven, Connecticut. Pastore described the community policing approach followed by his department. Prior to implementing this approach, police officers had little or no communication with health service providers in dealing with drug users in the New Haven community. More recently, through cooperation and joint training programs with Yale University, police officers have become a "credible part of the extended family" and collaborate actively with both providers and consumers. Making personal contact with drug users and getting to know them by name are encouraged, since problems can be dealt with on a more individualized basis. The community police slogan, according to Pastore, is "Humanize, don't demonize."

Pastore described a conference he had attended in 1995 at the Hoover Institute at Stanford University, which brought together over 100 police chiefs from around the country to discuss drug reform from the police perspective. Many police chiefs are critical of the current drug war, Pastore reported, and are supportive of harm reduction efforts that include community policing efforts. He said that future police departments adopting this approach will pride themselves on having a lower, not higher, arrest rate for drug users. Many drug problems on the street can be worked out on an interpersonal basis between police officers and users, instead of the police resorting to arrest procedures, he concluded.[4]

Walter Adkins, chief of detectives with the Police Department in San José, California, was the next to speak on the afternoon panel. In addition to his support for community-based policing described by Pastore, Adkins recommended the use of "drug courts" as an alternative to incarceration for many nonviolent drug offenders. In drug courts, defendants who have been charged with drug possession make a kind of plea bargain. Judges set aside a formal trial, along with criminal charges and sentences, while defendants undergo treatment and court-monitored supervision. Defendants can be jailed by the judge if they violate the terms of the treatment plan. If treatment is completed and the defendant becomes free of drugs, drug charges may be dismissed or sentences may be reduced.[5]

Next to speak was Joyce Rivera, the founder and executive director of St. Ann's Corner of Harm Reduction in Bronx, New York. As one of the "pioneers" of U.S. harm reduction, she spoke eloquently of the political nature of the movement, describing it as an "emerging and controversial field" that offers an alternative to the existing political domination associated with both the current drug war and the traditional disease model of addiction. Rivera identified the grassroots stage of the harm reduction movement as primarily social in origin and emotional in expression. Noting that the movement cannot be controlled from the top, since it is rapidly evolving and involves a diversity of opinions and leadership, she stated that the next step will be to provide operational definitions of harm reduction and to build regional alliances between various leadership groups, such as the HRC and the Drug Policy Foundation. In the meantime, she urged the leadership to "ride the wave of the emotional reactions" that often characterize this emerging social movement.

The final speaker for the afternoon panel was Ellen Fishman, representing the International Coalition for Addicts' Resources and Enlightenment (ICARE) in New York. The ICARE group, she explained, was developed as an active drug user support group and is currently involved in "user organizing" to provide "voices" for active addicts who wish to have a say in drug treatment and policy matters. Fishman urged an end to the stereotypical view of addicts as "gutter junkies." Addicts should have a more active stake in speaking out about their needs and "coming out of the closet," instead of remaining marginalized by society. Drug users should be more actively "involved in the dialogue" when it comes to establishing policy and programs, Fishman concluded.

HARM REDUCTION WITHIN
RECOVERY/ABSTINENCE CULTURES

During the afternoon of the first day of the conference, several "breakout" sessions were held simultaneously on various topics, including reaching women with harm reduction strategies; syringe exchange programs designed for specific populations; provision of group psychotherapy and other mental health services to drug users; conflict and cooperation between law enforcement and community providers of harm reduction; integration of harm reduction into methadone services; infectious disease prevention and harm reduction as a basic public health approach; and access to holistic health services (e.g., acupuncture, nutrition, massage) for drug users. Space does not permit a detailed description of all these breakout sessions, but one of the sessions deserves special mention here: the one on harm reduction in the context of recovery/abstinence cultures.

This session was facilitated by Roger Gooden of the National Association of People with AIDS (NAPWA). He introduced the first speaker,

Beri Hall, the community education coordinator for NAPWA, who described herself as "a black woman living with HIV, a recovering addict, a certified addictions counselor, and a harm reductionist." Hall told the audience that she had been in recovery for the past 6½ years and attributed her successful abstinence to participation in Twelve-Step recovery groups. Later, as an addictions counselor in a methadone maintenance program, she received training in harm reduction from the Chicago Recovery Alliance, a sponsor of needle exchange programs and other services for active drug users (and the group that designed the T-shirt I bought). "It wasn't until later that I came to realize that not only had I been practicing harm reduction in the methadone program as a counselor, but that it was through harm reduction that I had made it from hard-core drug usage to abstinence," she said. At first she was resistant to alternatives to abstinence for drug users, but came to redefine recovery as including "any positive change" (see Table 1.1). Hall also pointed out the link between drug use and HIV among infected users, emphasizing several important considerations:

1. There is a need to acknowledge drug use among many people who are HIV-positive.
2. Active drug users need to be aware of how drug use affects HIV disease.
3. Drug use may have an impact on compliance in adhering to prescribed medication for HIV disease.
4. Drug use may influence the attitude and spiritual connection of persons with HIV.
5. Primary care providers need to be aware of harm reduction strategies to help individuals who both use drugs and are HIV-positive.

As a final point, Hall said that all approaches to reduce harm are based on what the drug user is willing to do first—from participating in a needle exchange program to a total commitment to abstinence.

The next panelist was John de Miranda, a substance abuse specialist with the Peninsula Health Concepts group in California. de Miranda is the former western U.S. community development coordinator of Join Together, a resource center for community substance abuse prevention funded by a grant from the Robert Wood Johnson Foundation. Introducing himself as a recovering alcoholic who has worked for many years in the traditional substance abuse field, de Miranda said that he first heard of harm reduction when he was told by his colleagues in a traditional substance abuse treatment program to avoid making statements such as "The goal of our program is to reduce problems associated with alcohol and drug abuse," so as not to be confused with those who support harm reduction. He then began to hear more about harm reduction as "the enemy" of traditional substance abuse treatment providers.

de Miranda presented what he concluded to be two opposing "world views." First, he characterized harm reduction as a humanistic world view, founded on basic principles of public health, in which the primary focus is on the consumer or client. In contrast, he described the world view of traditional substance abuse programs as being based on a "power relationship" in which the professional caregiver holds power (access to treatment and recovery) over the patient; here the focus is on the program rather than on the client (a "take it or leave it" attitude).

Whereas harm reductionists are nonjudgmental and encourage any positive change, traditional substance abuse professionals are more likely to be judgmental and parochial in their approach to clients and to insist on abstinence as the only acceptable goal, de Miranda observed. He also noted that whereas harm reduction tends to be based more on research findings (e.g., empirical evidence documenting the effectiveness of needle exchange programs), the traditional field of substance abuse is based more on practice concerns and anecdotal clinical lore. As such, supporters of this approach tend to ignore research findings that contradict their beliefs. Despite these basic differences, de Miranda urged the two sectors to seek areas of overlap and common ground, rather than to view themselves as mutually exclusive camps. One possible area of overlap is that both approaches might agree on some common goals, such as acceptance of methadone maintenance, designated driver practices, and responsible beverage serving training programs, de Miranda concluded.

In the audience discussion that followed, panelist Hall posed the following question: "If one is now sober, and starts to use again, is that harm reduction?" "Absolutely not!" one audience member strongly replied. "That would be a relapse, not harm reduction."

SUBSTANCE USE MANAGEMENT

On the second morning of the Oakland conference, a plenary session was held on the topic of "Substance Use Management: Drugs and Drug Use." The facilitator was Dan Bigg of the Chicago Recovery Alliance. Bigg pointed out that the term "substance use management" refers to harm reduction programs and policies that help active users to manage their ongoing drug use. He emphasized the point that many drug users are capable of making positive changes on their own, including giving drugs up altogether, without the assistance of formal treatment—despite the "myth" held by many critics of harm reduction that addicts are incapable of changing their behavior without coerced treatment or incarceration.

People need to change their attitudes toward addicts "from persecution and collaboration to respect and collaboration," Bigg said. There is a need to replace the uniformity myth that "all addicts are the same" with one that appreciates the uniqueness of each individual drug user. Finally, Bigg concluded, there is a need to move beyond offering drug users a single choice between abstinence or punishment (i.e., "Abstain, or be busted and go to jail") or between abstinence or no treatment at all (i.e., "Abstain, or get out of our treatment program"). Progress can be made in harm reduction by offering users a wide variety of choices for any positive change, instead of just a single option.

The next speaker was Richard Elovich of the Gay Men's Health Crisis Center in New York City. He described a prevention program developed at his center that is geared to gay men who are HIV-negative. The program in Substance Use Counseling and Education adopted the following slogan: "Stay Negative—It's Not Automatic." Elovich noted that most harm reduction prevention programs (e.g., needle exchange) have focused on the link between injection drug use and risk of HIV infection. In the gay community, however, there is a high incidence of noninjection use of such substances as alcohol or cocaine, which increase the risk of engaging in high-risk sexual behaviors and thus of possible HIV infection. Traditional substance abuse programs that equate any substance use with addiction fail to reach many in the gay community who do not or will not accept the label of "addict" or "substance abuser." Elovich also stated that traditional treatment often emphasizes a confrontation-of-denial approach. That is, it demands that all clients must accept the program's model of addiction and requirement of total abstinence, or be refused services.

In contrast to traditional substance abuse treatment that is based on a dichotomous disease model (in which patients are seen either to have or not to have an addictive disease) Elovich adopts a model that places both substance use and its associated risks along a continuum ranging from minimum to extreme levels. Because many who are at risk for HIV in the gay community are not aware of their risk or are otherwise unmotivated to change their behavior, the program is open-ended and nondirective. Drawing upon the stages-of-change model first proposed by Prochaska, DiClemente, and Norcross (1992), Elovich stated that many gay men are in the "precontemplation" stage of behavior change. With these "precontemplators," the program's goal in the early stages is to keep them from dropping out, rather than insisting upon active behavioral change. "Dropout prevention, not action, is the goal," Elovich concluded. The prevention program includes both individual and group counseling, as well as outreach services.

Jon Paul Hammond of Philadelphia Street Outreach Services, the next speaker, presented a talk on harm reduction for crack cocaine smokers ("pipers"). Hammond began by noting that when the Prevention Point needle exchange program was first introduced in Philadelphia in 1991, workers came into contact with many crack smokers, in addition to the main targeted group of injection drug users. Although most crack smokers do not inject cocaine and are thus at lower risk for HIV transmission, many of them have other major health problems, including respiratory and other lung disorders, as well as oral infections or sexually transmitted diseases. Many crack users who approached the needle exchange program for other services (e.g., provision of condoms and swipes) complained that few treatment options were available for crack addicts, other than traditional abstinence-only treatment programs. Such programs are reluctant to meet crack users "where they are at," according to Hammond. The Philadelphia program workers thus began to offer educational information on harm reduction techniques for crack smokers, including information on harmful versus safer drug use administration; encouragement of smoking less often with lower drug dose levels, and of smoking in less harmful environments or settings; and information on how to get help in cutting back or quitting. Hammond concluded with his observation that since many crack smokers also use other substances (e.g., alcohol, prescription drugs, injection drugs), a general harm reduction approach for polydrug users is both necessary and important.

After this talk, Bigg as moderator reminded the audience that abstinence is also a form of drug use management. He noted that "abstinence" has many meanings, and does not always mean permanent and lasting abstinence. For some, abstinence may apply only in specific settings, such as work or school; for polydrug users, it is also possible to abstain from one or more drugs.

Next to speak was Charlton (Chilly) Clay, a health educator and ethnographer with the Seattle–King County Department of Public Health. The title of his presentation was "Methamphetamine and Harm Reduction among Gay and Bisexual Men." Having formerly met Clay on several occasions in Seattle, I was aware of his impact as coordinator of Project NEON (Needle and Sex Education Outreach Network), a community-based harm reduction project that promotes safer anal sex and injection practices among gay/bisexual men who also inject crystal methamphetamine ("crystal meth"). Clay spoke about this group as being particularly at risk for HIV infection. He reported that in Seattle, although 19% of men who have sex with men (MSM) and who do not use injection drugs are HIV-positive, fully 40% of the MSM group who also shoot crystal meth are HIV-positive.

After epidemiologists discovered this combination of risk factors in 1993, Clay was asked to conduct an ethnographic study of this high-risk group. His sample consisted of 28 men who were both MSM and crystal meth injectors. These men described crystal meth as a very seductive drug, with effects that can last up to 16 hours. The drug induces a prolonged state of euphoria (the effects can make one very "sexy and horny"), during which long-term sexual activity often occurs. Some men who lose erectile functioning because of the drug effects are more likely to assume a passive sexual role ("switching from top to bottom"), thereby placing them at greater risk for unprotected anal transmission of HIV. Because these men are simultaneously engaging in two taboo behaviors—high-risk sex and injection drug use—they often see themselves as "double outlaws" in terms of the gay community's own social norms. Such norms serve as "regulatory schemes," and a man's behavior is seen as being in alignment with or in transgression of that community's values, Clay observed.

Project NEON was established as a harm reduction community outreach program to provide services for this high-risk group. A new needle exchange program was set up especially for crystal meth injectors. The exchange was established in collaboration with Seattle's Stonewall Recovery Services, a group that offers both harm reduction and abstinence-based counseling for gay and lesbian substance users. Project NEON relies mainly on peer educators who provide outreach and educational harm reduction services, including promotion of safe sex practices (e.g., encouraging use of the "female condom" for anal receptive intercourse). They also publish preventive educational material in the form of a specialized magazine (*Amphetazine*). At the end his talk, Clay recommended harm reduction as a humane antidote to the homophobic and moralistic views that characterize many public attitudes toward the group of "double outlaws":

> It is all too easy for those standing at the sidelines of the HIV/AIDS epidemic to merely place blame on individuals for getting or transmitting HIV, for being pathological drug addicts, for being "irresponsible." The war on drugs has further fostered the use of language in which drug users are described in terms of their supposed weak character, their moral failings, their genetic predispositions or diseases, and their criminality. All of these vocabularies focus on the pathology of the individuals and overlook the critical effects of social context in shaping drug use patterns and the transmission of HIV. They overlook the processes by which individuals, for better or worse, internalize and transform cultural messages and deal with the effects of oppression. The vocabularies of pathology prejudice our perceptions. They preclude an ability to listen to drug users with more open ears. They preclude an ability to recognize the capacities drug users possess to become creative partners in addressing social problems. I believe harm reduction is an antidote to the toxic effects of judgment and moralism that frames our thinking and actions on the issues of drugs and drug users. (Clay, 1997, p. 21)

The final speaker for this plenary session was Kristen Ochoa, who works in the UCSF Department of Epidemiology and Biostatistics at the University of California at San Francisco; she develops HIV testing protocols and training for homeless groups in the San Francisco area. She described a harm reduction program that she helped develop in Mexico City for street youth who abuse inhalants—that is, who sniff glue, solvents, gasoline, and other intoxicating vapors. The project, called *Proyecto Reduccion de Dano* (Project Harm Reduction), employs street youth as outreach workers. Workers engage in outreach work in various community settings, including church meetings, concerts, and the streets. Ochoa also stressed the need to expand harm reduction services beyond the problem of inhalant abuse to meet a variety of basic needs, such as providing food, shelter, and employment opportunities.

MEDICINAL MARIJUANA

The controversial topic of medicinal marijuana was discussed on the afternoon of the second day of the conference. The opening talk was presented by Todd Mikuriya, a psychiatrist in private practice who serves as the medical coordinator for the Northern and Southern California Committees for Compassionate Use, and for the Cannabis Buyers Clubs (CBCs) located in San Francisco, Oakland, and Santa Cruz. Mikuriya told the audience that cannabis was prescribed for a variety of medicinal purposes in the United States until 1937, when it was removed from prescriptive availability. Mikuriya's own opinion about the medicinal value of cannabis is that is "a powerful immunomodulating drug that appears to calm the immune system in autoimmune conditions." In particular, it provides relief from nausea and promotes appetite in patients with AIDS.

Mikuriya also recommended the use of marijuana as a possible substitute for people who are addicted to more harmful drugs, such as alcohol or opiates. He stated, "Pharmacologically, cannabis substitution for drugs with undesired or harmful side effects, prescribed, over the counter, or illicit, is harm reduction"; he added that in some cases, marijuana can be considered a "gateway drug" leading addicts back to less harmful substance use. Mikuriya spoke of the growth of CBCs in California and in other states, where individuals who have been medically diagnosed with an illness that may respond favorably to the medicinal properties of marijuana can purchase marijuana for their personal use. People who attend CBCs benefit from the nonjudgmental and accepting attitude of those providing the service, he concluded.

The cofounders of the Oakland CBC, Jeff Jones and Liana Held, spoke on the same panel. They founded the Oakland CBC in 1995 and patterned it after the San Francisco CBC, founded by Dennis Peron. CBCs were established as an alternative means for patients to obtain marijuana for medicinal purposes after the U.S. government (during the Bush administration) shut off the federal supply of medicinal marijuana in 1988. Patients attending the Oakland CBC require a physician's letter recommending marijuana as medicine for a particular disorder and are asked to participate in an intake interview. Those purchasing marijuana at the Oakland CBC are not allowed to consume it on the premises, but are advised to administer it in privacy and not in the presence of children. Held said that the CBC was established as a safe, clean place for patients to obtain medicinal marijuana, as opposed to buying it on the street from dealers, who may try to sell buyers additional hard drugs such as cocaine or heroin.

Joanne McKey, founder of Seattle's Green Cross Patient Co-op, also gave a presentation on the panel. She admitted that she has smoked marijuana since 1987, after a physician recommended it for the treatment of her painful muscle spasms associated with a spinal cord injury. Speaking from her wheelchair, McKey said that she began sharing some of her home-grown marijuana with AIDS patients in 1993, and later provided it to more than 100 people with various diseases and conditions (e.g., glaucoma, multiple sclerosis, AIDS, and back injuries). Letters from physicians recommending medicinal marijuana for their patients are required. Growing marijuana specifically for Green Cross use was discontinued in 1995 after McKey was arrested (a narcotics team seized more than 130 plants from her trailer on Bainbridge Island, near Seattle). Although the charges were later dismissed, Green Cross workers are now forced to purchase marijuana from street dealers in order to provide it to patients in need.

The final speaker on the medicinal marijuana panel was Vic Hernandez, a Harvard-trained epidemiologist who is now working with the AIDS Prevention Action Network, and is the founder of Cannabis Helping Alleviate Medical Problems (CHAMP) in San Francisco. Hernandez spoke of the need for a harm reduction approach to pain management for people with HIV/AIDS. He described the problem faced by many AIDS patients who are also in recovery from substance abuse: How are they to medicate debilitating pain effectively and improve their quality of life, without at the same time relapsing into substance abuse? Hernandez observed that "participation of people in group action and dialogue efforts directed at community targets, such as particulars about pain management among people with HIV/AIDS in recovery, enhances control and beliefs in the ability of individuals to change their lives."

DRUG-USING YOUTH AS HARM REDUCTION PROVIDERS

Another afternoon breakout session focused on the topic of drug-using youth as harm reduction providers; this session was chaired by Heather Edney of the Santa Cruz Needle Exchange Project. First to speak was Angela Rodrigues, of the New York Peer AIDS Education Coalition. Rodrigues acknowledged Edith Springer as her trainer in providing harm reduction outreach services. She described her life a year prior to beginning her outreach work—a year in which, in her own words, she was "homeless, drug-addicted, and all fucked up." She contrasted her present role as a peer educator who is also an active drug user with the image of other professional outreach workers, who are not drug users and, in her experience, often misinform people about the real risks of drug use and HIV infection. As a peer educator, on the other hand, she can identify with drug users; she can reach out and "give it to you raw."

In Rodrigues's view, professional workers define themselves as "normal" people and see addicts as "fucked-up" people. She put it this way:

"My motto is 'Everyone fucks up, and I'm here to help you if you need me to.' " Whereas professional outreach workers try to push people into treatment, Rodrigues adopts a harm reduction approach. For example, if she meets a crack user who smokes eight vials a day, she tries to get the person to cut back to six a day, and later four vials a day, and so on until the user reaches the point where he or she wants to quit. As a peer outreach worker, her message to active drug users at risk for AIDS is this: "I've been there, and I accept you as you are."

Three young women (ages 18, 19, and 21), representing the Street Survival Project of the Center for Young Women's Development in San Francisco, then gave a presentation entitled "Hiring Youth Who Use: A Smart Harm Reduction Approach." A summary of their contribution, published in the abstract booklet for the conference, states:

> Izzy, Nelly and Erica are three young women who work in various areas of service-providing around issues of drug-related harm. We work with the Street Survival Project, a youth-run organization based on the philosophy of harm-reduction that employs and trains young women to be peer educators and to bring survival information and necessities to other young women in their communities. We're also involved with a youth needle exchange site and a research project out of the San Francisco Dept. of Public Health AIDS Office on young people in the street economy. We are going to talk about the importance of hiring users to work in their own communities, and the complex issues surrounding it. We will talk about the contradictions of being a user and provider, especially in one's own community, of accessing services in the same community we're working in, and of the importance of not only having a more immediate trust with the participant, but of creating a contradiction to the traditional roles of drug user/service provider, making more visible the self-determination we as drug users have to do work in our own communities. ... Throughout our presentation we will speak of our own experiences and those of our outreach and exchange participants to help bring a first-hand perspective of young women, service providers and active drug users to this conference. (Smith, Velasco, & Berman, 1996, p. 14)

Some of the concerns expressed by both panelists and members of the audience about hiring active drug users as outreach workers included fears that active users would get "high" on the job and would be unreliable workers, along with fears that such a hiring policy would lead to legal problems that would undermine funding support. In response to these concerns, the panelists noted some potential benefits of recruiting drug users as outreach workers. First, users can provide more accurate information on the risks of drug use and ways to cope with drug-related problems (based on their personal experience in problem solving) and can recommend a range of potential services. The panelists also noted that drug users (including those on methadone maintenance) need jobs as much as anyone else, and that working as outreach workers encourages them to take more responsibility for their drug use (e.g., not coming to work "high"). Moreover, access to prospective clients is likely to increase, since "our clients are our friends," as one panelist put it. Finally, active users are more likely to have a compassionate attitude toward other drug users, and thus they may serve as a "bridge between youth who use and the health community," said another participant.[6]

INTEGRATING HARM REDUCTION AND DRUG TREATMENT

"Moving Drug Treatment: The Integration of Harm Reduction and Drug Treatment Models" was the title of another panel at the conference, facilitated by Howard Josepher of the ARRIVE/Exponents program in New York City. The first speaker was Reda Sobky, an internist associated with Humanistic Alternatives to Addiction Research and Treatment (a group in Alameda County, California), who is well known for his work in obtaining addiction treatment services for low-income Medicaid patients, including access to methadone. He described methadone as a medicine that relieves suffering, regardless of the source of the suffering. Sobky also spoke of the spiraling increase of overdose deaths among heroin users. Because addicts are forced to buy street drugs of unknown purity and potency, they run the risk of a fatal overdose. Since the ultimate purpose of harm reduction is saving lives, Sobky noted, greater access to opiate agonists such as naloxone (Narcan) may save the lives of many users who would otherwise die from overdose. If someone sees an addict "turning blue" from a potential overdose, administration of naloxone can precipitate immediate withdrawal (through its blocking effects on opiate receptors) and may reverse the overdose effects. Dr. Sobky urged needle exchange programs to offer naloxone as a readily available first-aid agent that is likely to reduce the number of overdose deaths.

Emmett Velten, a psychologist with the Bay Area Addiction Research Treatment center, was the next speaker. Velten pointed out that traditional addiction treatment programs often rely on spiritual recovery programs based on the Twelve-Step philosophy. He advocated offering a wider range of self-help groups, in addition to the Alcoholics Anonymous or Narcotics Anonymous approaches, so that treatment retention will be enhanced and fewer dropouts will occur. Velten described a variety of existing alternative groups, including secular self-help organizations such as Women for Sobriety, the Secular Organization for Sobriety, Rational Recovery, Self-Management Recovery Training, and Moderation Management (all but the last of these is abstinence-based). No single approach is best for everyone, he said, concluding that "when clients are given the choice of treatment, they do better than if they are assigned treatment by someone else."

Lurend Cray was next to speak on the panel. She described the ARRIVE/Exponents program in New York City, which began offering low-threshold, harm reduction services to injection drug users with criminal justice histories in 1988. Cray, the training coordinator of this program, described it as an ongoing series of 24 classes given over an 8-week period (and repeated five times a year). The classes are offered to provide assistance to individuals and their families who are undergoing difficult life transitions: from incarceration to life in the outside community, from addiction to recovery, from homelessness to finding shelter, and from welfare to work. The classes provide basic training in life skills, job training, coping skills, stress management, nutrition information, and parenting skills. To date, over 5,000 substance abusers and family members have registered for the ARRIVE/Exponents program, and no one is ever mandated or coerced to attend. Ms. Cray said that she and the other program staff attempt to "meet people where they're at," to reduce harm, and to help them to make the decision to help themselves by providing a supportive and nonjudgmental attitude.

INTEGRATING HARM REDUCTION AND PSYCHOTHERAPY

Another panel at the Oakland conference was entitled "Integrating Harm Reduction into Psychotherapy Approaches." First to speak was Andrew Tatarsky, a personal friend and colleague, who is a licensed clinical psychologist and certified substance abuse counselor in New York State; he is presently in private practice with PsychologicA, a treatment and training institute in New York City. Tatarsky spoke of his 14 years of experience in traditional substance abuse treatment centers, where he reported feeling frustrated by the low overall success rate for clients based on the sole outcome criterion of continued abstinence (only about a third of the clients ever reached this goal). He began wondering how to reach the vast majority of people with addiction problems who are not receiving any type of treatment, and concluded that harm reduction psychotherapy could serve as a bridge or link for this larger population of active substance users. Tatarsky spoke of an important philosophical parallel between harm reduction and the practice of psychotherapy: "Harm reduction places engagement of the individual in a potentially healing, self-affirming relationship at the forefront of any intervention; and that's what good psychotherapy has always been about." In harm reduction, as in psychotherapy, the choice of goals is client-driven and supported by the therapist. The aims of harm reduction psychotherapy are to find methods that work for the client in terms of his or her goals, and not to blame the client for failure to change.

Tatarsky described the clinical rationale for engaging in harm reduction psychotherapy as follows. First, this approach acknowledges the diversity of the population of people who use substances: A wide range of differences exists in this clientele, including types of drugs used, different motivational stages of change, and various psychiatric comorbidities that may be present. Second, there are the benefits of the therapeutic alliance between therapist and client, and the shared acknowledgment of the client's goals as the starting point of therapy. Third, substance use is viewed by the therapist as the client's attempt to cope with various life stressors. Finally, there is the assumption in psychotherapy that complex behaviors change incrementally, consistent with a harm-reduction approach.

Debra Rothschild, also a clinical psychologist in New York City and cofounder (with Tatarsky) of PsychologicA, a group practice specializing in harm reduction psychotherapy, described herself as an analyst who sees actively addicted clients in her clinical practice. She noted the "huge rift" that exists between the recovery community and the therapy practice community, and attributed it in large part to the perpetuation of the medical model in addiction treatment. The medical model reinforces the traditional doctor–patient relationship when addiction is treated as a disease, Rothschild said. In this model, the patient is expected to follow the doctor's orders, which are prescribed in an authoritarian or even dictatorial manner.

Psychotherapy, on the other hand, does not usually follow the medical model in treating clients with addictive behavior problems, Rothschild observed. Most of her clients come to her in a state of conflict about their drug use: They often report that although their use sometimes seems to help, at other times it causes major life problems. A therapist helps a client explore the source of the conflict, such as what feels good or bad about drug use, or the pros and cons of engaging in that behavior. By allowing the client to understand his or her own conflict about drug use, the therapist is better able to avoid being placed in the role of the authority who demands change on the part of the client. Rothschild also said that if the client projects onto the therapist the client's own desire or intent to stop using drugs, such "splitting" will reinforce the client's identification as a drug user. Instead, the therapist's aim should be to help the client accept and work on resolving his or her internal conflicts. In the published abstract for her presentation, Rothschild states: "The harm reduction model is one which embraces the more traditional psychotherapeutic stance of acceptance and empathy and which is, in fact, far more successful with anyone who misuses substances and desires assistance" (1996, p. 64).

Next to speak was Jeffrey Kragh, a doctoral candidate in counseling psychology at New Mexico State University. Kragh and his coauthor and advisor, Charles Huber, presented a paper showing that harm reduction has many similarities with counseling psychology and rational–emotive therapy. They pointed to the following parallels: Both harm reduction and the counseling psychology field adopt a "strengths and assets" approach to clients, rather than focusing on patient psychopathology; both adopt a "growth as process" approach to individual development over the lifespan; both recognize the importance of individual differences and the need for tailored treatment approaches; and both support a pragmatic and nonjudgmental approach to working with clients.

Bruce Liese, a clinical psychologist who is professor of family medicine and psychiatry at the University of Kansas Medical Center, was the last to speak. He described the application of cognitive therapy in the treatment of people with substance use problems. Cognitive therapy focuses on the role of automatic thoughts and cognitive distortions as they affect addictive behavior. Clients often experience drug-related beliefs that are activated by specific cues in high-risk situations. Therapists can help clients explore these thoughts and feelings and develop alternatives to excessive substance use, Liese noted. He described an ongoing group that he has led in Kansas City since 1992, called the Cognitive Therapy Harm Reduction Group. According to the published abstract,

> Through participation in the group, members have made substantial changes in their lives (including reduced drug use and other significant lifestyle changes), despite the fact that there is no pressure to maintain abstinence from addictive behaviors. . . . In each session, group members discuss hopes, goals, beliefs, and struggles regarding their addictions and abstinence. Group members are taught coping skills for dealing more effectively with relationship and career problems, depression, anxiety, and addictive behaviors. (Liese, 1996, p. 65)

Many of these points about harm reduction therapy were also emphasized in a plenary address given by another colleague and friend of mine, Patt Denning, a clinical psychologist and founder of Addiction Treatment Alternatives, an innovative psychotherapy program for substance users. During her talk, entitled, "Clinical Psychology and Substance Use Management," Denning criticized the dominant disease model ideology: "We as clinicians have been abandoning our patients and our principles to the disease model," she noted. Harm reduction therapy, on the other hand, utilizes approaches that are common among various psychotherapy approaches:

> Another important thing in clinical models, adaptive models, is that people who use drugs and people who don't use or abuse drugs, or people who are addicts, are all understandable by the same concepts that we use to treat other people. There is no difference between people who use and people who don't except for their behavior. The psychological principles do not need to be special in order to understand people who get into problems with drugs. (Denning, 1997, p. 14)

Denning also emphasized that harm reduction is consistent with the Hippocratic Oath, the fundamental statement of medical ethics:

Harm reduction reminds me of the Hippocratic Oath which states—and physicians take this oath— "Do no harm." That is the first principle in medicine, and embedded in the rest of that oath is the agreement that you will actually help. So, do no harm and actively help: that's precisely what harm reduction does. (Denning, 1997, p. 15)

Denning concluded her talk with a reminder that people with drug problems are best considered as consumers, rather than as victims of a biological disease beyond their control:

Finally, harm reduction is based on an awareness that [users] may have other, more pressing needs than drug abuse. They may have housing needs. They may have funding needs, or child care needs. [Users] may have all sorts of other things that they need and want to talk about. This is the basis of consumer-driven services: that we as workers have the responsibility of developing a needs hierarchy for the people under our care that is based on THEIR assessment of their needs more often than OUR assessment of their needs. (Denning, 1997, p. 15)

Following Dr. Denning's talk, I gave a plenary presentation entitled "Controlled Drinking and Behavioral Psychology." I described examples of harm reduction programs for people with alcohol problems, including the controlled-drinking controversy in the alcoholism treatment field. I also discussed the promising results of our harm reduction program for adolescents and young adults who are at risk because of "binge drinking" and its negative consequences. The details of this area of research are presented in Chapter 4 of this book.

OTHER TOPICS COVERED

Over the course of the conference, many more panels and talks were held on a wide range of topics related to harm reduction. Topics included scientific evaluations of syringe exchange programs; legal and policy issues; harm reduction in relation to speed and crack cocaine; treating the dually diagnosed users (i.e., applications of a harm reduction approach to individuals with concomitant substance use problems and mental disorders); concerns of families and communities affected by drug use; addressing issues of harm reduction in communities of color; sexual abuse and harm reduction (understanding the correlation between drug use and histories of sexual trauma); drug user activism and integration in harm reduction efforts; harm reduction in transgender communities; harm reduction in working with issues of domestic and sexual violence; integrating harm reduction into AIDS housing programs; harm reduction in prisons and with parolees; providing harm reduction support and services for sex workers; methadone as a legitimate treatment alternative; peer education as a harm reduction strategy; developing outcome measures for harm reduction interventions; and the uses of culture and the mass media in sending harm reduction messages.

THE CLOSING CEREMONY

After 4 days of meetings, the conference finally came to an end. The closing ceremony was led by Ram Dass, a spiritual leader and principal author of a well-known book on helping others, *How Can I Help?* (Ram Dass & Gorman, 1991). He thanked people in the large audience for attending the conference and for their willingness to listen to one another across so many cultural boundaries. In the controversial issue of drugs, all parties need to be listened to, from drug users to treatment professionals, he emphasized.

"I look at harm reduction as relieving the maximum amount of suffering," Ram Dass observed. Much of this suffering stems from the isolation of the human heart because people are cut off from what they need in terms of basic spiritual nurturance, he continued. Any interaction with another human being, no matter how brief or trivial, can either bring people closer together or set them apart. Much of the separation is due to people's overattachment to their particular roles in society and to their psychosocial identities, Ram Dass noted. People need help in freeing themselves from being trapped in specific roles. He began with this example: "It's perfectly fine if you are an administrator to administrate; just don't get caught in thinking you are an administrator!" He continued, "If you are a junkie, God bless you, but don't get caught in being a junkie! It's not interesting enough—there is no role identity which is THAT interesting. If you are recovering, recover, by God, recover! But don't get caught up in the drama of being a recoverer!" he exhorted the audience members, to their laughter and delight.

Ram Dass then spoke of the importance of people's getting beyond specific role attachments and meeting each other simply as fellow souls, listening to each other so that both sides are heard and accepted. As harm reductionists, we can recognize that we are a group of human beings who are facing a complicated social problem—one that causes "spinoffs" that end up hurting a lot of people, he said. Our goal is to optimize the relief of suffering, beginning with respect for fellow human consciousness as a basic human right. The "drug war" mentality, on the other hand, promotes suffering because of its attitude of righteous judgment toward others. This separation and suffering can be relieved by meeting our fellow human beings on a heart-to-heart basis. "Don't close your heart to the other human being," Ram Dass concluded, "Play your role impeccably, but don't get lost in it." On that note, the conference came to a close.

NOTES

1. Further information about the First National Harm Reduction Conference is available in the form of a published 126-page abstract booklet and/or set of audiotaped presentations available from the conference's sponsor, the Harm Reduction Coalition (HRC), 22 West 27th St., 9th Floor, New York, NY 10001. Several papers presented at the meeting were published in the Winter 1996 and Spring 1997 issues of the HRC's newsletter, *Harm Reduction Communication*.

2. In October 1990, the first U.S. conference on needle exchange took place in Tacoma, Washington, which is now the headquarters for the North American Syringe Exchange Network (address: 535 Dock St. Suite 112, Tacoma, WA 98402).

3. It should be noted in passing that Patrick Vanzo and the King County Division of Alcohol and Substance Abuse Services issued a policy statement in August 1994 on harm reduction services as part of the continuum of alcohol and drug services. I quote from this statement:

> It is our belief that services designed from client points of view are best and that traditional alcohol and drug services, exclusive of harm reduction, reach only 1 in 10 in need. Abstinence-governed models may initially repel some help seekers and, in a contemporary hierarchy of needs, the need to attend to the potential for premature death due to communicable diseases such as AIDS compels us to diversify our approaches to alcohol and drug afflicted populations. In this context then, we call for a full and informed discussion about the relative value of incorporating harm reduction formally in our continuum of care, with all the benefits, privileges, and responsibilities of any other accepted modality.
>
> In a harm reduction environment the care giver meets the patients where they are—accepts that pragmatically and using special intervention skills, engages help seekers in an ongoing process of defining their needs and obtaining help in meeting these. All of this occurs within the context of abstinence as the optimal, eventual goal. En route the help seeker may relapse and progress will be stymied; however, the care giver will continue to support the help seeker in defining needs and seeking further help. (King County Division of Alcohol and Substance Abuse Services, 1994, pp. 1–2)

4. Other U.S. cities have adopted the community policing programs similar to the one in New Haven described by Pastore. In Seattle, for example, Police Chief Norm Stamper was expanding the community policing program in 1996:

> In all four of Seattle's precincts, citizens, neighborhood groups and the specially designated community cops have been forging close relationships for about seven years. The community officers have been doing that not by spending their days in their squad cars responding to 911 calls but rather by getting out of their cruisers, walking their beats and getting to know by name the men, women and children who live there so that together they can get at the root of pressing problems.... [This] has meant meeting neighbors and merchants for coffee at places like the Savanh Cafe near South Edmunds Street, or getting to know people by name at Angie's Tavern, a block away. (Brown, 1996, p. A1).

5. According to an article (Navarro, 1996) on the status of drug courts in the United States, about 28,000 defendants were participating in over 100 drug courts or had graduated from them—a small fraction of the more than 700,000 offenders arrested on drug possession charges each year. As of 1996, drug courts were active

in 44 states, with an additional 8 courts scheduled to open and 77 in the planning stages. The article continued:

> Despite increasing emphasis on tougher punishment, drug courts have thrived because of frustration with so-called revolving-door justice and the onslaught of felony drug cases that are choking courts and crowding jails. . . . While Justice Department figures show that at least 44% of those convicted of drug possession are rearrested for similar offenses within three years, drug courts report recidivism in the range of 4 to 28%. (Navarro, 1996, p. A25)

6. On a sad note, Nelly Velasco, one of the young panelists from the Street Survival Project, died of an overdose of heroin shortly after the completion of the Oakland conference. A paper she presented at the conference was subsequently published in *Harm Reduction Communication,* the newsletter published by the HRC. Here is an excerpt:

> So why do I need support? . . . People seem to think that the only user who needs or deserves support is the one who's trying to quit. This really makes you feel alone and it's hard to get shit accomplished when you're one of the few people who believes in you. This idea of accepting more than just one heroin lifestyle is so radical, it's like swimming against the current. I need you to be aware how much my life and others like me is a contradiction. (Velasco, 1996, p. 7)

In the same newsletter, another woman who spoke on the same panel as Nelly, Erica Berman, gave this eulogy:

> Nelly Velasco, a 19-year-old Mexican IDU [injection drug-using] chick, overdosed and died on October 9, 1996, shortly after the First National Harm Reduction Conference in Oakland where her piece that appears here was presented. Nelly was very ambitious, and very much alive. Her death certainly was not planned. Why did Nelly leave us? And why have countless other harm reduction workers gone? Who knows the answers to these questions—I know I don't. What I do know is that people are dying, and we're in such early stages of this movement that as we continue to move on in the direction we're going—where people are beginning to feel as though they can start an honest dialogue about use—we also really need to watch each other's backs, and we really need to start creating more and more options for each other and for the people we work with. What Nelly was missing was more than one place to work that supported her fully, more people in her life that accepted where she was at and supported and loved her for all that awesome talent and sincere empathy and caring for a hell of a lot of people. If I could see anything good coming out of this fucked up, shitty death, it's that within the movement we begin to organize around and address the issue of death among us, and how we can begin to take better care of ourselves and each other. (Berman, 1996, p. 7)

See also Anonymous (1997, p. 10).

REFERENCES

Anonymous. (1997, Spring). On the death of Nelly Velasco. *Harm Reduction Communication*, No. 4, p. 10.

Berman, E. (1996, Winter). Editorial comment on Nelly Velasco's death. *Harm Reduction Communication*, No. 3, p. 7.

Bertram, E., Blachman, M., Sharpe, K., & Andreas, P. (1996). *Drug war politics: The price of denial.* Berkeley: University of California Press.

Brown, C. E. (1996, November 23). Seattle plans to expand community policing. *The Seattle Times*, p. A1.

Clay, C. (1997, Spring). Getting high and "getting well": Gay and bisexual crystal meth injectors in Seattle. *Harm Reduction Communication*, No. 4, pp. 18–21.

Clear, A. (1997, Spring). Welcoming address: First National Harm Reduction Conference. *Harm Reduction Communication*, No. 4, pp. 1–13.

Denning, P. (1997, Spring). Clinical psychology and substance use management. *Harm Reduction Communication*, No. 4, pp. 13–15.

Harm Reduction Coalition (HRC). (1996). *Mission and principles of harm reduction* [Brochure]. Oakland, CA: Author.

King County Division of Alcohol and Substance Abuse. (1994, August 23). *Policy statement on harm reduction services.* Seattle, WA: Author.

Liese, B. S. (1996). The cognitive therapy harm reduction group. *The First National Harm Reduction Conference Abstract Booklet.* Oakland, CA: Harm Reduction Coalition.

Navarro, M. (1996, October 17). Experimental courts are using new strategies to blunt the lure of drugs. *The New York Times*, p. A25.

Prochaska, J. O., DiClemente, C. C., & Norcross, J. C. (1992). In search of how people change: Applications to addictive behaviors. *American Psychologist, 47,* 1102–1114.

Purchase, D. (1997, Spring). Do unto others. *Harm Reduction Communication*, No. 4, pp. 1–22.

Ram Dass, & Gorman, P. (1991). *How can I help?* New York: Knopf.

Rothschild, D. (1996). Harm reduction and psychotherapy. *The First National Harm Reduction Conference Abstract Booklet.* Oakland, CA: Harm Reduction Coalition.

Smith, I., Velasco, N., & Berman, E. (1996). Hiring youth who use: A smart harm reduction approach. *The First National Harm Reduction Conference Abstract Booklet.* Oakland, CA: Harm Reduction Coalition.

Springer, E. (1991). Effective AIDS prevention with active drug users: The harm reduction model. *Journal of Chemical Dependency Treatment, 4*(2), 141–157.

Springer, E. (1996, Winter). The spectrum of harm reduction. *Harm Reduction Communication*, No. 3, pp. 20–21.

Velasco, N. (1996, Winter). Nelly is in control. *Harm Reduction Communication*, No. 3, pp. 5–7.

Woods, I. (1997, Spring). My journey to harm reduction. *Harm Reduction Communication*, No. 4, pp. 4–6.

CHAPTER TWO

Harm Reduction around the World

A Brief History

G. ALAN MARLATT

Harm reduction is an international movement that arose in response to the growing AIDS crisis in the 1980s (see DesJarlais & Friedman, 1993), although the origins of this approach to drug problems can be traced back to the 19th century (Berridge, 1992). In the past decade, many countries have recognized the need for more pragmatic and adaptive strategies to reduce the risk of HIV transmission among injection drug users. The success of innovative public health approaches introduced in Europe (particularly in the Netherlands and the United Kingdom) and in Australia, such as syringe exchange programs and the medical prescription of addictive substances, further spurred the development of the harm reduction model (known in the United Kingdom as "harm minimization").

The growing worldwide interest in harm reduction led to a series of international conferences that began in Liverpool, England, in 1990; the proceedings of the first conference were published in 1992 (O'Hare, Newcombe, Matthews, Buning, & Drucker, 1992). Annual international conferences have taken place in the intervening years in Barcelona, Spain (1991), Melbourne, Australia (1992), Rotterdam, the Netherlands (1993), Toronto, Canada (1994), Florence, Italy (1995), Hobart, Australia (1996), Paris, France (1997), and São Paulo, Brazil (1998). In addition to the volume published after the Liverpool conference, two further volumes of proceedings have since been published—one from the Melbourne meeting (Heather, Wodak, Nadelmann, & O'Hare, 1993), and the most recent from the 1994 Toronto conference (Erickson, Riley, Cheung, & O'Hare, 1997).

The purpose of this chapter is to provide a brief history of harm reduction as it has evolved outside the United States. First to be presented is the model of harm reduction practiced in the Netherlands. Next is the seminal work on harm minimization strategies (e.g., medical prescription of "hard" drugs in addiction treatment) developed in the United Kingdom. The chapter concludes with a description of selected harm reduction policies and programs in other European countries and in Australia and Canada. We return to a discussion of recent developments concerning harm reduction in the United States in Chapter 10 of this book. For now, let us begin our armchair travels with the development of the harm reduction model in Holland.

THE DUTCH MODEL

Foreign visitors to Amsterdam and other major cities in the Netherlands are often struck with what appears to be a liberal and permissive approach to drugs and sex. Special "coffee shops" sell marijuana and hashish, which can be consumed in the shop or taken home. In the red-light district, prostitutes can be viewed sitting in their parlors along many streets, beckoning to prospective clients. Prices for sexual services are fixed and condom use is mandatory. Pornography shops and "live sex" shows are predominant throughout the district, where police officers on bicycles patrol the streets, providing protection for both prostitutes and their customers. In another part of the city, one of several mobile vans known as the "methadone bus" is parked on a side street, servicing addicts who line up for oral methadone, condoms, and clean hypodermic syringes (given in exchange for their used needles). How did all this come to be?

In the summer of 1990, I was invited to Holland to give a series of workshops on relapse prevention to the staff at the Jellinekcentre (named after E. M. Jellinek, a prominent U.S alcoholism scholar) in Amsterdam. Thanks to the expertise of the Director, psychologist Jan Walberg, and his professional staff, I learned the basic elements of the Dutch model of harm reduction. This approach is based on a pragmatic philosophy and embraces a public health view of drug problems, as stated by the Dutch sociologist E. M. Engelsman (1989), a leading proponent of this perspective:

> The Dutch being sober and pragmatic people, they opt rather for a realistic and practical approach to the drug problem than for a moralistic or over-dramatized one. The drug abuse problem should not be primarily seen as a problem of police and justice. It is essentially a matter of health and social well-being. (p. 212)

Holland, a country with just over 15 million inhabitants, began to make radical changes in national drug policy in the 1970s in response to growing drug problems in the late 1960s. Prior to drug policy reform, stiff sentences were meted out to those caught possessing illicit drugs, including prison terms of 1 year or more for the possession of marijuana (van de Wijngaart, 1991). One Dutch expert gives the following historical perspective:

> Although the use of drugs and especially of opiates was not at all a new phenomenon for the Netherlands, the roots of the present-day drug problem are located in the late sixties. It was the time of student and youth protests, the questioning of the established social order and the search for new (sub-)cultural values. As part of this search people began to experiment with drugs like cannabis and hallucinogens. In 1972 heroin became widely available in the Netherlands. The initial reaction of national and local authorities did not differ much from the reaction we nowadays still see in many other countries, which in simple words says: 'This is an undesired phenomenon. We must get rid of it by all means!' 'All means' meant a repressive judicial policy and . . . a [rapidly] growing drug free treatment movement. (Grund, 1989, p. 993)

Changes in this traditional, repressive drug policy began to occur in the Netherlands as early as 1972 (Cohen, 1997). In that year, the Narcotics Working Party published a document concluding that the basic premises of drug policy should be congruent with the extent of the risks involved in drug use. This policy change led to the adoption of a revised Dutch Opium Act in 1976, which made a distinction between drugs of "unacceptable risk" (heroin, cocaine, amphetamines, and LSD) and drugs with lower risk, such as marijuana and hashish (van de Wijngaart, 1991). Commenting on this distinction, Engelsman notes: "In this regard the Dutch prove very pragmatic and try to avoid a situation in which consumers of cannabis suffer more damage from the criminal proceedings than from the use of the drug itself" (1989, p. 213).

Another goal of this policy change was to separate the markets in which "hard" drugs and "soft" drugs circulate. Individuals purchasing cannabis products in designated "coffee shops" are not exposed to dealers who would otherwise promote the sales of such drugs as cocaine or heroin. Although the distinction between types of drugs based on their harmful effects is consistent with the philosophy of harm reduction, the term "harm reduction" itself was not introduced until 1981 in a publication issued by the State Secretary for Health and Environmental Protection. Engelsman (1989) describes this trend:

> In the eighties a new treatment philosophy emerged. . . . Increasing encouragement by the Government has been given to forms of aid which are not primarily intended to end addiction as such, but to improve addicts' physical and social well-being and to help them to function in society. At this stage the addicts' (temporal) inability to give up drug use was being accepted as a fact.

This kind of assistance may be defined as harm reduction or more tradition- ally: secondary and tertiary prevention. Its effectiveness can only be ensured by low threshold facilities and accessible help, which are the key concepts in Dutch drug policy. This takes the form of: field work on the street, in hospitals and in jails; open-door centres for prostitutes; the supply of the medically prescribed substitute drug methadone; material support; and social rehabilita- tion opportunities. (p. 216)

This movement toward a more humane and pragmatic approach was stimulated in large part by direct input from Dutch drug users and addicts themselves. In 1980 the *Junkiebond* (Junkie League) was established in Rotterdam as a kind of trade union for concerned hard drug users. There are now local groups in most major cities, with national representation in the Federation of Dutch Junkie Leagues. As described by van de Wijngaart (1991),

The starting point of the 'Junkiebond' is to look after the interests of the drug users. The most important thing is to combat the deterioration of the user or, to put it another way, to improve the housing and general situation of the addict. Their philosophy is that drug users themselves know best what their problems are. The work of the 'Junkiebond' involves consultations with government officials about matters like the distribution of methadone, the availability of free sterile syringes, the policy of the lawmakers and police, and housing problems. (p. 39)

Input from addicts associated with the *Junkiebond* led to the develop- ment of the first needle exchange program in Amsterdam in 1984. The Municipal Health Service delivered disposable needles and syringes in large quantities once a week to the *Junkiebond* for distribution and collection of used needles. As AIDS and the risk for HIV infection through shared needles increased in the mid-1980s, the number of exchanged needles and syringes rose from 100,000 in 1985 to 720,000 in 1988 (Brussel & Buning, 1988). Overall, the evidence supporting the importance of needle exchange and related harm reduction programs in reducing HIV infection in the Netherlands is strong (Buning, Brussel, & Santen, 1992).

These and other related developments led to the adoption in 1985 of a revised drug policy that provided the framework for the current emphasis on "normalization" of the drug problem in Holland. The normalization policy is summed up by Engelsman (1989) as follows: "The Dutch policy of normalization seems to have produced a context where the addict more resembles an unemployed Dutch citizen than a monster endangering soci- ety" (pp. 216–217). Dorn (1989) elaborates on this:

The Dutch position as outlined by Engelsman and his compatriots is summa- rized in the term 'normalization.' This is presented as a pragmatic policy position lying in between the War on Drugs, on the one side, and Legalization, on the other. Normalization is primarily attentive to the needs of the drug user and to the desirability of reducing to a minimum all the forms of harm that may stem from control responses, as distinct from the drug use per se. Normalization is not, however, a giving up of law enforcement. It is the fine tuning of law enforcement so as to avoid stigmatizing labeling of drug users . . . and it is the attempt to separate drug markets in unacceptably dangerous drugs from those in less dangerous drugs. . . . Of course, this version of pragmatism (and it is only one version among many) would be like a red flag to a bull as far as 'zero tolerance' policy makers in any country are concerned. (p. 995)

Low-threshold programs based on the principles of harm reduction have greatly augmented the range of treatment services available to the Dutch population of drug users over the last 20 years. The Dutch treatment system has expanded from a mainly abstinence-oriented model to a multiple-option approach, ranging from low-threshold (e.g., methadone maintenance) to high-threshold (e.g., drug-free therapeutic communities) programs, thus making help accessible to a majority of addicts.

During my visit to the Jellinekcentre in Amsterdam, I observed the range of treatment programs available, from low-threshold outreach projects (e.g., the mobile "methadone bus") to high-threshold abstinence-based inpatient programs (e.g., therapeutic communities and long-term residential care). Harm reduction programs include fieldwork with addicts in the streets, in hospitals, and in jails; open-door health centers for sex workers; and extensive needle exchange programs. In contrast with the high-threshold programs, the low-threshold programs do not require a commitment to abstinence or drug testing as a prerequisite for admission. All they ask of the addict is a willingness to show up and (it is hoped) to begin taking steps in the direction of reducing harm.

On one afternoon during my visit to Amsterdam, I traveled as a visitor on one of the two "methadone buses" run by the Jellinekcentre—an experience that allowed me to see how the low-threshold approach works in actual practice. Addicts can obtain methadone in the bus only if they have regular contact with a medical doctor and are enrolled in the central methadone registration file (both of which can be easily arranged). The staff on the bus consisted of a driver and two male nurses, who knew most of the addicts by name and exchanged social pleasantries with them during their brief visits. During the 2 hours that the bus was parked in one downtown area known to have a large addict population, approximately 50 addicts came by for their daily dose of oral methadone (no "take-home" doses are allowed). Used needles were dropped in a receptacle and were promptly replaced with new, sterile needles. The nurses also handed out condoms and first-aid supplies upon demand.

In one exchange with a young couple and their child, the staff agreed to provide help with fixing the couple's apartment, which was badly in need of repair. An arrangement was made to send a team of volunteers (including a plumber) to assist the family later in the week. Later it was explained to me that once public health officials make contact with addicts in this helpful and respectful manner, bridges can be built that may lead these persons to seek help in the future (Marlatt & Tapert, 1993).

One of the most significant results of this easy-access, low-threshold treatment philosophy is that the Dutch claim to be in contact with a majority of the addict population: "In Amsterdam about 60–80% are being reached by any kind of assistance. This percentage is certainly higher in less urbanized regions" (Englesman, 1989, p. 217). Such a high rate of contact is very helpful in terms of AIDS prevention and other public health programs. Data are available that support the effectiveness of the harm reduction approach with injection drug users. One study showed, for example, that the average age of these users is rising (in Amsterdam, from 26.8 to 30.1 years between 1981 and 1987), and that people who use injection drugs for the first time tend to be older (Brussel & Buning, 1988).

Similar encouraging results have been reported on the effects of the Dutch law regarding cannabis use. As noted above, the amended Opium Act in 1976 created a *de facto* decriminalization of the use of marijuana and hashish. This change in policy does not seem to have led to increased use of cannabis products among the Dutch citizenry. According to a 1985 report by the Dutch Ministry of Welfare, Health and Cultural Affairs, "In 1976, 3% of young people aged 15–16 and 10% of the 17–18 age group had occasionally used hashish or marijuana. In 1985 these figures were 2% and 6% respectively" (p. 2). Other data sources indicate that a decreasing number of adolescents in the Netherlands smoke cannabis products. A survey by Sijlbing and Persoon (1985) showed that 12% of high school students in the Netherlands had used cannabis at least once in their lifetimes—considerably less than the 59% found for the same group at the same time in the United States (Johnston, O'Malley, & Bachman, 1985). These same two surveys showed that current use (monthly prevalence) in the same population was lower in Holland (5.4%) than in the United States (29%). As van de Wijngaart (1991) has concluded in his review of this literature, "De facto decriminalization of cannabis does not produce more cannabis use and appears to be successful" (p. 126).

The striking differences between Dutch and U.S. drug policies were pointed out to me during my visit to Amsterdam by another international visitor to the Jellinekcentre, a drug specialist from India who was visiting drug treatment centers in both the United States and Europe. During one conversation, he summarized his impressions to me as follows:

> In America, you have a big government hierarchy with the Drug Czar at the top of the heap who tells the addicts what to do and what not to do, and if the addict fails to comply, he is put in prison or jail. In Holland, in comparison,

the approach is quite different; someone from this center sits down next to the addict on the park bench and asks, "How can we help you to return to a productive life in this society?" (Quoted in Marlatt & Tapert, 1993, p. 257)

Any attempt to apply the Dutch model of drug policy to other countries is a difficult matter, given all of the cultural differences involved (MacCoun, Saiger, Kahan, & Reuter, 1993). Can the Dutch model be a model for changes in U.S. drug policy? One Dutch expert feels that it cannot be:

> There is absolutely no guarantee that attempts to imitate Dutch drug policy in other countries would meet with success. . . . Crucial elements of the Dutch context appear to be: a strong belief in equal rights; belief in the possibility and legitimacy of social intervention; and a sound system of welfare and health care provisions. By comparison, some aspects of the American situation which appear to be important determinants of the nature of the "drug problem" in that land (the existence of strong social polarities, the lack of adequate welfare provisions, and the sheer geographical size of the country) do not apply in the Dutch context. (van de Wijngaart, 1991, p. 129)

On the other hand, others have argued that the Dutch position on drugs is relevant to the development and modification of drug policy in other countries (Duncan & Nicholson, 1997; Leuw & Marshall, 1994). Kaplan, Haanraadts, Vliet, and Grund (1994) state:

> In our view, the Dutch experience (with some local adaptations of course) is indeed a markedly relevant example to the world. Support for our view stems from a number of local, national and international movements which are rallying under the banner of public mental health/crime prevention reforms to respond to a perceived failure of the international control system. . . . If Dutch drug policy is indeed the rational outcome of conscious political decision-making and problem-solving, then Dutch drug policy could be an example to the world. Dutch drug policy is an example to the world insofar as Dutch society is a forerunner in the "shift to different goals" strategy for solving social problems. (p. 311, 329–330)

The Dutch have received considerable criticism for their unique drug policy, particularly from the United States and from European countries with more prohibitionistic policies (e.g., France and Sweden). Within the Netherlands itself, public opposition has increased in reaction to the growing number of "drug tourists" from neighboring countries, who come to Holland to purchase drugs for their own consumption and who often constitute a public nuisance for citizens (Korf, 1994). A related problem involves the smuggling of drugs purchased in Holland for resale in other countries. Cannabis products are widely available and constitute a major attraction for many international visitors. As of 1994, more than 1,000 "coffee shops" selling hashish existed in the Netherlands, with more than 300 of them located in Amsterdam alone (Jansen, 1994).

In response to both international and local opposition to the problems of drug tourists and the public nuisance issue, the Dutch Ministry of Public Health announced a revised drug policy in a 1995 report entitled "Continuity and Change"(see also Maris, 1996a, 1996b). Although no radical changes are instituted, the new policy is "geared to tackling and containing the nuisance drug-use causes society" (Dutch Ministry of Public Health, 1995, p. 2). In order to prevent large purchases of cannabis products (for possible resale outside the Netherlands), the maximum quantity that "coffee shops" may sell to an individual has been reduced from 30 grams to 5 grams. Also, although individuals may grow up to 10 marijuana plants (in Dutch, *nederweed*) for their own use, large-scale production will be prosecuted. The report notes that the "steppingstone" theory (i.e., the theory that use of soft drugs is the gateway to hard drug use) is not supported, based on the current ratio of about 650,000 Dutch soft drug users to a stable population of 25,000 hard drug users. The report also recommended that heroin maintenance programs be explored with hard-core addicts (similar to the current trial of heroin maintenance conducted in Switzerland from 1993 to 1996; see below). In a commentary on the new policy, Kerssemakers (1995) concluded:

> . . . the foundation the Dutch drug policy is based upon has remained in place. . . . The policy paper mainly seems to be written for the world outside the Netherlands. There has been a great deal of pressure in this connection from abroad. Sweden and to an even larger extent France, where Public Health Minister Hubert called the Dutch drug policy "devastating," are exerting considerable pressure. The Netherlands lacks the wherewithal to face up to it with conviction. We are a small country and can not afford to have troubled relations with our most important partners. As far as that is concerned, perhaps it is time for the torch of drug policy innovation to be taken over by other European nations. (p. 4)

One such other European country to explore innovative policies for drug use and harm reduction is the United Kingdom, which is discussed next.

THE U.K. (MERSEYSIDE) MODEL

The first international conference on harm reduction was held in Liverpool, England, under the sponsorship of the Merseyside Health Authority, in 1990 (O'Hare et al., 1992). The United Kingdom pioneered the "medicalization" approach, in which drug abusers can be prescribed drugs such as heroin and cocaine on a maintenance basis. The prescribing of drugs to addicts dates back to the Rolleston Committee of the 1920s, in which a group of prominent British physicians recommended that in certain cases addicts be prescribed narcotics in order to reduce the harm of their drug use and to help them lead useful lives (Rolleston, 1926). Although prescribing drugs for addicts fell into disfavor over the ensuing years, this policy continued to be practiced by the Merseyside Health Authority, serving the population around the city of Liverpool (Marks, 1991).

In the Merseyside harm reduction model, addicts are offered a wide range of services, including needle exchange and outreach education; prescription of drugs such as heroin and cocaine; and counseling, employment, and housing services. Pharmacists fill prescriptions for smokable drugs and prepare these as "reefers" (cigarettes into which drugs such as heroin and methadone are injected). In addition to reefers, pharmacists dispense drugs in ampoule, liquid, and aerosol forms (Riley, 1994).

As described by Marks (1991), all addicts who register with the Drug Dependency Service in the Merseyside area are initially offered treatment for their addiction, including inpatient detoxification. Only about 10% are interested in treatment geared toward cessation of drug use:

> If treatment is resolutely refused by the patient, a policy of harm-reduction is adopted where the individual ceases to be a patient and becomes a client, maintaining his or her habit but minimizing the danger to himself or herself and the damage to the rest of society. This essentially comprises a ration of drugs. . . . From the standpoint of mutual trust, it is possible to begin to engage the client in a rational, reflective evaluation of his or her lifestyle and behaviour. (Marks, 1991, pp. 307, 310)

Decisions about each addict's treatment or drug maintenance goals are made by members of an interdisciplinary team, including physicians, social workers, nurses, and other therapists. As such, the medicalization program is not directed only by the physician who writes prescriptions:

> Despite the fact that the prescription is formally signed by the doctor, he or she is not the recognized leader of the team; each team member is seen as having equal status and any change in treatment (or the decision to maintain treatment) is agreed by the whole team or, in cases of dispute, by a majority. (Marks, 1991, p. 310)

In a commentary on the role of drug prescriptions for addicts, Strang (1990) has noted five potential functions of this approach:

1. The prescription as a means of relieving withdrawal symptoms (the major function methadone prescriptions serve for opiate addicts).

2. The prescription as bait to capture the drug taker. Strang compares this procedure to the marketing strategy of providing "loss-leaders" to potential consumers (offering below-cost or even free items to engage the interest of a wider purchasing group):

Low-threshold prescribing programs or the provision of other benefits (e.g., free legal aid or needles and syringes) might be regarded as loss-leaders; thus, one measure of their value would be the extent to which they encouraged recruitment and subsequent flow on to the next level in the journey of treatment. (1990, p. 145)

3. The prescription as adhesive to improve retention. Here the purpose is to enhance retention and prevent treatment dropouts, since the continued prescribing of drugs increases the probability of continued attendance.

4. The prescription as promoter of change. Prescribing drugs may offer an "intermediate goal" in the process of habit change—in other words, a short-term goal that may facilitate further advances if the addict begins a step-down program of reducing the harm of drug use:

> If treatment is seen as working through a cascade of processes of change (either sequentially or simultaneously) with the end state of each process acting as one of a hierarchy of goals, then the beneficial impact of the prescription could be gauged according to its effectiveness in achieving these intermediate goals. Some of the intermediate goals within the cascade or hierarchy might reasonably be seen as particularly important, such as the cessation of sharing injecting equipment, and the move from injectable to oral-only drug use. (Strang, 1990, pp. 146–147)

The importance of intermediate goals in the harm reduction model is also emphasized by Allan Parry (1989), a leading pioneer figure in the Liverpool program:

> Harm reduction takes small steps to reduce, even to a small degree, the harm caused by the use of drugs. If a person is injecting street heroin of unknown potency, harm reduction would consider it an advance if the addict were prescribed safe, legal heroin. A further advantage if he stopped sharing needles. A further advance if he enrolled in a needle-exchange scheme. A much further advance if he moved on to oral drugs or to smoked drugs. A further advance in harm reduction if he started using condoms and [engaging in] safe sex practices. A further advance if he took advantage of the general health services available to addicts. A wonderful victory if he kicked drugs, although total victory is not a requirement as it is in the United States. (p. 3)

5. The prescription as the end state. The possibility exists that some addicts who are unwilling or unable to achieve abstinence can be maintained on prescribed drugs indefinitely (e.g., methadone or heroin maintenance).

The police force plays a critical role in the Merseyside harm reduction approach (Chappell, Reitsma, O'Connell, & Strang, 1993). Police representatives sit on health authority drug advisory committees to improve drug prevention and treatment programs. They routinely refer arrested drug offenders to treatment services and provide public support for needle exchange programs. A key feature of the police program is its "cautioning policy," in which first-time drug offenders are cautioned or warned that any further unlawful possession of drugs will result in prosecution. These first-time offenders are not given a criminal record; instead, they are given information about treatment services and needle exchange programs. If a drug user then registers with the appropriate service agency, he or she is then legally entitled to carry drugs for personal use.

How effective is this approach? Although controlled outcome trials have yet to be conducted on the Merseyside model, health and crime statistics for this region tend to provide support, especially concerning the rates of HIV infection among injection drug users (IDUs in the following quote):

> At the end of June 1991, Mersey Region had the second lowest rate of HIV-positive IDUs of all 14 English regions: eight per million population compared with an English national rate of 34, and a top rate of 136 per million in North-West Thames; the rate for the UK as a whole was 51, with Scotland registering a rate of 183 HIV-positive IDUs per million population. The Merseyside programs have also been successful in reducing crime. In 1990 and 1991, the Merseyside police were the only force in the UK to register a decrease in crime rates. (Riley, 1994, p. 5)

Beyond the Merseyside program of drug medicalization described above, the United Kingdom has had a long history of prescribing injectable heroin to opiate addicts (Strang, Ruben, Farrell, & Gossop, 1994). Since 1926, as noted earlier, British physicians have had the freedom to prescribe any available pharmaceutical drug to their addicted patients:

> Whilst the prescribing of heroin, cocaine, and dipipanone (Diconal) is now restricted to those doctors who hold a special license (in practice, the doctors who work in National Health Service drug treatment centres), any qualified medical practitioner can prescribe oral or injectable methadone, morphine, or any other available pharmaceutical drug. (Strang et al., 1994, p. 193)

Although it has been controversial within the United Kingdom, the practice of drug medicalization has received additional impetus from the advent of the AIDS crisis. Programs for the exchange of needles and syringes for injecting addicts were introduced under the rubric of "harm minimization"—the British term for harm reduction (Stimson, 1994). Despite these advances, opposition to prescribing drugs to addicts (particularly noninjectable drugs such as cannabis, hallucinogens, and cocaine) remains strong in many parts of the United Kingdom:

> ... whilst the threat of HIV has legitimized risk reduction and harm minimization measures vis-à-vis drug injecting, there has been little parallel

development concerning harm minimization with other (that is, non-inject-able) drugs. Even in the present favorable climate, it is likely that those who advocate harm minimization for the use of Ecstasy or other commonly used drugs, will find short shrift from the drug and political establishments. (Stimson, 1994, p. 255)

Nevertheless, in an editorial in the journal *Addiction*, Gerry Stimson, director of the Centre for Research on Drugs and Health Behavior at the University of London, stated that the U.K. system has been effective in preventing an epidemic of HIV infection among drug injectors:

> Since the mid-1980s there have been major changes in syringe-sharing risk behaviour, and evidence that specific preventive interventions have been successful: a plausible case can be made for the success of public health interventions in averting a potential public health disaster. . . . The key target was current injectors who were unable or unwilling to stop injecting. Ideas of service accessibility, flexibility of service delivery, multiple and intermediate goals for treatment and—most significantly—of harm minimization, were introduced. (Stimson, 1996, p. 1085)

For comprehensive reviews of the U.K. System of dealing with drug addiction from a harm minimization perspective, two edited volumes are available on this topic (Strang & Gossop, 1994; Strang & Stimson, 1990). A book reviewing harm minimization programs targeted at alcohol use in the United Kingdom is also available (Plant, Single, & Stockwell, 1997).

POLICIES AND PROGRAMS IN OTHER EUROPEAN COUNTRIES

European countries are divided on issues of harm reduction and legalization of drugs, despite the movement toward a common European market economy. Some countries, particularly France (Aeberhard, 1996) and Sweden (Yates, 1996), have rejected the more open policy advocated by the Dutch and the Swiss (Klingemann, 1996). By contrast, several European cities (Amsterdam, Zurich, Frankfurt, and others) have joined together in an alliance to promote harm reduction practices for their high-risk urban drug users.

A report on one such city, Frankfurt, Germany, was presented by Werner Schneider, Frankfurt's drug policy coordinator, at the Ninth International Conference on Drug Policy Reform (sponsored by the Drug Policy Foundation and held in Santa Monica, California, in October 1995). Started in 1990, the Frankfurt program has become a model of harm reduction for large European cities. Services offered include mobile vans for providing counseling and needle exchange services to addicts; needle exchange access in city pharmacies; low-threshold methadone programs; overnight shelters for homeless addicts; four crisis centers to provide medical care (via "contact cafés"); and three "health care rooms" (safe areas where addicts can inject drugs). Schneider (1995) presented data showing the positive effects of this program (e.g., a drop in the number of annual drug overdose deaths, from 140 in 1991 to only 22 deaths in 1994).

In another presentation at the same conference, several medical researchers from Switzerland (headed by Ambros Uchtenhagen, director of psychiatry at the University of Zurich) reported on "the Swiss experiment"—a seminal harm reduction program aimed at hard-core drug users (Uchtenhagen, Dobler-Mikola, & Gutzwiller, 1996). In 1993, Switzerland began conducting a 3-year scientific drug policy study that combined the provision of hard drugs to addicts with medical and social service programs (Karel, 1993). Although the Swiss formerly provided addicts with a safe environment for drug injectors, known as the *Fixerstuebli* (shooting room) (Haeming, 1992), they had less success with the *Plastzpitz* (Needle Park) project, in which addicts were allowed to purchase and use drugs in a public arena. Swiss authorities closed down Zurich's Needle Park in 1992, after pursuing a hands-off policy since the park was first permitted to operate in 1987. Officials considered an alternative approach: that of decentralizing services and making heroin and other injectable drugs available to hard-core addicts on a prescription basis. In this new program, which was available in eight Swiss cities, addicts who qualified were provided with medical access to heroin, morphine, and injectable methadone, along with services including lodging and help in finding employment, treatment for somatic and psychiatric conditions (including HIV), and counseling for familial and lifestyle problems. Although Switzerland is a small country with a population of only 6 million, an estimated 30,000 to 40,000 are addicted to hard drugs.

The program was designed to involve a total of 700 addicts. In the summer of 1995, 340 Swiss heroin addicts received a legal supply of heroin each day from one of the prescribing programs. Smaller numbers of addicts were prescribed injectable morphine or methadone. The program accepted only "hard-core junkies"—those who had a long history of injecting and who had failed in previous attempts to quit. Several important questions were addressed by this study, including the following: Can addicts stabilize their drug use by being assured of a legal, safe, and stable source of heroin? Will this policy lead to a reduction in crime? Will addicts on the program be able to hold a legal job? Are they healthier and less likely to be infected with HIV? Will overdose deaths be reduced? The preliminary results were promising, as summarized by Nadelmann (1995):

> In late 1994, the Social Welfare Department in Zurich held a press conference to issue its preliminary findings: 1) Heroin prescription is feasible and has produced no black market in diverted heroin. 2) The health of the addicts in

the program has clearly improved. 3) Heroin prescription alone cannot solve the problems that led to the heroin addiction in the first place. 4) Heroin prescription is less a medical program than it is a social-psychological approach to a complex personal and social problem. 5) Heroin per se causes very few, if any, problems when it is used in a controlled fashion and administered in hygienic conditions, with clients controlling their dose. (p. 12)

HARM REDUCTION IN CANADA AND AUSTRALIA

Harm reduction was first recommended as the framework for Canada's national drug strategy in 1987 (Riley, 1994), although subsequent changes may have weakened the impact of this policy (Fischer, 1997; Fischer, Erickson, & Smart, 1996). In March 1994, Canada hosted the Fifth International Conference on the Reduction of Drug-Related Harm in Toronto—the first of these conferences to be held in North America. The published proceedings of the Toronto conference (Erickson et al., 1997) reflect the range of topics covered at the meeting: 26 chapters are included on a wide range of topics, such as national drug policy comparisons (Canadian vs. U.S. policies), harm reduction for special populations (pregnant women who use drugs, street youth, prostitutes, and prison populations), human rights issues (e.g., drug legalization vs. the "temperance mentality"), the definition and measurement of harmful versus helpful drug effects, and harm reduction intervention programs (with target populations ranging from binge-drinking college students to older adults with alcohol and drug problems).

The Canadian harm reduction model has been described by Diane Riley (1994) of the Canadian Centre on Substance Abuse:

> The first priority of harm reduction is to decrease the negative consequences of drug use. By contrast, drug policy in North America has traditionally focused on reducing the prevalence of drug use. Harm reduction establishes a hierarchy of goals, with the more immediate and realistic ones to be achieved as first steps toward risk-free use or, if appropriate, abstinence.
>
> Drug-taking behaviours result in effects that are either beneficial (as in the case of life-saving medication), neutral or harmful. Assigning a positive or negative value—a benefit or harm—to such effects is subjective and open to controversy, but a harm reduction framework at least offers a pragmatic means by which consequences can be objectively evaluated. (p. 1)

In her report, Riley (1994) reviews a number of areas in which harm reduction programs have been applied, including injection drug use (e.g., needle exchange programs and methadone maintenance), prevention of alcohol problems (moderate drinking programs), and health promotion and education. In regard to the health promotion and education programs, Riley states:

The harm reduction approach to education focuses on non-judgmental information about different drugs, their properties and effects, about the law and legal rights, about how to reduce risks, and where to get help if needed. It helps youth to develop a wide range of skills in assessment, judgment, communication, assertiveness, conflict resolution, decision-making and safer use.

Harm reduction education is based on humanitarianism, pragmatism and a scientific public health approach. The principles of harm reduction drug education are that drug use is normal; it is associated with benefits as well as risks; it cannot be eliminated altogether, but the harms can be reduced; many young people grow out of drug use; education should be non-judgmental; it requires an open dialogue with the young and respect for people's right to make their own decisions; and it emphasizes positive peer support, not divisiveness. (1994, p. 11)

The Canadian approach to reformulating drug education and prevention programs in terms of harm reduction is also advocated in Australia. In a critical review of traditional drug education programs that emphasize only the harmful effects of drugs and espouse a "just say no" approach to resisting any drug use, O'Connor and Saunders (1992) recommend an alternative approach based on harm reduction principles:

... it is proposed that for illicit substances a new perspective should be adopted. The concept of drug education as some type of useful "inoculation" against drug use and its imputed problems needs to be reassessed. It is advocated that future educational endeavors are supplemented by training. That is, the training of those who use drugs to do so well and wisely. While not encouraging drug use, there is little value in perpetuating a perspective that emphasizes DON'T but persuades few not to, while simultaneously ignoring those that do. . . . The focus of education needs to be shifted from the drug-free sanctuary of the classroom to venues of drug use. Concomitant with this reorientation is the need to accept that drug use, which has been an integral part of human history, is here to stay and that the task at hand is to strive, by all means possible, to reduce to an absolute minimum the levels of harm that are associated with use. The goal of drug education becomes one of harm reduction, not drug use elimination. (p. 178)

Australia was the first country to introduce harm reduction formally into its national drug policy (Crofts & Herkt, 1995; Hawks & Lenton, 1995; Herkt, 1993; Wodak, 1992). In 1992, Australia hosted the Third International Conference on the Reduction of Drug-Related Harm (Heather et al., 1993). At the conference, Australian Minister for Health Services Peter Staples stated:

Since its inception in 1985, Australia's National Campaign Against Drug Abuse has specified that its underlying aim was 'to minimize the harmful effects of drugs on Australian Society.' Although some may consider this aim represents a 'soft option' in dealing with drugs, the Australian Government does not. The Australian Government does not condone the use and misuse of drugs and firmly believes that a harm-reduction approach is realistic. We do not consider that a drug-free society is an achievable goal. Furthermore, the Australian Government believes that our efforts will bear fruit in the long term and engender in our society a responsible attitude to drugs. (1993).

In the current Australian drug policy, tobacco and alcohol are included along with illicit drugs, in recognition of the fact that these two substances are responsible for the vast majority of drug-related harm in Australia (Crofts & Herkt, 1995). Australia has also considered conducting a trial of providing heroin and other opiates to injection drug users (Bammer, Douglas, Moore, & Chappell, 1993).

REFERENCES

Aeberhard, P. J. (1996). The politics of harm reduction in France. *International Journal of Drug Policy, (7)*1, 27–30.

Bammer, G., Douglas, B., Moore, M., & Chappell, D. (1993). A heroin trial for the Australian Capital Territory: An overview of feasibility research. In N. Heather, A. Wodak, E. Nadelmann, & P. O'Hare (Eds.), *Psychoactive drugs and harm reduction: From faith to science* (pp. 136–152). London: Whurr.

Berridge, V. (1992). AIDS, drugs and history. *British Journal of Addiction, 87*(3), 363–370.

Brussel, G., & Buning, E. C. (1988). Public health management of AIDS and drugs in Amsterdam. In L. S. Harris (Ed.), *Problems of drug dependence* (NIDA Research Monograph No. 90, pp. 295–301). Rockville, MD: U.S. Department of Health and Human Services.

Buning, E. C., Brussel, G. V., & Santen, G. V. (1992). The impact of harm reduction drug policy on AIDS prevention in Amsterdam. In P. O'Hare, R. Newcombe, A. Matthews, E. C. Buning, & E. Drucker (Eds.), *The reduction of drug related harm* (pp. 30–38). London: Routledge.

Chappell, D., Reitsma, T., O'Connell, D., & Strang, H. (1993). Law enforcement as a harm-reduction strategy in Rotterdam and Merseyside. In N. Heather, A. Wodak, E. Nadelmann, & P. O'Hare (Eds.), *Psychoactive drugs and harm reduction: From faith to science* (pp. 118–126). London: Whurr.

Cohen, P. D. A. (1997). The case of the two Dutch drug-policy commissions: An exercise in harm reduction, 1968–1996. In P. G. Erickson, D. M. Riley, Y. W. Cheung, & P. A. O'Hare (Eds.), *Harm reduction: A new direction for drug policies and programs* (pp. 17–31). Toronto: University of Toronto Press.

Crofts, N., & Herkt, D. (1995). A history of peer-based drug-user groups in Australia. *Journal of Drug Issues, 25*, 599–616.

DesJarlais, D. C., & Friedman, S. R. (1993). AIDS, injecting drug use and harm reduction. In N. Heather, A. Wodak, E. Nadelmann, & P. O'Hare (Eds.), *Psychoactive drugs and harm reduction: From faith to science* (pp. 297–309). London: Whurr.

Dorn, N. (1989). Sideshow: An appreciation and critique of Dutch drug policies. *British Journal of Addiction, 84*, 995–997.

Duncan, D. F., & Nicholson, T. (1997). Dutch drug policy: A model for America? *Journal of Health and Social Policy, 8*(1), 1–15.

Dutch Ministry of Public Health. (1995). Continuity and change: Dutch drug policy in the years to come. *Jellinek Quarterly, 2*, 2–3.

Dutch Ministry of Welfare, Health and Cultural Affairs. (1985). *Policy on drug use.* The Hague: Government Printing Office.

Engelsman, E. M. (1989). Dutch policy on the management of drug-related problems. *British Journal of Addiction, 84*, 211–218.

Erickson, P. G., Riley, D. M., Cheung, Y. W., & O'Hare, P. A. (Eds.). (1997). *Harm reduction: A new direction for drug policies and programs.* Toronto: University of Toronto Press.

Fischer, B. (1997). The battle for a new Canadian drug law: A legal basis for harm reduction or a new rhetoric for prohibition? A chronology. In P. G. Erickson, D. M. Riley, Y. W. Cheung, & P. A. O'Hare (Eds.), *Harm reduction: A new direction for drug policies and programs* (pp. 47–68). Toronto: University of Toronto Press.

Fischer, B., Erickson, P. G., & Smart, R. (1996). The new Canadian drug law: One step forward, two steps backward. *International Journal of Drug Policy, 7*(3), 172–179.

Grund, J. P. C. (1989). Where do we go from here? The future of Dutch drug policy. *British Journal of Addiction, 84*, 992–995.

Haeming, R. B. (1992) The street-corner agency with shooting room ('Fixerstuebli'). In P. A. O'Hare, R. Newcombe, A. Matthews, E. C. Buning, & E. Drucker (Eds.), *The reduction of drug-related harm* (pp. 181–185). London: Routledge.

Hawks, D., & Lenton, S. (1995). Harm reduction in Australia: Has it worked? A review. *Drug and Alcohol Review, 14*, 291–304.

Heather, N., Wodak, A., Nadelmann, E., & O'Hare, P. A. (Eds.). (1993). *Psychoactive drugs and harm reduction: From faith to science.* London: Whurr.

Herkt, D. (1993). Peer-based user groups: The Australian experience. In N. Heather, A. Wodak, E. Nadelmann, & P. O'Hare (Eds.), *Psychoactive drugs and harm reduction: From faith to science* (pp. 320–330). London: Whurr.

Jansen, A. C. M. (1994). The development of a "legal" consumers' market for cannabis: The "coffee shop" phenomenon. In E. Leuw & I. H. Marshall (Eds.), *Between prohibition and legalization: The Dutch experiment in drug policy* (pp. 169–181). New York: Kugler.

Johnston, L. D., O'Malley, P. M., & Bachman, J. G. (1985). *Use of licit and illicit drugs by America's high school students 1975–1984.* (DHHS Publication No. ADM 85-1394). Washington, DC: U.S. Government Printing Office.

Kaplan, C. D., Haanraadts, D. J., Vliet, V., & Grund, J. P. (1994). Is Dutch drug policy an example to the world? In E. Leuw & I. H. Marshall (Eds.), *Between prohibition and legalization: The Dutch experiment in drug policy* (pp. 311–335). New York: Kugler.

Karel, R. (1993, September 17). Switzerland to start innovative program to help addicts control illicit drug use. *American Psychiatric News*, p. 4.

Kerssemakers, R. (1995). Drug policy paper overlooks opportunities. *Jellinek Quarterly, 2*, 4.

Klingemann, H. (1996). Drug treatment in Switzerland: Harm reduction, decentralization and community response. *Addiction, 91*(5), 723–736.

Korf, D. J. (1994). Drug tourists and drug refugees. In E. Leuw & I. H. Marshall

(Eds.), *Between prohibition and legalization: The Dutch experiment in drug policy* (pp. 119–143). New York: Kugler.

Leuw, E., & Marshall, I. H. (Eds.). (1994). *Between prohibition and legalization: The Dutch experiment in drug policy.* New York: Kugler.

MacCoun, R. J., Saiger, A. J., Kahan, J. P., & Reuter, P. (1993). Drug policies and problems: The promise and pitfalls of cross-national comparison. In N. Heather, A. Wodak, E. Nadelmann, & P. O'Hare (Eds.), *Psychoactive drugs and harm reduction* (pp. 103–117). London: Whurr.

Maris, C. W. (1996a). Dutch weed and logic: Part I. *International Journal of Drug Policy, 7*(2), 80–87.

Maris, C. W. (1996b). Dutch weed and logic: Part II. *International Journal of Drug Policy, 7*(3), 142–152.

Marks, J. (1991). The practice of controlled availability of illicit drugs. In N. Heather, W. R. Miller, & J. Greeley (Eds.), *Self-control and the addictive behaviors* (pp. 304–316). Botany, New South Wales: Maxwell Macmillan Australia.

Marlatt, G. A., & Tapert, S. F. (1993). Harm reduction: Reducing the risks of addictive behaviors. In J. S. Baer, G. A. Marlatt, & R. McMahon (Eds.), *Addictive behaviors across the lifespan* (pp. 243–273). Newbury Park, CA: Sage.

Nadelmann, E. (1995, Summer). Beyond Needle Park: The Swiss maintenance trial. *Drug Policy Letter, 27,* 12–14.

O'Connor, J., & Saunders, B. (1992). Drug education: An appraisal of a popular alternative. *International Journal of the Addictions, 27,* 165–185.

O'Hare, P. A., Newcombe, R., Matthews, A., Buning, E. C., & Drucker, E. (Eds.). (1992). *The reduction of drug-related harm.* London: Routledge.

Parry, A. (1989). *Harm reduction* [Interview]. *Drug Policy Letter, 1*(4), 13.

Plant, M., Single, E., & Stockwell, T. (Eds.). (1997). *Alcohol: Minimising the harm—what works?* London: Free Association Books.

Riley, D. (1994). *The harm reduction model: Pragmatic approaches to drug use from the area between intolerance and neglect.* Ottawa: Canadian Centre on Substance Abuse.

Rolleston, H. (1926). *Report of the Departmental Committee on Morphine and Heroin Addiction.* London: His Majesty's Stationery Office.

Schneider, W. (1995). *Harm reduction in Frankfurt.* Paper presented at the Ninth International Conference on Drug Policy Reform, Santa Monica, CA.

Sijlbing, G., & Persoon, J. M. G. (1985). Cannabis among youth in the Netherlands. *Bulletin on Narcotics, 37*(4), 51–60.

Staples, P. (1993). Reduction of alcohol and drug-related harm in Australia: A government minister's perspective. In N. Heather, A. Wodak, E. Nadelmann, & P. A. O'Hare (Eds.), *Psychoactive drugs and harm reduction: From faith to science* (pp. 49–54). London: Whurr.

Stimson, G. V. (1994). Minimizing harm from drug use. In J. Strang & M. Gossop (Eds.), *Heroin addiction and drug policy: The British system* (pp. 248–256). New York: Oxford University Press.

Stimson, G. V. (1996). Has the United Kingdom averted an epidemic of HIV-1 infection among drug injectors? *Addiction, 91*(8), 1085–1088.

Strang, J. (1990). The roles of prescribing. In J. Strang & G. Stimson (Eds.), *AIDS and drug misuse* (pp. 142–152). London: Routledge.

Strang, J., & Gossop, M. (Eds.). (1994). *Heroin addiction and drug policy: The British system.* New York: Oxford University Press.

Strang, J., Ruben, S., Farrell, M., & Gossop, M. (1994). Prescribing heroin and other injectable drugs. In J. Strang & M. Gossop (Eds.), *Heroin addiction and drug policy: The British system* (pp. 192–206). New York: Oxford University Press.

Strang, J., & Stimson, G. (Eds.). (1990). *AIDS and drug misuse.* London: Routledge.

Uchtenhagen, A., Dobler-Mikola, A., & Gutzwiller, F. (1996). Medically controlled prescription of narcotics: A Swiss national project. *International Journal of Drug Policy,* 7(1), 31–36.

van de Wijngaart, G. F. (1991). *Competing perspectives on drug use: The Dutch experience.* Amsterdam: Swets & Zeitlinger.

Wodak, A. (1992). Beyond the prohibition of heroin: The development of a controlled availability policy in Australia. In P. A. O'Hare, R. Newcombe, A. Matthews, E. C. Buning, & E. Drucker (Eds.), *The reduction of drug-related harm* (pp. 49–61). London: Routledge.

Yates, J. (1996). The situation in Sweden. *International Journal of Drug Policy,* 7(2), 88–90.

CHAPTER THREE

Basic Principles and Strategies of Harm Reduction

G. ALAN MARLATT

From Chapters 1 and 2, most readers will have already drawn some conclusions about the nature of harm reduction and how it differs from traditional drug policies and treatment programs. At this point, let us review some of the central themes that emerge from this analysis, in order to summarize the underlying principles and strategies of harm reduction. After a discussion of five basic principles, based on an earlier paper on this topic (Marlatt, 1996a), several strategies and procedures are presented to exemplify how harm reduction can be applied.

BASIC PRINCIPLES, ASSUMPTIONS, AND VALUES

1. *Harm reduction is a public health alternative to the moral/criminal and disease models of drug use and addiction.* In the United States, views of drug use and addiction have been based on two competing and sometimes conflicting models: the moral model and the disease model. The moral model, as expressed in U.S. drug control policy, is that the use and/or distribution of certain drugs is a crime deserving of punishment. As an extension of the moral model (assumption: illicit drug use is morally wrong), the criminal justice system has collaborated with national drug policy makers in pursuing the "war on drugs," the ultimate aim of which is to foster the development of a drug-free society. The majority of federal funding for drug controls has been based on a "supply reduction" approach. The U.S. Drug Enforcement Agency is funded primarily to promote interdiction programs designed to reduce the supply of drugs coming into

the country (e.g., to destroy the supply of coca plants used to produce cocaine in Colombia and other Latin American countries). Other national agencies, as well as state and local police, are funded to arrest drug dealers and users alike in an attempt to reduce the supply of drugs further.

The second approach is to define addiction (e.g., alcoholism or heroin addiction) as a biological/genetic disease that requires treatment and rehabilitation. Here the emphasis is on prevention and treatment programs that focus on remediation of the individual's desire or demand for drugs—a "demand reduction" approach. Despite the apparent contradiction between viewing the drug user as a criminal deserving of punishment and as a sick person in need of treatment, the supply reduction and demand reduction models are in agreement that the ultimate aim of both approaches is to reduce and eventually eliminate the prevalence of drug use by focusing primarily on the drug user ("use reduction"). Further discussion and evaluation of the supply reduction and demand reduction approaches to illicit drug use can be found in Chapter 10.

Harm reduction, with its philosophical roots in pragmatism and its compatibility with a public health approach, offers a practical alternative to both the moral and disease models. Unlike proponents of the moral model—who view drug use as bad or illegal, and who advocate supply reduction (via prohibition and punishment)—supporters of harm reduction shift the focus away from drug use itself to the consequences or effects of addictive behavior. Such effects are evaluated primarily in terms of whether they are harmful or helpful to the drug user and to the larger society, not on the basis of whether the behavior itself is considered morally right or wrong. Moreover, unlike advocates of the disease model—who view addiction as a biological/genetic pathology, and who promote demand reduction as the primary goal of prevention and abstinence as the only acceptable goal of treatment—harm reduction offers a wide range of policies and procedures designed to reduce the harmful consequences of addictive behavior. Harm reduction accepts the practical facts that many people use drugs and engage in other high-risk behaviors, and that idealistic visions of a drug-free society are unlikely to become reality.

2. *Harm reduction recognizes abstinence as an ideal outcome but accepts alternatives that reduce harm.* The moral model and the disease model also share one strong common value: the insistence upon total abstinence as the only acceptable goal of either incarceration or treatment. Despite the harsh reality of high recidivism rates for released drug prisoners and the correspondingly high rate of relapse for treated addicts, there has been no relaxation of this absolute insistence upon abstinence. Contemporary U.S. drug policy is based on the ultimate criterion of "zero tolerance"—that is, the notion that *any* illegal drug use, including the occasional smoking of marijuana, is as intolerable as a daily pattern of intravenous heroin injection. The only acceptable goal of almost all U.S. alcohol and

drug treatment programs is lifelong abstinence, along with continued attendance at Twelve-Step recovery groups. In fact, abstinence is almost always required as a precondition for treatment, since most chemical dependence treatment programs refuse to admit patients who are still using drugs. The requirement that one must first abstain in order to receive treatment designed to maintain abstinence exemplifies a "high-threshold" approach, which often presents a barrier to those seeking help (Marlatt, Tucker, Donovan, & Vuchinich, 1997).

Consistent with a policy of total abstinence, the principle of zero tolerance establishes an absolute dichotomy between no (zero) use and any use whatsoever. This all-or-none dichotomy labels all drug use as equally criminal (or sick), and fails to distinguish between lighter and heavier drug use or degrees of harmful use. Along similar lines, individuals subjected to drug testing as a condition of employment often fail, because the tests (e.g., urinalysis, hair analysis, blood testing) are evaluated as either "clean" or "dirty." According to this pass–fail criterion, one is equally "dirty" if one smokes a single marijuana cigarette or smokes crack cocaine on a daily basis for months. U.S. drug policy is based on the assumption that there can be no acceptance of occasional or "casual" use of drugs; all use equals abuse.

Absolute abstinence is also emphasized as the only acceptable goal of prevention and treatment by those who subscribe to the disease model of addiction (Marlatt, 1996b). From this perspective, addiction is viewed as a progressive disease that cannot be cured, but only "arrested" by a lifelong commitment to abstinence. Any subsequent drug use is defined as a relapse back into the disease condition, an inevitable outcome determined by biological factors beyond the individual's control (craving and "loss of control" triggered by biological drug effects). The unwillingness of the U.S. alcoholism treatment community to accept moderate alcohol consumption as an alternative to abstinence is clearly evident in the intensity of feelings evoked by the controlled-drinking controversy (discussed in Chapter 4).

Harm reduction is *not* antiabstinence. Harmful effects of unsafe drug use or sexual activity can be placed along a continuum, much like the temperature range indicated on a thermometer. When things get too hot or too dangerous, harm reduction promotes "turning down the heat" to a more temperate level. This gradual, "step-down" approach encourages individuals with excessive or high-risk behaviors to take it "one step at a time" to reduce the harmful consequences of their behavior. The ultimate goal of abstinence greatly reduces or entirely eliminates the risk of harm associated with excessive drug use or unsafe sex. In this sense, abstinence is included as an ideal endpoint along a continuum, ranging from excessively harmful to less harmful consequences. By placing the harmful effects of drug use or sexual behavior along a continuum rather than by dichotomizing drug use as legal or illegal, or by diagnosing drug use as indicating the presence or absence of an addictive disease, supporters of harm reduction encourage any movement toward decreased harm as a step in the right direction (Marlatt & Tapert, 1993).

Harm reduction strategies also apply to the use of legal drugs, including tobacco and alcohol. For smokers who are unable to quit "cold turkey," nicotine patches, gum, and sprays are available as less harmful (i.e., involving a lower cancer risk) than smoking cigarettes. Although nicotine replacement therapies were initially designed as an aid to quitting, some people use these products to maintain a safer level of nicotine use (see details in Chapter 5). Similarly, the harmful effects of excessive drinking can be reduced by teaching moderation skills.

The same issues arise regarding goals for sex education (see Chapter 7). Although the potential harmful effects of unsafe sexual practices are well documented (e.g., increased teenage pregnancies, risk of sexually transmitted diseases), public opinion is sharply divided between those who insist upon sexual abstinence and others who urge condom distribution and education in safe sex for our youth. A comprehensive harm reduction approach can embrace both goals: Abstinence can be supported and encouraged as the safest practice, but safer sex can also be presented as a valid means of reducing potential harm for those who are already saying "yes" to sex. However, those who support sexual abstinence abhor alternative approaches that promote safe sex and condom distribution in schools. A *Time* magazine essay entitled "Fifteen Cheers for Abstinence" illustrates this view:

> What will keep today's young safe from the downward spiral—which is not only the familiar descent of children bearing children and disintegrated families and AIDS, but also the more general American sexual devolution, the swamp of the id? I offer 15 cheers for abstinence.... The young tend to fulfill expectations. Government-sponsored condom distribution announces that the society officially expects to get copulating dogs.... The mentality of abstinence demands a certain elementary moral metaphysics. Teach this: the more you indulge in anything, good or bad, but especially bad—in drugs, casual sex, violence, idiot music, stupidity, driving 90 m.p.h., bad manners, rage—the more you lose. The more you abstain, the more you gain. This is not cheap rhyming paradox but a good truth that in the past generation or two has been swept away by raw sewage. (Morrow, 1995, p. 90)

3. *Harm reduction has emerged primarily as a "bottom-up" approach based on addict advocacy, rather than a "top-down" policy promoted by drug policy makers.* Recall from Chapter 2 that needle exchange programs for injection drug users (IDUs) began in the Netherlands in response to input from addicts belonging to the *Junkiebond* group, who advocated for drug policy changes that would permit the legal exchange of needles in order to reduce the risk of HIV infection. Many of the harm reduction projects reviewed in this book have also originated at the local level; they have often been promoted through grassroots advocacy by those directly

involved in receiving and providing services. Many harm reduction programs have emerged from community-based public health interventions
that support substance users and their communities in reducing drug-related
harm.

Addiction and AIDS are problems that are so plagued with stigma and
tainted with moral condemnation that individuals who suffer from these
twin problems are often marginalized by society. Whereas those affected by
such disorders as cancer or mental illness have formed powerful lobbying
groups and "patient advocacy" societies (e.g., the American Cancer Society,
the National Alliance for Mental Illness), it is rare to find parallel advocacy
groups in the addictions field. Although the gay community has rallied in
support of advocating better prevention (e.g., safe sex programs) and
treatment services for those who are HIV-positive, until recently the U.S.
community of IDUs has had little or no impact on the provision of services
for addicts. There are some indications, however, that something similar to
the Dutch *Junkiebond* may be developing in the United States. An example
is the International Coalition for Addict Self-Help (P.O. Box 20882,
Tompkins Square Station, New York, NY 10009). This group publishes a
newsletter entitled *The Addict Advocate*. An article in a recent issue
discussed the "treatment on demand" issue, as viewed from the perspective
of active drug users:

> In its broadest sense, TOD [treatment on demand] has just two main compo-
> nents. They are, of course, "treatment" and "demand," but far from being
> clear and easily defined terms, they are ambiguous, convoluted, and subject to
> broad interpretation by persons of differing views. To begin with, what
> "treatment" are we speaking of? Upon whose "demand" shall this treatment
> commence? . . . Is it feasible that the addict will, one day, be permitted to be
> the final arbiter of whether he or she receives medical treatment on a demand
> basis, or is it hopeless naiveté to think so? Will addicts be permitted to
> determine which treatment modality suits their needs, and have ready access
> to it? (Sisko, 1995, p. 1)

Addict advocacy has led to the development of innovative harm
reduction strategies such as needle exchange. Such advances have developed
on a "bottom-up" rather than a "top-down" basis (see Chapter 7 for details
on needle exchange programs). Community-based local efforts have served
as the basis for such programs (Moore & Wenger, 1995). The impetus for
harm reduction programs has not come from the "top down"—neither the
White House Office on National Drug Policy nor the National Institute on
Drug Abuse has promoted or supported harm reduction as a national drug
policy. If anything, these approaches have been denigrated and criticized at
the federal level (see Chapter 10).

Since the mid-1980s, American AIDS prevention programs for active
IDUs have been based on a "provider–client" model often described as

"street-based outreach" (Brown & Beschner, 1993). In this approach, a number of outreach workers (OWs) who are not themselves drug users are hired to work with IDUs in their own community as clients, to provide AIDS prevention information and materials (e.g., bleach to clean needles, condoms), and to refer IDUs to available treatment programs. Until recently, active IDUs (the "clients") have rarely been called upon to play larger roles in helping themselves or their community. Since the advent of addict advocacy in establishing needle exchange programs in the United States, this picture is beginning to change.

In a special issue of the *Journal of Drug Issues* entitled "Drug Users as Risk Reduction Agents" (Czajkoski & Broadhead, 1995), several programs and projects that have utilized active IDUs as OWs are described. In an introductory editorial to the special issue, Broadhead (1995) notes:

> Despite their status as clients, research has documented that IDUs have responded very impressively to the outreach services they have received. IDUs have adopted many risk reduction measures at high rates, and they have significantly augmented OWs' efforts. For example, IDUs have been documented helping OWs prepare and distribute bleach kits, recruiting users who need help, helping OWs learn about new drug scenes and copping areas, and vouching for OWs who need help in becoming established. In short, in the United States, active drug users have proven themselves to be far more capable and responsive than outreach experts ever anticipated or allowed for in their intervention efforts. . . . Given the impressive response of drug users around the world in support of prevention efforts and health initiatives, alternatives to the traditional "provider–client" outreach model are sorely overdue in the United States, and it would be wise for governments in other parts of the world to expand their support for user-based initiatives and self-help organizations. (pp. 505–506)

The special issue of this journal contains a number of articles documenting programs that have recruited active IDUs to help street addicts to control, reduce, or stop their use of drugs (Levy, Gallmeier, & Wiebel, 1995); to provide AIDS prevention efforts for IDUs (Broadhead, Heckathorn, Grund, Stern, & Anthony, 1995); and to develop such citywide services for IDUs as the Prevention Point Needle Exchange in San Francisco (Moore & Wenger, 1995).

4. *Harm reduction promotes low-threshold access to services as an alternative to traditional, high-threshold approaches.* The street-based outreach programs described above provide an example of the low-threshold approach to harm reduction. Rather than setting abstinence as a high-threshold requirement or precondition for receiving addiction treatment or other assistance, advocates of harm reduction are willing to reduce such barriers—thereby making it easier for those in need to "get on board," to get involved, and to get started. Low-threshold programs do this by several

means: by reaching out and achieving partnership and cooperation with the targeted population in developing new programs and services; by reducing the stigma associated with getting help for these kinds of problems; and by providing an integrative, normalized approach to high-risk substance use and sexual practices.

First, supporters of a low-threshold approach are willing to meet the individual on his or her own terms—to "meet you where you are" rather than "where you should be" (Marlatt, 1996a). Input from members of the targeted population is encouraged and promoted, in an attempt to forge a partnership or alliance between those providing services and those receiving them (even when both groups consist of active drug users). New programs are developed in collaboration with those directly involved and affected. Through dialogue, discussion, and mutual planning efforts (e.g., use of "focus groups" to provide initial input and goal setting), innovative outreach programs and associated services will continue to emerge at the community level. Throughout the negotiation process, those affected are accepted as partners who are capable of assuming responsibility for making personal changes in their behavior and helping others to do the same. Any changes that a person feels capable of making and that are "steps in the right direction" to reduce harm are supported, so as to enhance self-efficacy for successful change (Marlatt, Baer, & Quigley, 1995).

A second component of low-threshold approaches involves reducing the stigma associated with problems of addiction, substance abuse, and high-risk sexual practices. As we have already noted, the moral and disease models often stigmatize individuals with these problems as either criminal/immoral addicts or victims of an incurable genetic or biological disease; neither of these positions is consistent with a user-friendly, low-threshold approach. But can this stigma be reduced? In a review of the literature on determinants of help seeking by individuals with substance use problems (Marlatt et al., 1997), we found that the primary factor that motivates people to seek treatment is their personal experience of the problematic consequences or harmful effects of using drugs. Therefore, problems in personal health, family and relationship difficulties, financial problems, and the like can become the focus for help seeking, instead of "substance abuse" itself. When the focus is shifted toward reducing the harm associated with drug use or high-risk sex, and away from labeling the problem as one of addiction or deviance, prospective help seekers are more likely to come "out of the shadows" and seek assistance. On this basis, a higher proportion of the population at risk should become registered in some kind of harm reduction program, as is currently the case in the Netherlands (see Chapter 2).

The third aspect of a low-threshold approach is the capacity for harm reduction to embrace and consolidate a variety of behaviors that span substance use and high-risk sexual behaviors. Drug use is rarely independent of other high-risk behaviors—not only unsafe sexual practices, but driving under the influence, aggression and violence, attempted suicide, and so forth. With a common focus on the harm such behaviors cause, rather than on pathologizing or condemning the persons who engage in these behaviors, doors can be opened that are currently padlocked by stigma and shame. Harm reduction normalizes these high-risk behaviors by placing them in the context of acquired habits—addictive behaviors that are strengthened by the influence of powerful reinforcers (Marlatt & Vanden-bois, 1997).

Harm reduction defines much drug use and other addictive behaviors as maladaptive coping responses, rather than as indicators of either physical illness or personal immorality. A comprehensive, low-threshold approach is designed to promote the development of more adaptive coping mechanisms and mechanisms of social support. Such problems are best conceptualized within an integrative, holistic perspective that views drug use and/or high-risk sexual behaviors as interdependent and reciprocally interactive components of personal lifestyle. By adopting a comprehensive health promotion response to lifestyle problems—one that encompasses substance use, sexual practices, exercise, nutrition, and other personal and interpersonal habits (both helpful and harmful)—harm reduction can offer an attractive low-threshold gateway to welcome anyone who is willing to "come as you are."

5. *Harm reduction is based on the tenets of compassionate pragmatism versus moralistic idealism.* A popular bumper-sticker of the mid-1990s proclaims: "Shit happens." As a pragmatic approach, harm reduction accepts this unpleasant fact of life as a basic premise. Harmful behavior happens—it always has, and it always will. Once this premise is accepted, the goal becomes one of compassionate pragmatism: What can be done to reduce the harm and suffering for both the individual and society? Pragmatism does not ask whether the behavior in question is right or wrong, good or bad, sick or well. Pragmatism is concerned with the management of everyday affairs and actual practices, and its validity is assessed by practical results. William James, a pioneer in developing the philosophy of pragmatism, put it this way:

> Pragmatism represents a perfectly familiar attitude in philosophy, the empirical attitude, but it represents it, as it seems to me, both in a more radical and in a less objectionable form than it has ever yet assumed. A pragmatist turns his back resolutely and once for all upon a lot of inveterate habits dear to professional philosophers. He turns away from abstraction and insufficiency, from verbal solutions, from bad a priori reasons, from fixed principles, closed systems, and pretended absolutes and origins. You see by this what I meant when I called pragmatism a mediator and reconciler ... that she "unstiffens" our theories.
>
> She has in fact no prejudices whatever, no obstructive dogmas, no rigid

canons of what shall count as proof. She is completely genial. She will entertain any hypothesis, she will consider any evidence. . . . Rationalism sticks to logic and the empyrean. Empiricism sticks to the external senses. Pragmatism is willing to take anything, to follow either logic or the senses, and to count the humblest and most personal experiences. She will count mystical experiences if they have practical consequences. . . . But you see already how democratic she is. Her manners are as various and flexible, her resources as rich and endless, and her conclusions as friendly as those of mother nature. (James, 1907/1975, pp. 43–44)

Unlike the moralistic idealism associated with drug policy designed to produce a "drug-free society," harm reduction accepts the fact that some people have always used drugs and will continue to do so, just as some people will continue to engage in high-risk sexual behaviors. Accepting that such potentially harmful behaviors occur "as a fact of life," however, does not mean condoning or promoting these behaviors or the people who engage in them. Rather than simply labeling the persons who engage in such behaviors as good or bad, harm reduction first asks this question: To what extent are the consequences of these individuals' behaviors harmful or helpful to the individuals and to others who may be affected? The next question is this: What can be done to reduce these harmful consequences? Moral idealists often cannot accept what harm reduction promotes as the means to this end. Needle exchange programs are viewed as an unaccept- able "means" to such critics because they believe that this approach "sends the wrong signal"—in other words, that it condones or even promotes injection drug use and addiction. For some critics, the practical outcome of such programs in saving the lives of drug addicts or their partners is devalued or rejected outright (e.g., "These addicts deserve what they get").

As an approach based on acceptance and compassion, harm reduction has parallels with other philosophies and schools of therapy. Harm reduc- tion adopts a humane approach to dealing with human suffering—a stance that is similar to humanistic psychology as espoused by Carl Rogers, Abraham Maslow, and others. Maslow (1968) described a hierarchy of human needs, with basic survival needs (food, shelter) as the base; one cannot begin to work with an individual's higher needs (psychological, social, and spiritual) until the basic needs have been met. This "needs hierarchy" approach is parallel to the pragmatism of harm reduction. The "client-centered" approach favored by Rogers (1951) is consistent with harm reduction's emphasis on establishing a partnership between clients and providers in which the clients' needs come first in developing programs or services. Harm reduction is also compatible with learning theory in psychology and its application in terms of cognitive and behavior therapies (reviewed in the next section).

On a spiritual level, harm reduction is congruent with the basic principles of Buddhist psychology, especially the teachings of the "Middle

Way"—a path between the extremes of indulgent excess and strict asceticism in dealing with craving and attachment (Marlatt, 1994). In a review article linking Buddhist theory with addiction, the underlying pragmatism of Buddhism is noted:

> Taking addiction as a form of attachment normally associated with craving, Buddhist teachings then constitute a rich source of etiological models and possible therapies for addictions, for Buddhism of whatever type proposes how craving and attachment arise, what forms they take and provides detailed accounts of strategies to deal with them. . . . The Buddha's attitude to the relevance of his teachings was one of pragmatism—if it helped, then use it. (Groves & Farmer, 1994, pp. 183–191)

Harm reduction is a compassionate approach because it does not denigrate people who engage in high-risk sexual or drug-taking behavior. Instead of using pejorative terms to label such people, harm reduction shifts the focus to the individuals' behavior and its consequences. For instance, the shift is from speaking of "drug abuse" to speaking of the "harmful use of drugs," or from labeling someone a "drug abuser" to calling him or her a "consumer" who experiences harmful or helpful consequences. The word "consumer" seems particularly apt, because people consume both substances and services; drug users also represent a significant economic consumer group (if we consider the high purchase costs of both licit and illicit substances, from tobacco to heroin).

PROCEDURES AND STRATEGIES

From descriptions of the methods and procedures of harm reduction, three basic strategies emerge: working with individuals or groups, modifying the environment, and implementing public policy changes. A helpful analogy that encompasses all three strategies is to think of a person learning to drive a car. Driving is a good example, because it is a high-risk behavior that most people engage in. To abstain from driving is safe but inconvenient. Three approaches are combined that can influence driving behavior and reduce harmful consequences: (1) driver education and training in responsible driving behaviors; (2) environmental availability of harm-reducing measures in both the car itself (e.g., seat belts, air bags, antilock brakes, working lights, a well-maintained engine, etc.) and the road it travels on (e.g., safer freeways and road conditions); and (3) laws and policies designed to regulate driving (e.g., speed limits, blood alcohol limits, no-passing zones, etc.) and to establish penalties for violators (fines, suspension of license, jail sentences). With this driving analogy as an organizing principle, the following discussion provides an overview of these three global methods of harm reduction.

Implementing Harm Reduction with Individuals and Groups

Just as high school students learn the rules of the road and the ways to operate an automobile safely in driver education classes, education and training are essential in the application of harm reduction to individuals and groups. Drivers-in-training first learn about driving regulations and rules by reading manuals and engaging in classroom discussions before they can take an exam to obtain a provisional license. Driving behaviors are then practiced on the road (exposure to high-risk environment and training in coping with emergencies) until the drivers are ready to take the final driver's license road test. Drivers who violate the laws related to driving (e.g., exceeding the speed limit) are often mandated to attend additional training sessions (e.g., a defensive driving course) in order to retain their licenses.

In a similar manner, harm reduction practices can be taught in educational programs designed to help people reduce the risks of engaging in such behaviors as drinking, smoking, eating, using licit and illicit drugs, and sexual activities. The goal of such training, whether it be for driving or for any of the behaviors just mentioned, is the prevention of harm.

In work with individuals, alone or in groups, *education* is the key to the prevention and minimization of harm related to high-risk drug use and sexual behavior. Unlike prevention programs for youth that focus exclusively on abstinence and promote a zero-tolerance, "just say no" approach, programs based on harm reduction are designed to accommodate those who have already "said yes" (or who are leaning in that direction) when it comes to experimenting with drugs and sex. Such programs can be structured in group settings (e.g., prevention programs in schools) to include discussion of *both* abstinence and drug use or sexual activity. The decision to become active or to remain abstinent can be informed by a discussion of the relative pros and cons of each choice.

As an example, members of our staff at the University of Washington Addictive Behaviors Research Center were asked to visit a private high school in Seattle to discuss drinking problems with members of the senior class (Somers, 1995). School officials invited us to put on a program similar to the one we developed to work with University of Washington freshmen (described in Chapter 4). Since most of the high school seniors were planning to attend college within a year, and since most of these students were already drinking, it was decided that a harm reduction approach was the best alternative to traditional abstinence programs.

When we met with members of the senior class (with no teachers present), we asked them what they thought we were going to talk about. One young woman, with a bored expression, replied: "Another 'just-say no' lecture. Well, while you're doing that, I'm going to be daydreaming about the big party coming up Friday night." After we explained that we were there to talk about drinking and its risks and benefits (as we did with college freshmen), the attitude shifted to one of animated discussion. All but 1 student in the class of 20 revealed that they were active drinkers; these students spoke freely about their experiences with alcohol, both positive and negative. In this interactive discussion, students raised numerous questions that could easily be addressed within the framework of harm reduction (e.g., how to respond to peer pressure to get drunk, how to help a friend who has overindulged, how males and females respond differently to alcohol, how alcohol affects sexual activity, etc.).

The one student who reported that he was an abstainer was challenged at first by some of the other students, one of whom accused him of being "holier than thou" and "looking down your nose" at students who were not abstinent. "Not at all," he replied. "I'm hoping to make the college sports teams in the fall, and I don't want to do anything like drinking that might interfere with my physical training or slow my reaction time." The ensuing discussion focused on the advantages and disadvantages of drinking, including the effects of alcohol on reaction time, with everyone actively involved. Toward the end of the meeting, several students thanked us for promoting such an open forum in which their views about drinking were accepted and discussed, even though alcohol consumption was illegal for these underage drinkers. Another student told us, "We should be doing this in junior high school, when most of us first started to experiment with alcohol. Maybe some of us seniors could lead the discussion with the ninth-graders, the way you did with us." Following this introductory meeting, school officials invited us to put on several harm reduction workshops for the graduating class. This program was found to reduce harmful drinking patterns significantly over the course of the school year (Somers, 1995).

Educational prevention programs based on a harm reduction model share several common elements. Input from participants (e.g., students) is sought when programs are first developed. This strategy avoids relying on materials developed by adult experts and administered in an authoritative, "top-down" manner, such as the Drug Abuse Resistance Education (D.A.R.E.) programs currently administered in many U.S. schools. D.A.R.E. and similar programs are often actively resisted or rejected by students. In harm reduction education, the program format is similarly interactive, with active discussion encouraged throughout. Information is exchanged on an interpersonal basis, and "lectures" by experts are avoided. Active role plays are used to practice coping skills and to rehearse what to do in high-risk situations. Alcohol and drug use can be integrated into discussions of sexual activity, rather than dealt with as separate, unrelated topics. A strong emphasis is placed on personal choice and responsibility, as is done in training young people to drive ("Once behind the wheel, you are responsible for your driving behavior and its consequences").

The overall goals of prevention programs based on harm reduction include enhancing awareness of high-risk behaviors and their consequences (helpful or harmful), training in coping skills to deal effectively with high-risk situations involving drugs or sex, and facilitating health-promoting and risk-reducing behaviors (e.g., training in moderation skills). Like driver education programs, prevention programs based on harm reduction principles are geared toward effective self-management, both on and off the "road."

But what happens if the driver does go off the road and ends up in the ditch? Or drives too fast under the influence of alcohol? Or is responsible for an accident that causes harm to the driver or others? Here the emphasis shifts from prevention to intervention. Many of the techniques discussed so far under the rubric of harm reduction represent intervention or treatment methods for individuals who have already developed an addiction problem or who are continuing to engage in unsafe or abusive sexual behavior.

The first goal of a harm reduction intervention is to attempt to stabilize a client's problem behavior and to prevent further exacerbation of harmful consequences. In this respect harm reduction is similar in purpose to tertiary prevention or relapse prevention: to enhance maintenance of behavior change and to keep the problem from getting worse (Marlatt & Gordon, 1985; Marlatt, 1996b). Once the target behavior is stabilized, the second goal of a harm reduction intervention is to encourage or facilitate reduction of harmful consequences, ranging from small decrements in risk to total cessation of the problem behavior.

Most familiar treatment approaches for addictive behaviors can be adopted within a harm reduction framework. Many of these treatment methods are discussed in Chapters 4 through 7, which are directed to specific high-risk drug use and sexual behaviors. Harm reduction interventions can be applied in the context of both individual and group therapy, including self-help groups (e.g., Moderation Management, a self-help group that helps problem drinkers reduce harmful drinking practices; see Chapter 4). Cognitive and behavior therapies are particularly well matched with a harm reduction approach, since they focus on behavior change based on the principles of learning and a continuum model of habit modification and coping skills training. Pharmacotherapies may also be useful in harm reduction programs, such as the use of naltrexone to reduce alcohol craving, prescriptions of oral methadone for injection heroin users, or the application of nicotine replacements (e.g., nicotine patches) to aid smokers who wish to cut down or quit. Recent treatment approaches for addiction to cocaine and other substances often combine pharmacotherapy with behavior therapies such as relapse prevention to reduce harmful drug use (Carroll, 1996).

In considering these therapies for possible inclusion in a comprehensive harm reduction program, it is important to seek collaborative input from clients or groups in establishing therapeutic goals and selecting helpful interventions. In congruence with the principles of harm reduction discussed above, the planning of prevention and treatment programs becomes a shared experience based on a partnership between providers and clients. Unlike many traditional interventions, harm reductionists do not apply externally developed techniques without collaboration and negotiation with the people who are the recipients of these services. Approaches that are "client-centered," or that attempt to meet clients where they are (e.g., the motivational interviewing approach developed by Miller & Rollnick, 1991), are very compatible with the philosophy of harm reduction. Clients who experience addictive behavior problems that co-occur with other mental health disorders (e.g., a client with comorbid alcohol dependence and depression) are best treated by therapists who are experienced in harm-reduction psychotherapy (Gordon, 1998; Marlatt & Roberts, 1998; Tatarsky, 1998).

Increasing Environmental Availability of Harm Reduction Measures and Procedures

In working with individuals in prevention and treatment programs as described above, the primary goal is similar to that of driver education—to train the "driver" to engage in safer, harm-reducing activities, such as reducing the frequency and intensity of substance use or high-risk sex. The emphasis is on helping people develop motivation and skills associated with improved self-management. Linked to the goal of enhancing self-management skills with high-risk individuals or groups is the goal of environmental change. Even the safest driver will be at risk for problems if he or she is driving an unsafe car (with no seat belts, worn-out tires, cracked windshield, etc.), or if the road itself is in bad shape (with no shoulders, no centerline, no traffic control signals, etc.). Similarly, if an IDU cannot gain access to clean needles or cannot find a safe place to inject, the motivation or skills required for harm reduction practices become irrelevant. A high school student on prom night may wish to be safe when it comes to sex, but if no condoms are available, the risks of unsafe sexual practices increase.

The goal of reduced harm cannot be met unless the environmental means are available. In many cases, public policy dictates what can and cannot be legally done in making harm reduction tools and techniques more widely available. The controversies surrounding harm reduction policies (e.g., legalization of drugs, controlled drinking, availability of condoms in schools, etc.) are addressed in greater detail in Chapter 10. For now, it is sufficient to note that environmental access to harm reduction methods is intrinsically linked to matters of public policy.

To take alcohol consumption as an example, policy dictates rules and regulations, such as establishing a legal drinking age, setting limits on blood alcohol levels for drivers, limiting outlets or hours of sale for alcoholic beverages, and so on. Harm reduction, although it does not condone underage drinking or consumption to the point of intoxication, poses a pragmatic question: If it happens, what can be done to reduce the harmful consequences? An example of such an environmental option designed to reduce the harm associated with excessive drinking was described in an article in *The New York Times* entitled "Resort Van Service Is Driving Them to Drink" (1995):

> Westhampton Beach, N.Y.—On a recent Friday night, Dawn Assnel and her housemates here in the Hamptons argued about who would be the designated driver for a night of bar-hopping. So the next night, they did what more than 1,000 other 20-somethings here do every Friday and Saturday: they called a van. "Now, I can get drunk and not have to worry," said Ms. Assnel, 26, a clothing designer in Manhattan. Since Westhampton Taxi added 14 vans to its fleet of two dozen cars two years ago, the police here say drunken driving arrests and late-night accidents have fallen sharply. . . . "Since they've begun operating the vans, it's cut down on our accidents, the 4 o'clock-in-the-morning accidents, and we have fewer D.W.I. arrests," Conrad Teller, Chief of the Westhampton Beach Village Police Department, said. Drunken driving arrests have dropped by two-thirds since 1992, Officer Joseph Caldora said. "Now, in one shot you have 20 people bombed out of their socks in vans instead of on the road," he said. Pointing to what appeared to be a drunken driving checkpoint, Melody Lamback, a 29-year-old advertising executive, dryly noted, "That's why we take these taxis." Jonathan Hargrove, 23, who works in construction, offered another explanation. "The real reason we take the cabs: We don't want to bury any friends," he said. "I just buried one in December."

This van service is but one example of an environmental measure to reduce harm among heavy drinkers. Another alcohol-related example is a program developed in Scotland, designed to replace bar glasses that shatter when broken with containers that crumble into less harmful pieces; this was done to reduce the risk of injuries linked to pub fights and brawls, in which broken glasses can be used as weapons (see Chapter 4).

The environmental availability of harm-reducing tools and settings for injection drug use represents a similar challenge. Availability of clean needles (e.g., from needle exchange programs, dispensing machines, or over-the-counter purchases from pharmacies) is associated with reduced risk of HIV infection. Having access to clean and safe places to inject drugs (such as those provided in Frankfurt, Germany; see Chapter 2) is associated with reduced risk of drug overdose deaths. Allowing addicts to register with physicians in order to obtain prescribed drugs, as is the case already in some European countries, is another example.

High-risk sexual behaviors also benefit from enhanced environmental availability of harm-reducing methods. Condom distribution programs are an obvious example; if condoms are not readily available to persons who are sexually active, the risk of unprotected sexual contact and thus of sexually transmitted disease is greatly increased. In cities like Amsterdam, red-light districts are permitted to offer access to sexual experiences ranging from watching a "live sex" show to seeking the services of sex workers, so long as they adhere to standards of safe sex and health promotion. When prostitution is legalized and permitted to take place in a controlled, safe environment, access to services and help from a public health perspective is enhanced. With the exception of Nevada, prostitution is illegal in the United States, and access to sexual services is illegal and driven underground as a result.

Reforming Policies to Accommodate Harm Reduction

Policies and laws set limits on driving behavior: speed limits, limits on passing ("safe passing zones"), limits on parking, age limits for obtaining driver's licenses, and so forth. There are also rules and regulations designed to enhance safety on the road and to reduce accidents (e.g., requirements to use seat belts and to have working headlights and brake lights). If accidents occur, legal responsibility is determined and various penalties can be applied, from license suspension to imprisonment. The same is true for policies affecting drug-taking and sexual behaviors.

As indicated above, public policies affect the environmental availability of harm-reducing agents, such as the provision of clean needles to IDUs or the distribution of condoms to sexually active young people. Throughout this chapter and elsewhere in this book, various public policy alternatives are described that would facilitate the reduction of harm for both substance use and its consequences. The most controversial policy topic, however, involves changing laws that regulate the consumption of illicit substances and provide penalties for those who break the law. Policies that exist in other countries, such as the distinction between "hard" and "soft" drug use and the decriminalization of cannabis use (the Netherlands) or the ability of physicians to prescribe drugs to addicts (the United Kingdom and Switzerland), are currently rejected in the United States (DuPont & Voth, 1995). The U.S. policy of zero tolerance underlies the war on drugs and its harsh penalties for those who violate prohibition (e.g., the fixed mandatory sentences for drug offenders). A more detailed discussion of U.S. drug policy and its implications for harm reduction is presented in Chapter 10.

REFERENCES

Broadhead, R. S. (1995). Introduction: Drug users as risk reduction agents. *Journal of Drug Issues, 25*(3), 505–506.

Broadhead, R. S., Heckathorn, D. D., Grund, J. C., Stern, L. S., & Anthony, D. L. (1995). Drug users versus outreach workers in combating AIDS: Preliminary results of a peer-driven intervention. *Journal of Drug Issues, 25*, 531–564.

Brown, B. S., & Beschner, G. M. (1993). *Handbook on risk of AIDS: Injecting drug users and sexual partners.* Westport, CT: JAI Press.

Carroll, K. M. (1996). Relapse prevention as a psychosocial treatment: A review of controlled clinical trials. *Experimental and Clinical Psychopharmacology, 4*(1), 46–54.

Czajkoski, E. H., & Broadhead, R. S. (1995). (Eds.). Drug users as risk reduction agents [Special issue]. *Journal of Drug Issues, 25*(3).

DuPont, R. L., & Voth, E. A. (1995). Drug legalization, harm reduction, and drug policy. *Annals of Internal Medicine, 123,* 461–469.

Gordon, J. R. (1998). Harm reduction psychotherapy comes out of the closet. *In Session: Psychotherapy in Practice, 4,* 69–77.

Groves, P., & Farmer, R. (1994). Buddhism and addictions. *Addiction Research, 2,* 183–193.

James, W. (1975). *Pragmatism: A new name for some old ways of thinking.* Cambridge, MA: Harvard University Press. (Original work published 1907)

Levy, J. A., Gallmeier, C. P., & Wiebel, W. W. (1995). The outreach assisted peer-support model for controlling drug dependency. *Journal of Drug Issues, 25,* 507–529.

Marlatt, G. A. (1994). Addiction, mindfulness, and acceptance. In S. C. Hayes, N. S. Jacobson, V. M. Follette, & M. J. Dougher (Eds.), *Acceptance and change: Content and context in psychotherapy* (pp. 175–197). Reno, NV: Context Press.

Marlatt, G. A. (1996a). Harm reduction: Come as you are. *Addictive Behaviors, 21*(6), 779–788.

Marlatt, G. A. (1996b). Models of relapse and relapse prevention: A commentary. *Experimental and Clinical Psychopharmacology, 4*(1), 55–60.

Marlatt, G. A., Baer, J. S., & Quigley, L. A. (1995). Self-efficacy and addictive behavior. In A. Bandura (Ed.), *Self-efficacy in changing societies* (pp. 289–315). New York: Cambridge University Press.

Marlatt, G. A., & Gordon, J. R. (Eds.). (1985). *Relapse prevention: Maintenance strategies in the treatment of addictive behaviors.* New York: Guilford Press.

Marlatt, G. A., & Roberts, L. J. (1998). Introduction to special issue on treatment of comorbid addictive behaviors: Harm reduction as an alternative to abstinence. *In session: Psychotherapy in practice, 4,* 1–8.

Marlatt, G. A., & Tapert, S. F. (1993). Harm reduction: Reducing the risks of addictive behaviors. In J. S. Baer, G. A. Marlatt, & R. McMahon (Eds.), *Addictive behaviors across the lifespan* (pp. 243–273). Newbury Park, CA: Sage.

Marlatt, G. A., Tucker, J. A., Donovan, D. M., & Vuchinich, R. E. (1997). Help-seeking by substance abusers: The role of harm reduction and behavioral–economic approaches to facilitate treatment entry and retention by substance abusers. In L. S. Onken, J. D. Blaine, & J. J. Boren (Eds.), *Beyond the therapeutic alliance: Keeping the drug-dependent individual in treatment* (NIDA Research Monograph No. 165, pp. 44–84). Rockville, MD: U.S. Department of Health and Human Services.

Marlatt, G. A., & Vandenbois, G. R. (1997). *Addictive behaviors: Readings on etiology, prevention, and treatment.* Washington, DC: American Psychological Association.

Maslow, A. (1968). *Toward a psychology of being* (2nd ed.). Princeton: Van Nostrand.

Miller, W. R., & Rollnick, S. (1991). *Motivational interviewing: Preparing people for change.* New York: Guilford Press.

Moore, L. D., & Wenger, L. D. (1995). The social context of needle exchange and user self-organization in San Francisco: Possibilities and pitfalls. *Journal of Drug Issues, 25,* 583–598.

Morrow, L. (1995, October 2). Fifteen cheers for abstinence. *Time,* p. 90.

Resort van service is driving them to drink. (1995, September 1). *The New York Times,* p. A7.

Rogers, C. R. (1951). *Client-centered therapy.* Boston: Houghton Mifflin.

Sisko, B. (1995). Treatment on demand: Realistic goal or impossible dream? *The Addict Advocate, 3*(1), 1.

Somers, J. M. (1995). *Harm reduction and the prevention of alcohol problems among secondary students.* Unpublished doctoral dissertation, University of Washington.

Tatarsky, A. (1998). An integrative approach to harm reduction psychotherapy: A case of problem drinking secondary to depression. *In Session: Psychotherapy in Practice, 4,* 9–24.

PART TWO

APPLICATIONS TO ADDICTIVE BEHAVIORS AND HIGH-RISK SEXUAL BEHAVIORS

CHAPTER FOUR

Harm Reduction for Alcohol Problems

Expanding Access to and Acceptability of Prevention and Treatment Services

MARY E. LARIMER
G. ALAN MARLATT
JOHN S. BAER
LORI A. QUIGLEY
ARTHUR W. BLUME
ELIZABETH H. HAWKINS

Harm reduction philosophy originally developed out of concern for the users of illicit drugs, but many of its principles and techniques are equally applicable to alcohol problems (Single, 1996). Alcohol is legal for adults; yet problem drinkers and illegal drug users face similar barriers, such as lack of access to appropriate prevention and treatment services. These barriers also include lack of consideration for client choice or level of problem severity in treatment planning, and insistence on absolute abstinence for entry into treatment (Marlatt, Larimer, Baer, & Quigley, 1993; Marlatt, Tucker, Donovan, & Vuchinich, 1997). Harm reduction seeks to broaden the availability of prevention and treatment services by lowering the threshold for entry into such services. Harm can also be reduced by teaching skills, modifying the environment, and promoting public policies to reduce the risks of drinking. Although harm reduction for alcohol problems has often been equated with controlled drinking, this approach is considerably broader than simply focusing on nonabstinent or reduced-drinking goals (Marlatt et al., 1993).

The present chapter first reviews the risks and benefits associated with drinking, and provides a rationale for a harm reduction approach to alcohol problems. Controlled drinking is integrated into the broader harm reduction framework; we provide a review of the available evidence regarding when and for whom controlled-drinking goals may be appropriate. Several other types of clinical approaches included under the general rubric of harm reduction are covered, such as brief interventions, guided self-change approaches, and prevention approaches emphasizing motivational enhancement and skills building. Recent pharmacological advances in treating alcohol problems are also described. Finally, harm reduction approaches at the policy and environmental levels are reviewed.

ALCOHOL USE: PREVALENCE, PROBLEMS, RISKS, AND BENEFITS

Alcohol use in the United States is widespread; it occurs at a rate far exceeding the rates of all illegal drug use combined. In the 1995 National Household Survey on Drug Abuse (National Clearinghouse for Alcohol and Drug Information [NCADI], 1997), 111 million Americans aged 12 and over reported alcohol use in the past month; 32 million reported engaging in "binge" drinking (consuming five or more drinks at least once in the past month); and 11 million people reported being heavy drinkers (consuming 5 or more drinks on five or more days in the past month). In 1993, there were 4.2 million new users of alcohol, and the rate of new users among the 12–17 age group increased from 125 per 1,000 persons (in 1991) to 172 per 1,000 (NCADI, 1995).

Alcohol use, especially when heavy, has been associated with a variety of harmful consequences. Excessive alcohol use has been associated with traffic accidents and fatalities (National Highway Traffic Safety Administration [NHTSA], 1994), unsafe sexual behavior (Strunin & Hingson, 1993), suicide (Chassin & DeLucia, 1996), domestic violence (Kantor, 1993), and crime (Collins & Messerschmidt, 1993). Health consequences of excessive alcohol consumption include liver disease (the 10th leading cause of death in the United States; National Center for Health Statistics, 1996), pancreatitis (Singh, 1991; National Institute on Alcohol Abuse and Alcoholism (NIAAA, 1993); cardiovascular complications such as cardiomyopathy, hypertension, arrhythmias, and stroke (NIAAA, 1993); certain cancers (Tuyns, 1990); and endocrine (including reproductive functioning) and neurological complications (NIAAA, 1993). In 1990 alone, the nation's estimated direct and indirect costs due to alcohol (i.e., for medical costs, lost productivity, etc.) totaled $99 billion (Hogan, 1993).

The fourth edition of the *Diagnostic and Statistical Manual of Mental Disorders* (DSM-IV; American Psychiatric Association, 1994) distinguishes two categories of alcohol problems. "Alcohol dependence" is characterized by a cluster of cognitive, behavioral, and often physical symptoms (tolerance and withdrawal; however, the specifier "without physiological dependence" may also be assigned) indicating that the individual has impaired control of alcohol use and continues use of alcohol despite adverse consequences. "Alcohol abuse," on the other hand, is a residual category applied to maladaptive patterns of alcohol use that have never met the criteria for dependence, including recurrent use of alcohol in situations when use is physically dangerous (e.g., driving while intoxicated). The DSM-IV definition of alcohol abuse is consistent with the definition of "hazardous alcohol consumption" proposed by the World Health Organization (WHO): "a level of alcohol consumption or a pattern of drinking that is likely to result in harm should present drinking patterns persist" (Edwards, Arif, & Hodgson, 1981, p. 225). One study estimated that 4.4% of U.S. adults in 1992 met DSM-IV criteria for alcohol dependence and that an additional 3% met criteria for alcohol abuse (Grant & Harford, 1995). Throughout this chapter, we use the terms "dependence" and "abuse" in accordance with the DSM-IV definitions unless otherwise indicated.

Despite the serious risks related to heavy alcohol consumption, research indicates that moderate consumption may have significant health benefits. For instance, considerable evidence suggests that moderate alcohol consumption (usually defined as one to two drinks per day) has beneficial effects, compared to either abstinence or heavy drinking (see Boffetta & Garfinkel, 1990; Coate, 1993; Gaziano et al., 1993; Moore & Pearson, 1986; Razay, Heaton, Bolton, & Hughes, 1992; Rimm et al., 1991; Rimm, Klatsky, Grobbee, & Stampfer, 1996; Stampfer, Colditz, Willett, Speizer, & Hennekens, 1988). Alcohol apparently protects individuals from cardiovascular disease by raising the concentration of high-density lipoprotein (Stampfer, Rimm, & Walsh, 1993).

Given that alcohol use can be both beneficial and risky, arguments have been presented on both sides concerning whether abstinence or moderation should be recommended to the public (Peele, 1993; Shaper, 1993; Holman & English, 1996). Concerns about how best to present the benefits of alcohol consumption to the U.S. public have been summarized in a commentary in the *American Journal of Public Health*:

> Is this a message for which the country ought to ready itself? If the medical and health establishments were to advocate regular drinking of small amounts of alcohol, would the risk of increased problem drinking outweigh the benefit of healthier hearts? Whose risk would increase and who would benefit? Can clinicians correctly identify patients for whom such advice would be contraindicated? (Stampfer et al., 1993, p. 802)

HISTORY OF APPROACHES TO ALCOHOL
PROBLEMS IN THE UNITED STATES

The debate regarding public health recommendations for moderate drinking versus abstinence is nothing new. Attitudes toward drinking in the United States have always been ambivalent. This ambivalence is particularly visible in the political arena, as illustrated by the following anecdote (quoted from Marlatt et al., 1993, p. 462).

> Former U.S. Senator Howard Baker has told the story of former Congressman Billy Mathews receiving a letter from one of his constituents asking, "Dear Congressman, how do you stand on whiskey?" Not knowing whether his correspondent was for whiskey or against it, Congressman Mathews framed this reply:
>
>> My dear friend, I had not intended to discuss this controversial subject at this particular time. However, I want you to know that I do not shun a controversy. On the contrary, I will take a stand on any issue at any time, regardless of how fraught with controversy it may be. You have asked me how I feel about whiskey. Here is how I stand on the issue.
>>
>> If when you say whiskey, you mean the Devil's brew; the poison scourge; the bloody monster that defiles innocence, dethrones reason, destroys the home, creates misery, poverty, fear; literally takes the bread from the mouths of little children; if you mean the evil drink that topples the Christian man and woman from the pinnacles of righteous, gracious living into the bottomless pit of degradation and despair, shame and helplessness and hopelessness; then certainly, I am against it with all of my power.
>>
>> But, if when you say whiskey, you mean the oil of conversation, the philosophic wine, the ale that is consumed when great fellows get together, that puts a song in their hearts and laughter on their lips, and the warm glow of contentment in their eyes; if you mean Christmas cheer; if you mean the stimulating drink that puts the spring in the old gentlemen's step on a frosty morning; if you mean the drink that enables the man to magnify his joy and his happiness and to forget, if only for a little while, life's great tragedies and heartbreaks and sorrows; if you mean that drink, the sale of which pours into our Treasury untold millions of dollars which are used to provide tender care for little crippled children, our blind, our deaf, our pitiful aged and infirm; to build highways, hospitals, and schools; then certainly, I am in favor of it. This is my stand, and I will not compromise. Your congressman.

As illustrated by Congressman Mathews's letter, Americans have found difficulty in reconciling alcohol's potential to produce both harmful and beneficial effects. Approaches to alcohol policy in the United States have tended to emphasize absolutes. For example, in the 19th century, the Women's Christian Temperance Movement redefined alcohol as bad ("demon rum") and drinking as immoral (Levine, 1978). The temperance ideology was codified into law with the passage of the Volstead Act in 1917, making alcohol illegal. Prohibition lasted until 1933, giving birth to organized crime attracted by profits from selling bootleg liquor.

Following the repeal of prohibition, U.S. attitudes shifted toward viewing the alcoholic, rather than alcohol, as the problem. The American Medical Association first defined alcoholism as a disease in 1956 (cited in Jellinek, 1960). In August 1992, the Joint Committee of the National Council on Alcoholism and Drug Dependence and the American Society of Addiction Medicine published its definition of alcoholism as a disease in the *Journal of the American Medical Association*:

> Alcoholism is a primary chronic disease with genetic, psychosocial, and environmental factors influencing its development and manifestations. The disease is often progressive and fatal. It is characterized by impaired control over drinking, preoccupation with the drug alcohol, use of alcohol despite adverse consequences, and distortions in thinking, most notably denial. (Morse & Flavin, 1992, p. 1012)

The disease model represents an advance over the earlier moral model (Brickman et al., 1982; Miller & Kurtz, 1994). However, both models view alcoholics as weak and/or as powerless to control their consumption, and emphasize total abstinence from alcohol as the only means of recovery. Both models believe in the benefits of (or even require) enforced abstinence because of alcoholics' temptation to drink (as in the moral model), or because of their denial or lack of touch with reality (as in the disease model) (Miller, 1993; Miller & Kurtz, 1994).

Defining alcoholism as a disease has had a major impact on the development of treatment and prevention approaches. When alcoholism is viewed as a "primary chronic disease," there is a tendency to view the "illness" as categorically present or absent. This dichotomous under-standing of drinking behavior tends to ignore or deemphasize conditions considered less serious than chronic alcoholism, such as problem drinking, heavy drinking, or episodic alcohol abuse (Fingarette, 1988). The term "primary chronic disease" also seems to rule out the possibility that excessive drinking may be a secondary reaction to a preexisting disorder or condition, such as depression or anxiety. In such cases, if the preexisting condition is alleviated by other means (e.g., psychotherapy or medication), drinking may return to normal levels. By contrast, if alcoholism is a primary chronic disease, it should continue unabated over time, regardless of external circumstances; only total abstinence should arrest its course. Finally, the definition put forth by the Joint Committee states that alcohol-ism "is often progressive and fatal," implying that no one diagnosed with alcohol problems can ever regain volitional control of his or her drinking. This "one size fits all" approach to alcohol problems may unintentionally discourage individuals with milder problems from participating in nonab-stinent treatment services more appropriate for their circumstances (Marlatt et al., 1997; Sanchez-Craig & Lei, 1986).

ADVANTAGES OF HARM REDUCTION
AS AN ALTERNATIVE TO TRADITIONAL
ABSTINENCE MODELS

Harm reduction, in contrast to the all-or-nothing approach implicit in the model of alcoholism as a progressive disease, provides an alternative model based on evidence that alcohol misuse represents a continuum of problems rather than a dichotomous disease state (Heather, 1995; Kahler, Epstein, & McCrady, 1995; Stockwell, Sitharthan, McGrath, & Lang, 1994). In addition, there is considerable evidence that alcohol problems, rather than being "progressive and fatal," are more likely to be intermittent or discontinuous, particularly among younger individuals (Alterman, Bridges, & Tarter, 1986; Vaillant, 1996). Alcohol problems may remit without formal treatment (Dawson, 1996; Sobell et al., 1996) and may continue at a stable level without progressing or worsening for many years (Vaillant, 1996).

Viewing alcohol problems as existing on a continuum and having a variable course serves to direct attention away from specialized, expensive, abstinence-oriented treatment services for severely dependent individuals and toward a broader range of treatment and prevention alternatives. Harm reduction facilitates movement along the continuum from greater to lesser negative consequences of alcohol use. Abstinence may be considered an anchor point of minimal harm, particularly for those at the more severe end of the continuum, but any incremental movement toward reduced harm is supported.

One of the primary advantages of harm reduction is the potential for increased participation in prevention and treatment services (Marlatt et al., 1997; Miller, Leckman, Delaney, & Tinkcom, 1992; Sanchez-Craig & Lei, 1986). Evidence suggests that up to 80% of U.S. alcoholics have never made contact with any self-help or professional treatment program (Institute of Medicine, 1990); there are an estimated 10 million untreated alcoholics in the United States (NIAAA, 1990). Proponents of the disease model often claim that untreated alcoholics are in chronic denial and will remain so until they "hit bottom" or are coerced into treatment (Morgan & Cohen, 1993). Alternatively, untreated individuals may be aware of what traditional treatment programs offer, but may reject the disease model and the requirement of absolute abstinence (Miller et al., 1992; Sanchez-Craig & Lei, 1986). If total abstinence is not a viable option and no other options seem available, there is no motivation for such individuals to make any changes in drinking behavior.

By contrast, offering a variety of treatment services—ones that include both moderation and abstinence as alternative goals—may result in many more untreated individuals' seeking help. Canada, Australia, and Europe offer controlled-drinking treatment programs that often attract clients uninterested in abstinence-based treatment (Miller, 1983). Offering a choice of treatment modalities and goals may enhance motivation to change alcohol use among problem drinkers who are in the "contemplation" stage of change (Prochaska & DiClemente, 1983). Moderate-drinking alternatives may help coax people "through the door," offering a low-threshold strategy consistent with the principles of harm reduction (Engelsman, 1989).

THE CONTROLLED-DRINKING CONTROVERSY

Early Findings on Controlled Drinking

Despite potential advantages, harm reduction is controversial because it tolerates nonabstinent outcomes for alcohol-dependent individuals. The so-called "controlled-drinking controversy" has raged for more than three decades, since Davies (1962) first published his account of 7 "normal" drinkers among a previously treated group of 93 male alcoholics in the United Kingdom. Davies's findings sparked a heated debate about the possibility—or impossibility—of alcoholics' ever drinking moderately. The occurrence of even a single case of controlled drinking by an alcoholic challenges the very definition of alcoholism as a disease.

Davies's findings were replicated by U.S. investigators from the Rand Corporation, an independent research firm. The first Rand report (Armor, Polich, & Stambul, 1978) found an improvement rate of 70% at an 18-month follow-up among men in 45 abstinence-based treatment centers over several different treatment outcome indicators. Controversy was sparked because not all of the improved patients were abstinent during the follow-up period. As the authors stated,

> . . . it is important to stress that the improved clients include only a relatively small number who are long-term abstainers. . . . The majority of improved clients are either drinking moderate amounts of alcohol—but at levels far below what could be described as alcoholic drinking—or engaging in alternating periods of drinking and abstention. . . . While the sample is small and the follow-up periods are relatively short, this finding suggests the possibility that for some alcoholics moderate drinking is not necessarily a prelude to full relapse, and that some alcoholics can return to moderate drinking with no greater chance of relapse than if they abstained. (Armor et al., 1978, p. 294)

A 4-year follow-up of the original Rand study (Polich, Armor, & Braiker, 1981) found that 18% of the patients reported drinking without problems or symptoms of dependence. The primary drinking pattern seemed to be in flux over time:

> When we examined longer time periods and multiple points in time, we found a great deal of change in individual status, with some persons continuing to improve, some persons deteriorating, and most moving back and forth be-

tween relatively improved and unimproved statuses. (Polich et al., 1981, p. 214)

Both the Davies (1962) findings and the Rand reports (Armour et al., 1978; Polich et al., 1981) indicated that continued but reduced drinking not only was possible following abstinence-based treatment for alcoholism, but in fact was likely. Although theorists who supported the disease model discounted the evidence, other researchers began to investigate moderate drinking as a viable goal for treatment.

Lovibond and Caddy (1970) published the first widely cited report of successful training for controlled drinking. Using a combination of behavioral treatment techniques, they reported that 24 of 31 alcoholics who received the experimental treatment were able to drink in a "controlled" manner 16–60 weeks after treatment. Although these results were promising, this study had significant limitations, particularly the lack of a control group. Therefore, two U.S. psychologists, Mark and Linda Sobell, conducted a study to systematically evaluate the effectiveness of a controlled-drinking program with 70 chronic male alcoholics at an inpatient treatment program (Sobell & Sobell, 1973, 1976, 1978). Patients ($n = 40$) judged to have a good prognosis were randomly assigned to receive controlled-drinking treatment (experimental group) or the traditional abstinence-oriented program offered by the hospital (control group). The other 30 patients were randomly assigned to either a behavioral program aimed at abstinence or a traditional abstinence-oriented treatment program.

The behavioral program for the controlled-drinking experimental group consisted of 17 sessions designed to help patients identify the functions served by their problem drinking (functional analysis) and to develop alternative and more appropriate ways of coping with problems. Specific treatment components included training in problem-solving and moderate-drinking skills, electrical aversion, patients' viewing videotapes of themselves intoxicated, and general education about alcohol and drinking behavior. In contrast, the control group received abstinence-oriented treatment, consisting of Alcoholics Anonymous (AA) meetings, group therapy, physiotherapy, and industrial training. Patients were contacted approximately every other month for 2 years; follow-ups also included information on each patient's progress from at least three collateral sources, including objective public records (e.g., hospital and jail admission records, driving records, etc.).

One-year follow-up results indicated that patients in the controlled-drinking experimental group were functioning well for a mean of 71% of all days, as compared to subjects in the abstinence-oriented control group, who were functioning well on only 35% of all days. At a 2-year follow-up, controlled-drinking patients were functioning well for 85% of days, compared to 42% for the control group. Despite these significant differences, patients in both groups experienced periods of hospitalization and incarceration during the 2-year follow-up (Sobell & Sobell, 1978). As an additional check on the validity of the Sobells' findings, independent investigators under the direction of Glen Caddy (Lovibond's coauthor in the 1970 report) conducted a 3-year follow-up of the same patients (Caddy, Addington, & Perkins, 1978). Although only 70% of the patients were contacted, the controlled-drinking participants continued their superiority to the abstinence-oriented control group on most measures of drinking and adjustment.

Criticism of the Sobells' Research

The collective results of this carefully conducted research were thrown into doubt by publication of a report by Mary Pendery, Irving Maltzman, and Jolyn West in the July 9, 1982 issue of the prestigious journal *Science* (Marlatt, 1983). Because the public read this report in local newspapers or viewed accounts on national news programs (e.g., the July 1, 1982 *CBS Evening News* program described the Sobells' original study as a "sham"), controlled drinking became tainted by the specter of scientific fraud. This view was reinforced by Maltzman's comment on the Sobells' study, quoted in *The New York Times*: "Beyond any reasonable doubt, it's fraud" (Boffey, 1982, p. A12). Negative media reports on the study continued for months (e.g., a highly critical segment aired on the *60 Minutes* television program on March 6, 1983).

At first reading, the *Science* article was indeed damning in its implications. The abstract reads in part:

> A 10-year follow-up (extended through 1981) of the original 20 experimental subjects shows that only one, who apparently had not experienced physical withdrawal symptoms, maintained a pattern of controlled drinking; eight continued to drink excessively—regularly or intermittently—despite repeated damaging consequences; six abandoned their efforts to engage in controlled drinking and became abstinent; four died from alcohol-related causes; and one, certified about a year after discharge from the research project as gravely disabled because of drinking, was missing. (Pendery et al., 1982, p. 169)

A careful reading of the Pendery et al. study, however, reveals a number of disturbing questions concerning the scientific credibility of the findings reported in the *Science* article. First and foremost, why were the results from the abstinence-oriented control group omitted from the article, despite the fact that these control group patients were contacted for Pendery's follow-up. A key strength of the Sobells' research design was that patients were randomly assigned to either the experimental controlled-drinking treatment or the abstinence-oriented control condition. The omission of outcome data for the control group is a critical flaw in the Pendery et al. (1982) study. These authors reported that 4 out of the 20 patients in the controlled-drinking group died during the 10-year follow-up, *without mentioning that in the abstinence-oriented control group, 6 out of 20 patients also died during the same time period* (Dickens, Doob, Warwick, & Winegard, 1982). The outcome for the controlled-drinking group can only be properly interpreted by comparing its progress with that of the abstinence-oriented control group.

In response to Maltzman's public allegations of professional misconduct and scientific fraud, the president of the Addiction Research Foundation in Toronto (where the Sobells were then employed) appointed a blue-ribbon panel of independent investigators chaired by Bernard Dickens, professor of law at the University of Toronto. The committee issued its final report in November 1982:

> The Committee has reviewed all of the allegations made against the Sobells by Pendery et al. . . . in their published *Science* article, and in various statements quoted in the public media. In response to these allegations, the Committee examined both the published papers authored by the Sobells as well as a great quantity of data which formed the basis of these published reports. After isolating each of the separate allegations, the Committee examined all of the available evidence. The Committee's conclusion is clear and unequivocal: The Committee finds there to be no reasonable cause to doubt the scientific or personal integrity of either Dr. Mark Sobell or Dr. Linda Sobell. (Dickens et al., 1982, p. 109)

The Dickens committee cleared the Sobells of all allegations of fraud. This finding was later confirmed by the Trachtenberg (1984) report, an independent investigation conducted at the request of the U.S. Alcohol, Drug Abuse and Mental Health Administration.

Continuation of the Debate

Unfortunately, the debate about the veracity of the Sobells' findings has continued (Marlatt, 1983). Maltzman (1989) even repeated allegations of scientific fraud against the Sobells, although several other papers strongly disputed his claims (Baker, 1989; Cook, 1989; Sobell & Sobell, 1989). Unfortunately, the mass media failed to highlight the findings of the Dickens committee, leaving the public with the continued impression that the controlled-drinking research conducted by the Sobells was fraudulent.

The continuation of this debate, 25 years after the original research was published and more than a decade after two independent committees cleared the Sobells, is a testament to the emotionality associated with the question of controlled-drinking in alcoholics. Dozens of articles and letters have been published on both sides of the debate, and proponents of both sides have claimed victory (e.g., Cook, 1985; Morgan & Cohen, 1993).

The Sobells have written in a recent editorial that, at least within the scientific community, there is now some consensus regarding the utility of controlled-drinking goals for some individuals under certain circumstances (Sobell & Sobell, 1995). Specifically, they conclude that, regardless of stated program goals, recovery for people with low levels of alcohol dependence typically involves moderate drinking, whereas recovery for more highly dependent individuals primarily involves abstinence. From a public health perspective, it makes sense to offer moderation-oriented programs to alcohol abusers and mildly dependent individuals as a means of increasing client recruitment and retention. Individuals who do not benefit from these programs can be "stepped up" to more intensive, abstinence-oriented services. The Sobells suggest that moderation-oriented programs for more severely dependent individuals should be much more limited, but may be acceptable as a harm reduction effort for those individuals who are completely unwilling or unable to abstain (Sobell & Sobell, 1995).

The various commentaries on the Sobells' editorial have largely disagreed with their conclusions, in some cases because of concern that the Sobells' view represents a false or premature consensus in the *conservative* direction—in other words, that controlled-drinking goals are actually appropriate under *more* circumstances than they have suggested (Duckert, 1995; Heather, 1995). In contrast, other commentators have expressed the more usual concern that controlled-drinking goals are being afforded too much credibility (Anderson, 1995; Buhringer & Kufner, 1995; Glatt, 1995; Hore, 1995). Because of the influence of traditional treatment programs on public opinion and research funding agencies, new controlled-drinking research in the United States, at least with severely dependent individuals, has become politically unpopular (Peele, 1992).

Despite the controversy, researchers have continued to examine the prevalence of nonabstinent drinking outcomes among alcohol-dependent individuals in abstinence-oriented treatment programs, as well as with alcohol-dependent and alcohol-abusing individuals specifically trained in controlled-drinking skills. In addition, considerable research has addressed the characteristics of people likely to succeed with controlled drinking as a goal, and the advantages of offering flexible goals or treatment options. The results of this research are reviewed in the following section.

MODERATE-DRINKING GOALS
FOR ALCOHOL-DEPENDENT INDIVIDUALS

From reviews of the research on controlled-drinking treatment and moderation training with alcohol-dependent individuals, we draw four main conclusions. Note that our conclusions are similar to those stated by the Sobells (Sobell & Sobell, 1995), but we also agree with those who hold that moderation goals may have wider applicability for alcohol treatment (Duckert, 1995; Heather, 1995; Ryder, 1996).

1. *Even in traditional abstinence-oriented treatment programs, some alcohol-dependent clients choose and achieve moderation goals.* Consistent with the Davies (1962) findings and the Rand reports (Armor et al., 1978; Polich et al., 1981), abstinence-oriented treatment outcome studies continue to find reduced, moderate, or nonproblematic drinking among patients. These results, though mixed, tend to support earlier findings. Even when treated with an abstinence goal, some alcohol-dependent individuals can and do engage in nonproblematic or "controlled" drinking during follow-up (Dawson, 1996; Finney & Moos, 1981; Helzer et al., 1985; Nordstrom & Berglund, 1987; Ojehagen & Berglund, 1989; Project MATCH Research Group, 1997; Sandahl & Ronnberg, 1990; Vaillant, 1996). Moderate-drinking outcomes vary widely, depending on the criteria used to define "moderation" and "abstinence," the original diagnostic criteria, the type of treatment utilized, and the follow-up period. However, long-term moderation tends to be as prevalent as continuous abstinence (Rychtarik, Foy, Scott, Lokey, & Prue, 1987; Vaillant & Milofsky, 1982). First reported by Armor et al. (1978), this finding has been documented in both moderate-drinking and abstinence-oriented outcome studies (Keso & Salaspuro, 1990; Project MATCH Research Group, 1997).

For example, Helzer et al. (1985) followed patients in 1977–1980 who met DSM-III criteria for alcohol dependence (American Psychiatric Association, 1980) and had been treated in four abstinence-based programs between 1973 and 1975. Former patients with no known alcohol problems during that time were contacted for interviews. Results indicated that 18.4% of participants engaged in some level of problem-free drinking during the 3-year period (1.6% were regular moderate drinkers, 4.6% were occasional moderate drinkers, and 12.2% were occasional heavy drinkers without alcohol-related problems). Self-reports were verified through contact with collateral informants and through examination of health records. Thus, the percentage of moderate drinkers (18.4%) actually exceeded that of participants who reported abstinence (15.1%) throughout the 3-year period.

Similarly, Nordstrom and Berglund (1987) found a higher percentage of social drinkers than of abstainers among patients with good social adjustment following alcohol treatment. The investigators examined hospital records of 324 living and 141 deceased patients treated for alcohol problems in Sweden between 1949 and 1967, and classified 70 patients (22% of the living subjects, 15% of the total sample) as having good social adjustment for a minimum of 15 years. These subjects were compared to an age-matched sample of 35 patients from the original 324 who were on disability pensions (an outcome strongly correlated with severe alcohol misuse in Sweden). Among the people previously identified as alcohol-dependent who had good social adjustment, 11 were abstaining, 21 were classified as social drinkers, and 23 were abusing alcohol (compared with 4, 1, and 24 subjects, respectively, in the disability group).

Data suggest that a large percentage of patients achieve neither continuous abstinence nor moderate drinking after discharge from abstinence-based alcoholism treatment centers (Helzer et al., 1985; Keso & Salaspuro, 1990; Norstrom & Berglund, 1987). Even when both abstinent and moderate-drinking outcomes are considered as legitimate forms of recovery from alcohol problems, only 20–40% of patients report long-term success with traditional treatment programs. Studies of the natural history of alcoholism and alcohol recovery further illustrate this point (Sobell et al., 1996; Dawson, 1996; Vaillant, 1996; Vaillant & Milofsky, 1982). For example, Vaillant and Milofsky (1982) followed 456 inner-city boys from age 14 to age 47, including 110 identified as having ever met DSM-III criteria for alcohol abuse. Although 49 men had been abstinent for at least 1 year during the follow-up period (defined as drinking less than once per month or having no more than 1 week of binge drinking), many subsequently returned to either moderate or abusive alcohol use. Eighteen men were considered stable moderate drinkers at age 47 (at least 2 years of drinking at least once per month with no alcohol-related problems), and 21 men were considered stable abstainers (3 or more years of abstinence).

A recent follow-up of these individuals at age 60, and a longitudinal sample of Harvard college students at age 70, suggested that a substantial portion of those diagnosed with alcohol abuse or dependence at age 47 remained alcohol abusers (Vaillant, 1996), although the percentage of individuals who were abstinent did increase over time. Interestingly, Vaillant (1996) defined "stable abstinence" as consumption of fewer than 12 drinks per year for the past 3 years, whereas "stable moderate drinking" necessitated consumption of more than 12 drinks per year without problems; these definitions make it difficult to distinguish true abstainers (no drinking at all) from occasional or light social drinkers. Despite this problem, stable moderate drinking was as prevalent as stable abstinence among the college student sample.

Studies of "natural recovery" (i.e., recovery from alcohol problems without reliance on formal treatment) have found that moderation outcomes are prevalent, even for individuals who clearly met DSM-IV criteria for alcohol dependence at one time (Dawson, 1996; Sobell et al., 1996). In one study, 75% of participants who reported previous drinking problems recovered without formal treatment, and 50% achieved stable moderate drinking (Sobell et al., 1996). Contrary to the progressive-disease model, these findings indicate that a majority of individuals with drinking problems recover on their own. These results also suggest that studies in abstinence-oriented treatment programs underrepresent the likelihood of moderation outcomes for alcohol-dependent and alcohol-abusing individuals.

2. *Even when they are trained in controlled drinking, many alcohol-dependent individuals choose abstinence. Over time, rates of abstinence (as compared to controlled drinking) tend to increase.* Since the debate

over the Sobells' study, relatively few studies have attempted to teach controlled-drinking skills to alcohol-dependent patients (Foy, Nunn, & Rychtarik, 1984; Foy, Rychtarik, O'Brien, & Nunn, 1979; Rychtarik et al., 1987). Considerably more research has been done with "problem drinkers" (individuals who meet criteria for alcohol abuse), although some studies have included subjects who met criteria for alcohol dependence (Miller et al., 1992).

The most frequently cited study of controlled-drinking training for alcohol-dependent individuals after the Sobell controversy is the work of Foy, Rychtarik, and colleagues (Foy et al., 1979, 1984; Rychtarik et al., 1987). In this research, male veterans received abstinence-oriented treatment, but half of the participants also received controlled-drinking treatment, with mixed results. At the 6-month follow-up, severely dependent subjects in the controlled drinking training group had slightly more days of abusive drinking than subjects who did not receive this training. However, this difference disappeared by the 1-year follow-up; at the 5- to 6-year follow-up, there were no significant differences between the two groups of patients. Participants who received controlled-drinking training were no more likely to relapse than those treated with an abstinence goal alone, and patients were slightly more likely to move from controlled drinking to abstinence than from abstinence to controlled drinking.

The findings described above are similar to those found among 99 out of an original sample of 140 problem drinkers treated with moderation goals who were followed up 3½, 5, 7, and 8 years after treatment (Miller et al., 1992). Fifty-two percent clearly met criteria for alcohol dependence, and all met criteria for alcohol abuse, at pretreatment. Miller and his colleagues summarized their results as follows:

> Over the long-run, patients who seek treatment with a goal of controlled drinking show increased rates of abstinence or non-remission. In our final located sample of patients treated with a goal of controlled drinking, the most common outcomes were abstinence (23%) and non-remission (35%). . . . A subset of patients do establish and maintain stable asymptomatic drinking. In our located sample, 14% were classified by very conservative criteria as asymptomatic drinkers, sustaining moderate consumption with no evidence of either negative consequences or symptoms of dependence. (1992, pp. 249, 261)

Analysis of long-term stability indicated that of 14 participants who were stable asymptomatic drinkers at follow-up, 12 (86%) achieved this status by the end of treatment, and all had achieved it by the 1-year follow-up. Many subjects who achieved moderate drinking early in their recovery later went on to become abstinent, so the percentage of abstainers increased in later follow-ups, consistent with the results of the Vaillant (1996) study. Failure to achieve stable moderation or abstinence by the end of the first year was associated with poor long-term prognosis.

3. *Offering a choice of goals tends to result in greater treatment retention and recruitment of a broader range of problem drinkers, without increasing the risk of relapse to uncontrolled-drinking states.* The Miller et al. (1992) results compare favorably with other treatment outcome studies of alcohol-dependent patients; they also highlight the usefulness of carefully monitored moderation trials as a pathway to abstinence for people who might otherwise not enter treatment (18% of subjects specifically mentioned this advantage of participation). Providing clients with opportunities for moderate drinking early in treatment is consistent with "low-threshold" harm reduction, compared to the "high-threshold" requirement of initial abstinence (Engelsman, 1989; Miller & Page, 1991).

Offering a choice of goals and inviting patients' involvement in treatment planning have been recommended to decrease dropout rates and to increase the likelihood of achieving treatment goals (Booth, Dale, & Ansari, 1984; Ojehagen & Berglund, 1989; Sanchez-Craig, Annis, Bornet, & MacDonald, 1984; Sanchez-Craig & Lei, 1986). For example, Ojehagen and Berglund (1989) followed 58 alcohol-dependent participants of a program that allowed patients to reevaluate and revise treatment goals and strategies every 3 months with their therapists. They found that 84% of their subjects initially chose abstinence, although by the 2-year follow-up only 67% had an abstinence goal. People oscillated between goals, but they were no more likely to relapse from an abstinence goal than from a controlled-drinking goal. Similarly, Miller et al. (1992) found that goal choice was not related to subsequent relapse. Since treatment dropout is a major threat to successful outcome (Marlatt et al., 1997; McLellan et al., 1996), the benefits of such flexibility are important harm reduction considerations.

4. *Client characteristics, goal choice, and severity of dependence may all be related to treatment outcome (abstinence, moderation, or relapse); when given a choice, individuals tend to choose the goal that is most appropriate for the severity of their problems.* Various studies have examined whether certain client characteristics, including demographic variables (age, gender, socioeconomic status, etc.), severity of alcohol dependence, or client choice of goals, can be used to predict or recommend moderate drinking versus abstinence. Rosenberg (1993) found that fewer prior episodes of treatment for alcohol problems were associated with successful moderation; this may reflect a lower level of dependence severity and higher flexibility of personal treatment ideology.

The relationship between pretreatment drinking pattern (i.e., episodic vs. continuous heavy drinking) and outcome have been mixed. Rosenberg (1993) concludes that moderation is more likely for individuals with a pattern of continuous drinking prior to treatment, whereas Dawson (1996) suggests that among "natural recoverers," moderation outcomes are more likely for those with a history of episodic drinking. These conflicting findings may reflect differences between those who seek treatment and those who recover on their own. Moderation has also been associated with shorter periods of abstinence prior to alcohol treatment, psychological and social stability, and higher level of education (Dawson, 1996; Rosenberg, 1993; Vaillant, 1996). Stable employment has generally been found to be predictive of good outcome, regardless of moderation or abstinence goals (Rosenberg, 1993).

Generally speaking, with some exceptions, younger individuals and women have been found to have greater success with moderation goals. Research concerning family history of drinking problems as a predictor of moderation has been mixed. Physician referral has been more predictive of successful abstinence than of moderation or relapse outcomes. Change of drinking situations and return to a recreationally oriented family have been associated with successful moderation, and ongoing AA participation has been shown to be predictive of successful abstinence. Regardless of treatment goal, early success at moderation or abstinence is associated with improved long-term outcome (Miller et al., 1992; Rosenberg, 1993).

Orford and Keddie (1986) studied 46 alcoholics in treatment to evaluate the relative contribution of severity of dependence and clients' beliefs and choices in predicting controlled drinking or abstinence. Dependence severity was measured by the Severity of Alcohol Dependence Questionnaire (Stockwell, Murphy, & Hodgson, 1983), the Rand criteria for "definite alcoholism" (Armor et al., 1978), estimated problem duration, family history of alcohol problems, extensive periods of abstinence or controlled drinking, and pretreatment drinking pattern. Clients' beliefs were measured by questionnaire, stated goal preferences, confidence in attaining goals, and previous exposure to AA or abstinence-oriented treatment.

Some clients were assigned to treatment in accordance with their stated goal preference, whereas other clients were randomly assigned to abstinence or controlled-drinking treatment. At a 1-year follow-up assessment, the severity-of-dependence hypothesis was not supported. Participants who were "mismatched" to treatment goal based on dependence indicators (e.g., severely dependent clients assigned to controlled-drinking treatment) did not have poorer outcomes than those who were "correctly matched" with their treatment goal. However, clients who received treatment in line with their beliefs were more likely to be classified as successful at the 12-month follow-up. Orford and Keddie (1986) concluded that these results

> ... offer more support for the idea that abstinence or controlled drinking outcomes of treatment depend upon the personal persuasion of a client, the persuasions of the treatment personnel, and the compatibility of the two, than they do to the idea that these outcomes are determined by the client's level of physical dependence. (p. 502)

Importantly, in the Orford and Keddie (1986) study, a simple treatment goal decision based on demographic data, severity of dependence, and treatment beliefs could be made for only about 40% of the cases. The investigators thus warned against rapid treatment goal decisions and recommended flexibility of goals. Using treatment progress to collect data and test options may lead to more informed clinical decisions regarding the likelihood of successful abstinence or moderation.

Similarly, the Miller et al. (1992) study supports the importance of goal choice as well as severity of dependence in determining outcome, further illustrating the need to be flexible in determining treatment goals. Although higher levels of alcohol dependence seemed related to long-term abstinence or nonremission (as opposed to long-term asymptomatic drinking), 10 of 14 asymptomatic drinkers in the study met DSM-III criteria for alcohol dependence at intake. Regardless of diagnosis (abuse vs. dependence), individuals who accepted abstinence as a goal were more likely to be abstinent, whereas those not accepting an abstinence goal were more likely to be asymptomatic drinkers.

Fears that opening the door to nonabstinent goals will lead to a stampede of clients choosing controlled drinking (Morgan & Cohen, 1993) do not appear to be supported by the data. In their study of the goal choices of alcohol-dependent clients, Foy et al. (1979) asked 63 alcohol-dependent male veterans about their long-term recovery goals after treatment. Approximately 70% of subjects chose abstinence as their long-term goal, with only 30% choosing controlled drinking. Ogborne (1987) reviewed the goal choices of 245 patients presenting for alcohol treatment in Toronto, and found that those with more severe levels of alcohol problems tended to choose abstinence as a long-term goal, whereas younger patients with fewer alcohol-related problems tended to choose moderation goals. Among alcoholic veterans, those choosing responsible controlled drinking over abstinence had a shorter history of abusive drinking (Pachman, Foy, & Van Erd, 1978).

CLINICAL INTERVENTIONS: ADVANCES IN THE ALCOHOL HARM REDUCTION FIELD

Having discussed the controversy about controlled drinking as an alternative for treatment of severe drinking problems, we now turn to moderation training as a secondary prevention strategy for drinkers who meet diagnostic criteria for alcohol abuse. We also focus on the expanded spectrum of prevention and treatment options available for those with a range of drinking problems.

In an influential report released by the Institute of Medicine (IOM, 1990), attention has been focused on a broader population of drinkers. The IOM report includes a diagram outlining the spectrum of possible responses to this continuum of alcohol problems in the general society; this diagram is reproduced here as Figure 4.1. On the left side of the figure, the base of the triangle contains the majority of people who either do not drink or are "social drinkers" not experiencing noticeable alcohol problems. Universal or primary prevention programs are directed toward this group, although such programs are likely to reach drinkers experiencing some problems as well. The middle section of the triangle includes individuals who show mild or moderate alcohol problems. Brief interventions to modify the drinking behavior and associated risks are recommended for this population: "The objective of brief intervention is to reduce or eliminate the individual's alcohol consumption in a timely and efficient manner, with the goal of preventing the consequences of that consumption" (IOM, 1990, p. 213). Finally, on the far right of the triangle are those individuals with substantial or severe problems. Specialized treatment programs already exist for people diagnosed as alcohol-dependent. Brief interventions have recently been

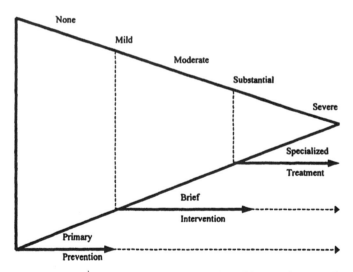

FIGURE 4.1. A spectrum of responses to alcohol problems. The triangle represents the population of the United States, with the spectrum of alcohol problems experienced by the population shown along the upper side. Responses to the problems are shown along the lower side (based on Skinner, 1988). In general, specialized treatment is indicated for persons with substantial or severe alcohol problems; brief intervention is indicated for persons with mild or moderate alcohol problems; and primary prevention is indicated for persons who have not had alcohol problems but are at risk of developing them. The dotted lines extending the arrows suggest that both primary prevention and brief intervention may have effects beyond their principal target populations. The prevalence of categories of alcohol problems in the population is represented by the area of the triangle occupied: Most people have no alcohol problems, many people have a few alcohol problems, and some people have many alcohol problems. From Institute of Medicine (IOM, 1990, p. 212). Copyright 1990 by the National Academy of Sciences. Reprinted by permission.

developed for individuals who meet the criteria for alcohol dependence or abuse, and for others with milder, less severe alcohol problems.

It is clear from inspection of Figure 4.1 that the overall number of drinkers decreases as one moves from left to right along the population triangle. The fewest number of drinkers (at the far-right apex) represent those with the most severe or substantial drinking problems. Figure 4.1 indicates that most people have few or no alcohol problems, many drinkers have some alcohol problems, and very few have many drinking problems. Yet the few drinkers with the greatest number of problems are those who receive the most attention and for whom specialized treatment programs are already available. It appears paradoxical to some observers (e.g., Kreitman, 1986) that the majority of individuals with some alcohol problems are the least likely to receive help—those in the midrange of the population triangle. From a public health perspective, this large segment of the drinking population should not be ignored—a recommendation strongly endorsed in the IOM report:

> If the alcohol problems experienced by the population are to be reduced significantly, the distribution of these problems in the population suggests that a principal focus of intervention should be on persons with mild or moderate alcohol problems. . . . The implications of this analysis are clear. There is a need for a spectrum of interventions that matches the spectrum of alcohol problems. It may be that, even prior to brief intervention, some work will be required to persuade individuals that even a mild or moderate problem exists; a stepwise progression into treatment interventions of graded levels of intensity should be possible. At present, in the absence of the capability for such a stepwise approach, an individual's denial that entry into, let us say, prolonged inpatient treatment is required is tantamount to a denial that any problem exists. (IOM, 1990, pp. 215–218)

Over the past two decades, particularly in the wake of the IOM (1990) report, there have been several developments in the alcohol field consistent with a harm reduction or public health approach (Single, 1996). Many of these developments serve to broaden the base of populations for whom effective interventions exist, as well as to provide real choices to alcohol-dependent or alcohol-abusing individuals wanting to be educated about or to reduce their harmful drinking, or even to abstain. These developments have led to an upsurge of interest in brief interventions (including brief physician advice), guided self-change approaches, and moderation-oriented self-help groups. Recent research on these developments is described below. In addition, several new pharmacological approaches to alcohol problems provide useful adjuncts to psychosocial interventions, for those individuals who choose to utilize them; these approaches are described in a later section.

Brief Interventions

Interest in brief interventions focusing on advice and motivational enhancement for reducing drinking was first stimulated by findings from abstinence-oriented treatment outcome research. In one key study, conducted in England by Edwards et al. (1977), 100 married men who were admitted to an outpatient clinic for the treatment of alcohol problems were randomly assigned to receive either a comprehensive treatment program or a single session of professional advice. The treatment group received a variety of interventions, including regular outpatient care, an introduction to AA, and admission to a 6-week inpatient unit if that seemed advisable. In contrast, the control condition consisted of a single session of professional advice, conducted conjointly with each man and his wife; the emphasis was on directing the husband toward abstinence, improving the marital relationship, and enhancing the husband's work record. A follow-up conducted a year later showed no significant differences in outcome between the two conditions. The overall results showed that a single session of advice appeared to be as effective as a much more extensive treatment. There also was evidence of a treatment-matching effect: Patients with more severe problems did better in the treatment condition, whereas those with less severe problems did better in the advice condition.

Chick, Ritson, Connaughton, Stewart, and Chick (1988) found mixed support for the efficacy of brief advice with more severely dependent drinkers. Over 150 subjects (80% male) were randomly assigned to one of three treatment conditions: simple advice (5 minutes, advice to stop drinking); amplified advice (30–60 minutes); or extended treatment (advice with the addition of detoxification, group treatment, social skills training, etc.). For both advice and extended-treatment subjects, informants, usually family members, were contacted by a social worker approximately once per month to monitor the patients' progress and to provide a "safety net" for those subjects who were not responding to treatment. At a 2-year follow-up, results of the comparison between the two advice conditions (including 21 patients who were removed because of a failure to respond to advice alone) and the extended-treatment condition indicated no differences in rates of long-term abstinence or problem-free drinking. However, there were slightly more short-term successful participants in the extended-treatment group than in the advice group. There were no significant differences in outcome between simple and amplified advice. Consistent with the findings of Edwards et al. (1977) regarding severity, failures in the advice group on average had had more previous treatment than other participants (Chick et al., 1988).

The Project MATCH Treatment Group (1997) compared a four-session version of individually administered motivational enhancement therapy (Miller & Rollnick, 1991; Miller et al., 1992) with 12 weekly sessions of cognitive-behavioral skills training or Twelve-Step facilitation therapy (individual counseling designed to increase utilization of AA and understanding of Twelve-Step philosophy) in the treatment of alcohol dependence. In all cases, the goal of treatment was abstinence. Results indicated that participants in all conditions showed substantial improvement, with no significant differences between the groups at 3-, 6-, or 12-month follow-up. In contrast to the results of earlier studies, participants with greater levels of dependence showed no difference in improvement rates, regardless of condition (i.e., brief motivational intervention vs. more extended counseling).

In each of the above-described studies, the stated goal for treatment was abstinence. Other studies of brief intervention have examined the goal of reducing harmful levels of alcohol consumption. The most extensive study of this kind was recently conducted under the auspices of WHO (Babor et al., 1994; WHO Brief Intervention Study Group, 1996). The core of this study, conducted at 10 treatment centers around the world, involved random assignment of heavy but nondependent drinkers to one of three conditions: no treatment (health screening only), minimal advice (5 minutes), or brief counseling (20 minutes plus a manual about reduced drinking). Results indicated that men who received advice about reducing or quitting drinking subsequently showed significantly greater reductions in drinking than did those subjects who received no treatment. These reductions did not seem to be associated with the intensity or duration of advice, in that a single 5-minute session was as effective as a 20-minute session combined with the manual. Similarly, there were no differences in drinking rates or patterns between subjects who received advice and those who received standard outpatient treatment. Women tended to reduce their drinking, regardless of condition.

Brief advice may be more beneficial for men than for women; 63% of men who received brief advice reduced their consumption by at least one drink per week, compared to 40% who reduced their consumption without intervention (Babor et al., 1994; WHO Brief Intervention Study Group, 1996). An alternative explanation for these findings might be that women may be more sensitive to the effects of *any* intervention, including the health screening utilized as a control group in this study. This interpretation would be consistent with other findings regarding the superiority of outcomes for women in moderation-oriented programs (Rosenberg, 1993; Sanchez-Craig et al., 1984; Sanchez-Craig, Spivak, & Davila, 1991).

Several additional secondary prevention studies have investigated brief outpatient treatment aimed at producing reduced alcohol consumption among "problem drinkers" without serious signs of dependence. Alden (1988) compared 12 weeks of behavioral self-management or developmental counseling with a goal of moderate drinking to a waiting-list control condition. Follow-up was conducted immediately following treatment and again 2 years later. Results indicated that subjects in both treatment groups significantly reduced their consumption, compared to the control group. At the 2-year follow-up, 50% of subjects in the behavioral self-management group and 44% of subjects in the developmental counseling group were drinking moderately. Reductions in drinking were associated with general improvements in health and mood.

Heather, Robertson, MacPherson, Allsop, and Fulton (1987) recruited "problem drinkers" via newspaper advertisements, and randomly assigned them to receive either a controlled-drinking behavioral manual or a standard alcohol information booklet in the mail. Participants who received the controlled-drinking manual significantly reduced their consumption by the 6-month follow-up, and generally maintained these reductions through the 1-year follow-up. Interestingly, the manual appeared to be most effective in helping the heaviest drinkers; heavy drinkers in the control group were more likely to require additional treatment than were heavy drinkers in the manual group.

Skutle and Berg (1987) also utilized newspaper advertisements in their study of behavioral treatments designed to prevent alcohol problems in early-stage problem drinkers. Participants received one of four treatment packages, including behavioral self-control training (manual or therapist-guided), coping skills training, or a combination. Results showed that participants in all groups significantly decreased their drinking, regardless of treatment condition; participants also showed a reduction in life problems related to alcohol use. These reductions in drinking and improvements in functioning were confirmed by interviews with collateral informants of good reliability. Similar results were found with low-dependence problem drinkers randomly assigned to receive either a cognitive-behavioral correspondence course or a minimal intervention consisting of information about alcohol misuse and instructions to record alcohol consumption. The cognitive-behavioral correspondence program produced significantly greater reductions in drinking than did the minimal-intervention control group; these reductions were maintained at a 12-month follow-up. However, individuals receiving the minimal intervention also evidenced changes in their drinking over time—a finding suggesting that even minimal contact may be sufficient to change drinking habits (Sitharthan, Kavanaugh, & Sayer, 1996).

Martha Sanchez-Craig and her colleagues at the Addiction Research Foundation in Toronto (Sanchez-Craig et al., 1984, 1991) have been at the forefront of the movement to provide brief cognitive-behavioral treatments for problem drinkers pursuing a moderation goal. Their treatment program (preceded by a comprehensive assessment) usually does not exceed six outpatient sessions. Counseling sessions include instructing clients in cognitive-behavioral strategies to achieve abstinence or moderate drinking, including goal setting, self-monitoring, identification of high-risk situations for drinking, and procedures to avoid drinking or excessive alcohol use. In one study, 70 early-stage problem drinkers were randomly assigned to abstinence or moderation goals; both groups maintained significantly reduced drinking levels over 2 years (Sanchez-Craig et al., 1984).

On the basis of these results, Sanchez-Craig and colleagues have developed the DrinkWise Program (Sanchez-Craig, Wilkinson, & Davila, 1995), a brief behavioral self-management approach designed for problem drinkers who are not severely dependent on alcohol. The program, available in group, individual, or telephone self-help formats, takes approximately 7 weeks to complete. Entry into the program is designed to be low-threshold. Initial results from 32 clients at a 3-month follow-up indicated an average reduction in alcohol use of 62% from baseline levels, and 94% of subjects were drinking at levels below those recommended for low-risk consumption (Sanchez-Craig et al., 1995). These findings suggest that problem drinkers who seek and receive moderation-oriented services show significant benefits.

A similar approach has recently been developed by the Sobells (Sobell & Sobell, 1993, 1995; Sobell et al., 1996) to provide skills training for problem drinkers who choose moderation goals. This self-guided approach emphasizes increasing both motivation to change and level of skills, while engaging the clients in active problem solving (via homework assignments, readings, etc.). Initial outcome data comparing this approach with and without the addition of a relapse prevention component indicated that subjects in both conditions demonstrated significant reductions in drinking rates and associated problems, with no differences in outcome between groups. Reductions in drinking rates averaged 53.8% from baseline to a 6-month follow-up; the number of alcohol-related problems decreased from an average of 4.1 negative consequences (in the year prior to treatment) to 1.7 at the 6-month follow-up.

Brief Intervention in the Primary Care Setting

Several recent studies and commentaries have focused on the effectiveness of physician-delivered brief intervention. The most comprehensive recent study evaluates the effectiveness of Project TrEAT (Trial for Early Alcohol Treatment; Fleming, Lawton, Baer, Johnson, & London, 1997). Project TrEAT was a randomized controlled trial of brief physician advice, conducted in 17 community-based primary care practices in Wisconsin. In all, 17,695 patients were screened for problem drinking. Those meeting criteria for problem drinking (482 men, 292 women) were randomly assigned to a control condition or an experimental condition consisting of two 10- to 15-minute counseling visits with their physician. Results indicated that those who received the advice showed significant reductions in average alcohol consumption, episodes of binge drinking, and frequency of excessive drinking. In addition, participants in the intervention group required fewer days of hospitalization during the 12-month follow-up period. These results suggest that significant benefits are associated with a relatively brief intervention within the context of other primary health care services.

Other physician-delivered interventions for problem drinkers have been associated with reductions in weekly alcohol use, particularly for male problem drinkers (Kahan, Wilson, & Becker, 1995). Support for reductions in alcohol-related mortality and morbidity associated with physician advice is more equivocal; however, it is possible that the relatively short-term follow-ups in the research reviewed by Kahan et al. obscured longer-term effects of alcohol reduction on morbidity and mortality indicators. Certainly, the potential advantages of incorporating alcohol risk reduction information into the primary care setting provide a rationale for continuing to pursue this line of research.

Brief Assessment

Another format for brief interventions is to offer people an opportunity to assess their drinking problems without specifying any particular treatment modality or treatment goal. One example of this approach is the "Drinker's Check-Up" described by Miller and his colleagues (Miller, Sovereign, & Krege, 1988; Miller & Sovereign, 1989). This intervention may be used to motivate drinkers to consider a choice of treatment options, including moderation and abstinence goals. By volunteering for a Drinker's Check-Up, individuals are offered an opportunity to evaluate their own drinking patterns and associated risks, and to take some remedial action as a result. The same principle has been used successfully in screening for hypertension risks (e.g., blood pressure assessment). Blood pressure monitoring devices are routinely available in settings such as medical clinic waiting rooms and other public places.

Technology is now available for the self-assessment of drinking patterns and associated health risks via computer software (Skinner, 1994). Similarly, Hester and Delaney (1997) have developed Windows software for assessing and providing feedback about alcohol use and its consequences. Opportunities for private self-assessment of one's own drinking behavior (i.e., at computer terminals in medical clinics, libraries, schools, etc.), with confidential feedback, may be utilized by otherwise unreachable or unmotivated problem drinkers.

Moderation-Oriented Self-Help Groups

The most recent development in the search for low-threshold alternatives to abstinence-based treatment has been the development of Moderation Management (MM), a self-help group founded by Audrey Kishline (1994), herself a former problem drinker. Based on empirical evidence of the effectiveness of cognitive-behavioral self-management approaches, MM self-help groups provide guidelines for moderate drinking; emphasize self-monitoring; and provide information about blood alcohol content, drink refusal skills, expectancy effects, and relapse prevention. The program guidelines suggest a 1-month period of abstinence prior to instituting moderate drinking; the return to moderate drinking is coupled with support and guidance from the group. MM is tailored to individuals with low to moderate levels of alcohol dependence. In contrast to the emphasis on lifetime attendance often promulgated by AA, MM guidelines stress using the group as needed. The guidelines also review the available information regarding the appropriateness of moderation goals.

Although no controlled outcome trials of MM are yet available, the group's founder has stated her support for research on the effectiveness of this approach. Local chapters of MM have formed across the United States, including an active group that meets daily "on-line" on the Internet. MM is thus a welcome addition to the available self-help resources for individuals attempting to resolve alcohol problems.

Brief Interventions for "Binge Drinking" in Young Adults

Brief interventions have increasingly been applied to prevention of alcohol-related negative consequences with adolescents and college students. Considerable research indicates that these populations are at elevated risk for problems because of their high alcohol consumption rates (Berkowitz & Perkins, 1986; Brennan, Walfish, & AuBuchon, 1986; Quigley & Marlatt, 1996). In a recent large-scale survey (Wechsler & Isaac, 1992), over half of college men (56%) and a third of college women (35%) had consumed five drinks or more in a row at least once in the past 2 weeks—a drinking pattern the authors identified as "binge drinking." Compared to non-binge-drinking students, binge drinkers were six times as likely to drive after consuming large quantities of alcohol, and twice as likely to ride with an intoxicated driver. Over one-third of the male and one-quarter of the female binge drinkers reported engaging in unplanned sexual activity, compared with only 10% of non-binge-drinking students of either gender. Despite the fact that the majority of students drink in a pattern associated with alcohol abuse (recurrent use in hazardous situations), few see themselves as having any problems with alcohol. Most students who drink do not meet the diagnostic criteria for alcohol dependence, nor do they consider themselves alcoholic.

An additional problem exists for most adolescent and college drinkers in the United States: They are engaging in the illegal behavior of underage drinking. Despite the fact that all states now have a minimum legal drinking age of 21, most individuals report their first alcohol use at a much younger age, typically in their junior high or high school years (e.g., Hawkins et al., 1997; Johnston, O'Malley, & Bachman, 1995). Although drinking rates among freshmen college students do show a marked increase over their drinking patterns in the senior year of high school (Baer, Kivlahan, & Marlatt, 1995), binge drinking is often established prior to college entrance. After the freshman year, however, there appears to be a gradual reduction in alcohol consumption over successive years of college. This "maturing-out" process characterizes most former college students, who report drinking less as they become older and are faced with increased life responsibilities (e.g., employment and family demands; Fillmore, 1987; Fillmore & Midanik, 1984). Most drinkers in U.S. society report their highest level of consumption during late adolescence, making the high school and college years a "high-risk window" for drinking-related injuries and problems.

In the United States, the policy of "zero tolerance" has been applied to underage drinking. Total abstinence is required, and programs designed to promote "responsible drinking" for underage drinkers are often deemed unacceptable. In response, many campuses have developed alcohol awareness programs based on a primary prevention philosophy (Braucht & Braucht, 1984)—providing information about the negative effects of drinking, and implying that students should simply not drink. Although such programs often lead to changes in alcohol-related knowledge and attitudes, few if any such programs have been found to produce changes in drinking behavior (Goodstadt, 1986; Moskowitz, 1989; Miller & Nirenberg, 1984). Specialized treatment programs are available for students who report alcohol dependence, but there is often no alternative for the majority of students who drink heavily but do not meet dependence criteria.

The reality is that most students drink. Harm reduction seeks to lessen the negative consequences associated with this choice. One example is our own work with students at the University of Washington. Our High Risk Drinkers Project is designed to test the effectiveness of an integrated approach to early intervention with college students. We have developed an alcohol skills training prevention program for high-risk college drinkers (Baer, Marlatt, & McMahon, 1993; Kivlahan, Marlatt, Fromme, Coppel, & Williams, 1990; Baer et al., 1992; Marlatt, Baer, & Larimer, 1995; Marlatt et al., 1998; Dimeff, Baer, Kivlahan, & Marlatt, 1998). College students who drank heavily were recruited in our first two studies (Kivlahan et al., 1990; Baer et al., 1992) to participate in an 8-week and a 6-week small-group program, respectively, to discuss alcohol use and related risks. The programs were nonconfrontational in tone, but nevertheless challenged students' assumptions about the effects of alcohol. In particular, we challenged the assumptions that "If some alcohol is good, more is better," and that "Alcohol consumption is necessary to improve social relationships and parties." These beliefs were challenged via information and class discussion of blood alcohol levels and the biphasic effects of alcohol (stimulant effects followed by depressant effects), as well as via homework assignments in which students experimented with drinking less. Results from the first study showed that students reported reductions in drinking rates of 40–50% over a 1-year follow-up period (Kivlahan et al., 1990).

In our second study, our group skills training intervention was compared to a single feedback-and-advice interview (Baer et al., 1992). In this feedback interview, a professional staff member met individually with students and gave them concrete feedback about their drinking patterns, risks (lower grades, blackouts, accidents), and beliefs about alcohol effects. Drinking rates were compared to college averages. Beliefs about alcohol effects were directly confronted through discussions of placebo effects and the nonspecifics of alcohol's effects on social behavior. Suggestions for risk reduction were outlined. In accordance with other studies of professional advice, the effects of this brief intervention were comparable to those achieved with the complete 6-week course (Baer et al., 1992).

In our third study, the Lifestyles Project (Baer et al., 1993, 1995; Marlatt et al., 1998), we evaluated the effectiveness of a prevention program based on motivational interviewing as the "first step" in a stepped-care program for reducing alcohol risks for students. Motivational interviewing (Miller & Rollnick, 1991) is designed to minimize resistance of those experiencing alcohol- and drug-related problems. Confrontational communications, such as "You have a problem and you are in denial," are predicted to create a defensive response. In contrast, placing the available evidence in front of the client and sidestepping arguments are facilitative and supportive of behavior change. This intervention is a good conceptual match to the risk factors and lifestyle of a college student population. Motivational interviewing is nonconfrontational and avoids the trap of labeling young people as "alcoholic" or "having a drinking problem" when they do not easily accept such labels. Furthermore, the technique is flexible; each interview is tailored to the specific history and risk factors of each individual. Issues of context (life in a fraternity or sorority), peer use, prior conduct difficulties, and family history of alcoholism can also be addressed. The highly variable nature of student drinking can be addressed with each interview. Motivational techniques also assume that clients are in a state of conflict or ambivalence, and need to come to their own conclusions regarding changing drinking behavior and reducing risks. The responsibility for change is left with the client. Since the client sets the goal (if any), it is considered a low-threshold intervention.

The specific intervention tested in the Lifestyles Project (Marlatt et al., in press) represented a combination of motivational interviewing with the alcohol skills training program described above. The program emphasized identifying students at risk for alcohol-related negative consequences; conducting a thorough assessment of their drinking habits, risks, and consequences; providing an initial feedback interview tailored from the assessment; and providing follow-up services if appropriate. Subjects were screened in the spring season preceding their first year of college, via a questionnaire sent to students while they were still in their senior year of high school. All incoming freshmen were invited to participate in screening. Assessment domains included drinking patterns, problems associated with alcohol, family history of drinking problems, and history of conduct-disordered behavior. Subjects were selected for inclusion in the study if they met either of two criteria: (1) self-reported consumption of at least five to six drinks on one occasion in the past month, or (2) self-reported history of three or more alcohol-related problems occurring at least three times in the past 3 years, as measured by the Rutgers Alcohol Problem Inventory (RAPI; White & Labouvie, 1989). This selection scheme identified approximately 25% of the sample (508 of 2,041 who completed screening) as at risk for drinking-related problems.

Of the 508 identified high-risk students, 348 were successfully recruited. These 348 subjects were randomly assigned to the prevention condition (motivational interviewing) or an assessment-only control group. All subjects completed a 45-minute baseline interview to obtain more detailed information about risk factors, and participants were asked to monitor their drinking on a daily basis for 2 weeks. Information from this assessment was used to guide individual feedback sessions for those in the experimental group.

In the feedback sessions, the interviewer met individually with students; reviewed their alcohol self-monitoring cards; and gave them concrete feedback about their drinking patterns, risks, and beliefs about alcohol effects. Participants' self-reported drinking rates were compared to college averages, and risks for current and future problems (grades, blackouts, accidents) were identified. Beliefs about real and imagined alcohol effects were addressed through discussions about placebo effects and the nonspecific effects of alcohol on social behavior. The biphasic effects of alcohol were described, and students were encouraged to question the "more alcohol is better" assumption. Suggestions for risk reduction were then outlined. In contrast to more confrontational approaches, interviewers simply provided assessment findings to the students and avoided moralistic judgments and arguments. Interviewers encouraged students to evaluate their situation and to begin contemplation of the possibility of change. "What do you make of this?" and "What surprised you about this?" were common questions raised in an effort to facilitate conversations about risk and the possibility of behavior change.

The specific goals of behavior change were left up to each student and not directed or demanded by the interviewer. Every student left the interview with a personalized summary feedback sheet (comparing his or her responses with college norms, and listing reported problems and risk factors), along with a generic "tips" page describing biphasic responses to alcohol, placebo effects, and suggestions for techniques of reduced risk drinking. Each contact ended with the statement, "We are always happy to meet with you to discuss issues about alcohol use or any other lifestyle concern." Students were encouraged to use our staff as a resource, and to make follow-up appointments as desired, but the primary responsibility for change was left with the students.

During the winter term of the second year of the study (1 year after the individual feedback interviews), members of the motivational intervention group were mailed graphic feedback pertaining to their reports of drinking at baseline and at the 6- and 12-month follow-ups. Each feedback sheet contained individualized bar graphs depicting baseline and subsequent levels of drinking quantity, drinking frequency, and alcohol-related problems. Every intervention student was given a summary paragraph of individualized feedback about his or her level of risk, and was encouraged to seek assistance if help was desired. Students with particularly high-risk profiles were also contacted by phone to offer assistance and encouragement to reduce their risks associated with alcohol use. If a student was interested, an additional follow-up interview was scheduled (this procedure resulted in 34 additional motivational interviews during the winter and spring of the second year of the study).

Statistical comparisons for treatment effects were completed on those high-risk students providing complete data at the 1- and 2-year follow-ups. Analysis of self-reports of typical drinking quantity, frequency, and peak consumption indicated that, compared to those in the control condition, treatment group students reported drinking significantly less frequently over time, consuming less per drinking occasion, and consuming a lower peak quantity over time. Despite a general maturing-out trend for all subjects, students in the treatment group reported significantly greater decrements in drinking at both the 1- and 2-year follow-up assessments than control subjects.

Analysis of alcohol-related problems with both the RAPI (White & Labouvie, 1989) and the Alcohol Dependence Scale (ADS; Skinner & Horn, 1984) revealed similar significant effects favoring those receiving the motivational intervention. For example, 2 years after having completed the motivational interview in their freshman year, treatment subjects reported a significant decrease in harmful consequences (as assessed by the RAPI) over the previous 6 months, compared to participants in the high-risk control group. Similar significant reductions were noted with the measure of alcohol dependence (the ADS): Using a cutoff score of 11 on the ADS, we found that only 11.0% of those in the motivational intervention group were classified as showing mild dependence at the 2-year assessment, compared to 27% of those in the control condition.

Other analyses have been completed on these data that are too lengthy to elaborate upon here. Treatment appeared to be associated with changes in perceived norms for alcohol use and with greater motivation to change drinking habits. A number of risk factors were also associated with drinking, such as living in a fraternity or sorority and having a personal history of conduct problems. These risk factors, however, did not interact with treatment response. Data from the 4-year longitudinal study of these students will allow us to assess whether changes in drinking result in changes in alcohol-related problem scores and in the development of alcohol dependence. In addition, we will assess whether these changes persist over time, whether control samples "catch up" in terms of drinking rates, and how other life changes (e.g., changes in living situation, dropping out of college, or graduation) affect changes in drinking behavior. Clearly, the preliminary results of this research indicate that harm reduction is a promising strategy in the secondary prevention of alcohol problems in young adults.

PHARMACOLOGICAL INTERVENTIONS FOR ALCOHOL PROBLEMS

The decade of the 1990s has produced new pharmacological adjuncts to psychosocial interventions for alcohol problems (Anton, Kranzler, & Meyer, 1994; O'Brien, 1996; Schuckit, 1996). In 1995, naltrexone (ReVia) became the first medication other than disulfiram (Antabuse) to receive Food and Drug Administration (FDA) approval for treatment of alcoholism. In addition, clinical trials of acamprosate are underway; acamprosate is already in use in many European countries, where preliminary evidence suggests that it shows considerable promise as an aid to preventing or limiting relapse episodes (Litten, Allen, & Fertig, 1996; O'Brien, 1997; Schuckit, 1996). Buspirone (BuSpar) has similarly shown promise in recent trials with anxious alcoholics (Kranzler et al., 1994; Tollefson, Montague-Clouse, & Tollefson, 1992). Other medications, such as fluoxetine (Prozac), have shown limited promise, primarily among individuals with dual or multiple disorders.

Despite promising research results, the use of these pharmacological treatments is controversial. In this section, we review the research evidence for several common pharmacological interventions, discuss their use within a harm reduction context, and briefly discuss controversies associated with their use.

Disulfiram

Disulfiram (Antabuse) has a long history as a treatment for alcohol problems (Litten et al., 1996; Schuckit, 1996; O'Brien, 1997). Disulfiram works by interfering with the production of aldehyde dehydrogenase, the enzyme responsible for breaking down alcohol acetaldehyde. When an individual on disulfiram drinks alcohol, the buildup of acetaldehyde causes an extremely unpleasant reaction, ranging from sweating and rapid heartbeat to more serious complications such as difficulties in breathing (Litten & Allen, 1991; Schuckit, 1996). The use of disulfiram, then, is hypothesized to provide additional motivation for the alcoholic to avoid drinking, in order to avoid this aversive reaction (Litten et al., 1996).

Disulfiram is widely used in the United States as an adjunct to abstinence-oriented treatment; many programs strongly recommend that alcohol-dependent individuals take disulfiram as an indication of their commitment to abstinence. Unfortunately, the limited outcome data available on disulfiram suggest that it is not superior to placebo in double-blind studies; moreover, compliance with disulfiram treatment is markedly low, due in part to its unpleasant and potentially serious side effects (Fuller et al., 1986; Litten et al., 1996; Schuckit, 1996; O'Brien, 1996).

The success of disulfiram seems to stem primarily from the fact that those who are willing to accept and comply with the regimen are often highly motivated to maintain abstinence. In his recent review of the literature, Schuckit (1996) suggests that there is not currently sufficient support for the widespread or coerced use of disulfiram for the average alcohol-dependent client. In fact, insistence on disulfiram compliance may represent a significant barrier to treatment utilization for individuals who are not willing to take this risky medication. Disulfiram may, however, be useful for some clients who choose to take it as a means to reach their goal for abstinence, provided that their daily dosing is monitored in conjunction with psychosocial treatment.

Naltrexone

Naltrexone (ReVia), an opiate antagonist, was initially developed as an adjunct to treatment for opiate abuse (O'Brien, 1996). The drug binds to opiate receptor sites in the brain, blocking the effects of opiates and leading to the onset of withdrawal in active users. Unfortunately, naltrexone has been considerably less useful than anticipated in the treatment of opiate abuse, primarily due to low motivation for naltrexone treatment and lack of compliance with taking the medication (O'Brien, 1996).

Despite its limited success in opiate treatment, naltrexone has generated considerable interest as an alcohol treatment adjunct. Two double-blind controlled trials have shown naltrexone to be superior to placebo in increasing time to first drink following treatment, decreasing the number of drinking days, and decreasing the amount consumed per drinking day (O'Malley et al., 1992; Volpicelli, Alterman, Hayashida, & O'Brien, 1992). Several smaller studies have shown similar findings, resulting in FDA approval of naltrexone as an adjunct to alcohol treatment in 1995 (Schuckit, 1996). Research on naltrexone suggests that it may reduce craving and pleasure or positive reinforcement from alcohol, and may also increase personal sense of control when drinking (Litten et al., 1996; O'Brien, 1997; O'Malley et al., 1992; Volpicelli et al., 1992; Volpicelli, Clay, Watson, & Volpicelli, 1994). Decreased craving and greater latency to drink have been found not only with alcoholics taking naltrexone, but also with social drinkers (Davidson, Swift, & Fitz, 1996). Six-month follow-up of alcohol-dependent patients treated with naltrexone suggests that many of these effects persist even after the medication has been discontinued, although naltrexone appears to have no advantage over counseling only in its effects on long-term abstinence rates (O'Malley et al., 1996).

Since naltrexone reduces the severity and frequency of drinking episodes, but does not increase rates of long-term abstinence, some have suggested that the utility of naltrexone may be greatest for those individuals who drink after treatment, since it may cause them to experience decreased reinforcement from the effects of alcohol (e.g., O'Brien, 1997; *Alcohol and Drug Abuse Weekly,* 1997). The possibility that Naltrexone represents a "controlled-drinking" treatment, rather than an abstinence adjunct, has resulted in considerable opposition to its use by some providers of traditional abstinence-oriented treatment. In addition, many within the abstinence-oriented recovery movement question the use of *any* medication in the treatment of drug or alcohol dependence (O'Brien, 1993, 1997). However, naltrexone reduces the intensity and severity of drinking episodes; this makes its use a viable harm reduction strategy for those who choose to take it.

Acamprosate

Acamprosate (calcium acetyl homotaurine) has been shown in both animal and human trials to reduce alcohol consumption. Several studies in Europe have indicated that alcohol-dependent individuals who receive acamprosate in conjunction with counseling have longer latency to first drink, more abstinent days, and lower dropout rates than do subjects receiving a placebo (O'Brien, 1997; Sass, Soyka, Mann, & Zieglgansberger, 1996; Schuckit, 1996). Based on the results of these European trials, clinical trials are now underway in the United States (O'Brien, 1997).

The mechanism of action of acamprosate is less well understood than that of naltrexone or other opiate antagonists. The compound is similar to the neurotransmitter GABA; increasing levels of this compound in the brain may block some of the reinforcing effects of alcohol (Littleton, 1995; O'Brien, 1993; Schuckit, 1996). It has also been suggested that acamprosate may decrease "craving" for alcohol (Littleton, 1995). Interestingly, despite hypothesized similarities in the effects of naltrexone and acamprosate on decreased use of alcohol, acamprosate has not generally been shown to reduce the intensity of drinking episodes; rather, it seems specifically to reduce the frequency of drinking, as well as to increase overall abstinence (Paille et al., 1995). This suggests that acamprosate may be a better choice for individuals who wish to abstain from alcohol, whereas naltrexone may be better suited to those wishing to moderate their alcohol intake.

Selective Serotonin Reuptake Inhibitors

Considerable interest exists in the application of antidepressant medications to the treatment of alcohol and substance abuse. In part, this interest has been generated by reports of substantial comorbidity between depression and substance abuse. Whereas earlier trials focused more on the effects of tricyclic antidepressants (Litten et al., 1996), more recent work has focused on the class of antidepressants known as selective serotonin reuptake inhibitors (SSRIs), particularly fluoxetine (Prozac) and sertraline (Zoloft). There is reason to believe that SSRIs may have a positive impact on alcoholics. Chronic alcohol abusers tend to have lower levels of serotonin than "normal" individuals (Linnoila & Verkkunen, 1992), and alcohol increases serotonin release, raising the possibility that drinking may represent an attempt to self-medicate endogenous depression (Schuckit, 1996). Although there are numerous flaws in this research, particularly difficulties in distinguishing the cause and effect of low serotonin in alcoholics, preliminary trials of SSRIs as adjuncts to alcohol treatment have been promising for those alcohol-abusing individuals who also experience significant depressive symptoms (Cornelius et al., 1995).

Buspirone

Antianxiety medications, particularly buspirone (BuSpar), have been applied to the treatment of alcohol problems for reasons very similar to those supporting the use of SSRIs. Specifically, the comorbidity of alcohol dependence and anxiety disorders is high; alcohol's sedative effects may serve to lessen anxiety symptoms, thereby negatively reinforcing excessive use of alcohol as a self-medicating strategy. Evidence does not currently support the use of buspirone to treat alcohol dependence in low-anxiety individuals (Litten et al., 1996; Schuckit, 1996), but it may be an effective adjunct to treatment when alcohol-dependent individuals present with clinical levels of anxiety (Kranzler et al., 1994; Tollefson et al., 1992).

The use of buspirone or an SSRI to treat alcohol-dependent or alcohol-abusing individuals with concomitant anxiety or depressive disorders is consistent with a harm reduction approach: Alcohol use is placed within the larger context of an individual's life problems, rather than being viewed as the primary problem. If medication and/or therapy can reduce the depressive or anxious symptoms, this may be sufficient to reduce alcohol use to nonproblematic levels.

HARM REDUCTION POLICIES

In addition to the types of clinical and pharmacological interventions covered here, public policies can reduce (or, conversely, can increase) alcohol-related harm. The policy arena is complicated; various constituents have conflicting interests and needs, all of which are affected by alcohol-related policies (Gordis, 1996; Plant, Single, & Stockwell, 1997). In addition, policy makers must often make decisions on the basis of incomplete information about the likely effects of policy changes. Despite these challenges, increasing attention is being focused on evaluating and implementing policies that can be demonstrated to reduce alcohol-related harm (Gordis, 1996; Musto, 1997; Rehm

& Fischer, 1997; Toomey, Rosenfeld, & Wagenaar, 1996). As Single (1996) points out, policies or interventions must *actually* reach the goal of reducing harm if they are to be considered effective.

Policy measures designed to reduce harm resulting from alcohol use tend to focus on restricting access to alcohol (e.g., the minimum legal drinking age, controls on the locations and operating hours of liquor stores, alcohol sales restrictions, and price increases via taxation) or on outlawing specific harmful behaviors (e.g., drunk-driving laws and server liability laws). These policies aim to decrease harm through reducing hazardous consumption.

Minimum Legal Drinking Age

Since the 1970s, considerable research has focused on whether a minimum legal drinking age of 21 is effective in preventing alcohol-related harm, particularly alcohol-related traffic accidents. Studies comparing the rates of accidents and arrests for drunk driving in states with higher versus lower drinking ages, as well as pre–post studies of states that have raised or lowered the drinking age, have consistently demonstrated a decrease in drunk-driving accidents and fatalities with an age-21 law (Wagenaar, 1983; Wagenaar & Holder, 1991; Toomey et al., 1996). As a result of these consistent findings, the federal government in 1985 began to put pressure on all states to raise their minimum drinking age to 21, in order to create uniformity across states and reduce accidents caused by younger individuals driving to and returning intoxicated from neighboring states where drinking was legal. Using the threat of withholding federal highway funds for noncompliance, the federal government was able to achieve compliance in all 50 states by 1988 (Toomey et al., 1996).

Despite the body of evidence demonstrating the efficacy of age-21 laws for reducing traffic accidents and fatalities among younger drivers, considerable controversy exists regarding this policy (Toomey et al., 1996). In particular, the overall efficacy of these laws is in question, since research indicates that the majority of individuals under the age of 21 are still able to obtain alcohol; in fact, for many people, the heaviest period of drinking occurs prior to age 21 (Johnston et al., 1995). Despite the widespread lack of compliance with age-21 laws, research suggests that these laws do result in less underage drinking than would result with a lower drinking age (O'Malley & Wagenaar, 1991). Furthermore, the evidence suggests that limiting access to alcohol for those under the age of 21 results in less drinking after age 21 as well, contrary to speculation that drinking would be heavier in an attempt to "make up for lost time" (Toomey et al., 1996). In fact, studies suggest that delaying the age of onset of drinking, and reducing consumption at an earlier age, are related to decreased risk for alcohol-related problems during college and beyond (Hawkins et al., 1997; Gonzalez, 1989)

Age-21 laws have also been linked to lower levels of alcohol-related injuries other than driving fatalities (Jones, Pieper, & Robertson, 1992). However, the extent to which the illegality of drinking contributes to certain increased risks for underage individuals is unclear. There may be less monitoring of such individuals' behavior because of their need to conceal consumption and to drink more on fewer occasions rather than less on more frequent occasions (as is more typical of adult consumption patterns). In fact, alcohol restrictions may have a potentially deleterious effect on patterns of alcohol consumption for minors; this possibility requires further exploration (George, Crowe, Abwender, & Skinner, 1989; Kilmer et al., 1998).

One documented unintended negative consequence of age-21 laws is the large number of young people cited for underage possession and consumption of alcoholic beverages, as compared to the small number of licensed establishments cited for providing alcohol to minors (Wagenaar & Wolfson, 1994). The intent of these laws is to discourage the sale or provision of alcohol to underage drinkers, but instead, the alcohol beverage industry has lobbied to shift primary enforcement of the law to target underage users themselves (Mosher, 1995). This is an inefficient system for enforcing the law (customers are much harder to identify than retail outlets); it also results in significant harm to underage drinkers (e.g., legal costs), while failing to decrease the number of underage drinkers (Wagenaar & Wolfson, 1994; Mosher, 1995). Toomey et al. (1996) have suggested that increased enforcement of laws designed to discourage the sale of alcohol to minors should result in even greater harm reduction benefits. In fact, decriminalizing underage possession and consumption of alcohol, while increasing enforcement of restrictions on sale or provision of alcohol to minors, could address many of the unintended harms resulting from minors' attempting to conceal illegal alcohol use.

Drunk-Driving Laws

In addition to laws setting a minimum legal drinking age, a variety of other legislation has attempted to discourage individuals from driving after drinking. These include "per se intoxication" laws (i.e., blood alcohol limits above which a driver is deemed to be intoxicated, regardless of other evidence indicating impairment); administrative license suspension laws (immediate suspension of one's driver's license at the time of arrest, prior to trial); zero-tolerance laws (making it a criminal offense to drive after any drinking if one is under the legal minimum drinking age); and mandatory jail sentences for drunk driving.

The number of alcohol-related traffic fatalities has shown a marked decline since the early 1980s (NHTSA, 1989). Although many factors may have contributed to this reduction, research suggests that tougher drunk-driving laws, particularly intoxication laws and administrative license suspension, have had a definite positive impact, despite problems with enforcement and detection of intoxicated drivers. At the same time, however, organizations such as Mothers Against Drunk Driving (MADD) and Students Against Drunk Driving (SADD) have instituted massive public education campaigns about the risks of driving after drinking, which may also have contributed to the decrease in accidents.

Despite these successes, evidence suggests that many individuals continue to drive after drinking, and only 23% of respondents to a 1995 survey reported they thought it was very likely that when drinking and driving they would be stopped by the police (NHTSA & NIAAA, 1996). In fact, these perceptions are fairly accurate: The number of drivers cited for driving under the influence, as compared to those who report having driven after drinking, is estimated to be only 1 for every 300 to 1,000 trips (Voas & Lacey, 1989). Moreover, arrests for driving under the influence have actually declined in recent years. In addition, public knowledge about changes in drunk-driving laws is lacking, which probably decreases the potential beneficial impact of these policies (Hingson, 1996).

Policies designed to increase enforcement of drunk-driving laws, such as sobriety checkpoints and alcohol sensors (noninvasive sensors that can detect the presence of alcohol on the breath when held in the vicinity of a driver), may substantially increase compliance with the laws (Wells et al., 1997; Lacey, Jones, & Fell, 1996). In addition, education or treatment programs for first-time offenders, in conjunction with (rather than instead of) legal sanctions such as mandatory license suspension, have been shown to help reduce recidivism rates (Wells, Bangert, McMillen, & Williams, 1995; Hingson, 1996). Interestingly, there is little support for the efficacy of mandatory jail sentences for drunk-driving offenders; in fact, there is some evidence that recidivism rates may be increased by longer jail sentences (Hingson, 1996; NHTSA & NIAAA, 1996; Mann, Vingilis, Gavin, Adlaf, & Anglin, 1991). It appears that increasing initial detection of drunk driving, and decreasing courts' discretion regarding license revocation (thereby increasing the perception that consequences will be swift and certain), have greater potential for reducing harm from drunk driving than increasing the length of jail sentences does.

Server Liability Laws

Server liability laws generally prohibit the service of alcohol to intoxicated individuals and to minors. Servers and/or establishments can be held liable for damages resulting from their failure to refuse service in such cases. These laws often apply not only to licensed establishments, but also to private individuals who provide alcohol at social functions (social host laws). Despite the widespread existence of server liability laws, evidence regarding their effectiveness is mixed, and research generally fails to support their efficacy in reducing alcohol-related harm (McKnight, 1993; 1996). As previously mentioned, few individuals or establishments that provide alcohol to minors are ever prosecuted (Wagenaar & Wolfson, 1994). Similarly, few establishments are ever cited for providing alcohol to intoxicated patrons (McKnight, 1996). Many social hosts are not even aware of their potential liability, since these laws are often not well publicized. Finally, servers often have little awareness of or training in recognizing intoxication and responding to it in compliance with server liability laws.

Several recent studies have tested whether increased training regarding identification and response to intoxicated patrons can increase compliance with server liability laws. Results generally demonstrate increases in server awareness, but little impact on servers' refusal to serve research confederates feigning to be intoxicated or underage drinkers (McKnight, 1993). Research does suggest that increased enforcement of server liability laws results in increased compliance with these laws, which in turn corresponds with decreased alcohol-related harm (McKnight, 1996; McKnight & Streff, 1994). Levy and Miller (1995) found that for every dollar spent nationally on enforcement of responsible alcohol service laws, there was a return of $90 in decreased costs to the states for alcohol-related harms. Unfortunately, McKnight (1996) concludes that increased public support for enforcement of these laws is necessary before changes will occur.

Restrictions on Liquor Sales and Outlets

Considerable research has been conducted to evaluate the effects on alcohol consumption and related harm of increasing or decreasing restrictions on alcohol sales (e.g., restricting the hours of operation, the number of alcohol outlets in a particular area, and the kinds of establishments that may sell alcohol). The evidence is mixed regarding access restrictions. For example, Wagenaar et al. (1996) surveyed underage drinkers and found that while their most common sources of alcohol were parents or older adults, 21% of those aged 18–20 had purchased alcohol directly from a retail source (generally a convenience store) where identification was rarely checked. Only 14% had purchased alcohol from a bar or liquor store, where identification was more routinely required for purchase. These findings suggest that the availability of alcohol at convenience stores and grocery stores may increase the harm associated with underage drinking, although improved enforcement may mitigate this problem.

There are mixed findings concerning whether greater alcohol availability increases overall consumption among adults of legal drinking age. Several studies have found increases in consumption associated with increasing the number of alcohol outlets, particularly increasing sales in grocery and convenience stores (Wagenaar & Langley, 1995; Wagenaar & Holder, 1995). Other studies have suggested that beer and wine sales may increase following a loosening of restrictions on sales, but that there is a corresponding decrease in sales of alcohol from other outlets such as liquor stores, resulting in net stability of consumption (Adrian, Ferguson, & Her, 1996).

Restrictions on availability of alcohol may increase harm to some subsets of users. For example, one study indicated that when restrictions were placed on liquor stores' hours of operation in some urban areas, the consumption of nonpotable alcohol (i.e., rubbing alcohol, grain alcohol) increased. Consumption of these substances substantially increases harm to users. These restrictions were subsequently lifted; in fact, hours were extended in an attempt to decrease the consumption of nonpotable alcohol (Single, 1996). This represents an example of a harm reduction strategy that does not attempt to reduce overall consumption, but still targets the reduction of harm.

Evidence suggests that increased density of alcohol outlets within a given geographical location (e.g., the downtown core in large cities) is associated with greater consumption and attendant harm within that district (Gruenewald, Millar, & Roeper, 1996; Scribner, MacKinnon, & Dwyer, 1994). Although it is difficult to separate cause from effect in these studies, the findings suggest that alcohol outlets should be distributed throughout communities rather than located in one district. Broader distribution of alcohol outlets may also actually serve to decrease drunk driving, as individuals will have shorter distances to travel in order to purchase or consume alcohol.

Taxation and Price Increases

Throughout history, taxation of alcoholic beverages has been used as a source of revenue (Godfrey, 1997; Musto, 1997; Gruenewald et al., 1996). More recently, however, taxation of alcoholic beverages has also been used as a means of decreasing consumption via increased prices. Research indicates that the demand for alcoholic beverages is somewhat elastic; an increase in price is met with a corresponding decrease in consumption per capita (Gruenewald et al., 1996). Taxation of alcohol in the United States is relatively low by international standards, but several Scandinavian countries rely heavily on taxation and price controls as a means of minimizing alcohol consumption and related harm.

Although the research on taxation clearly indicates that consumption decreases with increasing taxes, there are several areas of controversy regarding the harm reduction potential for this type of policy. First, the extent to which price controls may reduce consumption among heavy, binge, or problem drinkers is unclear. Some studies have indicated that underage drinkers (who are more likely to be binge drinkers) are particularly sensitive to price controls; higher alcohol taxes may be an effective means of reducing harm among this population. However, other studies have indicated that moderate drinkers reduce consumption more than heavy drinkers do when alcohol prices go up (Manning, Blumberg, &

Moulton, 1995). An additional concern is introduced if the price of legally obtained alcohol becomes too high: This may create a black market for smuggled alcohol and may increase illegal home distillation. Since smuggling and home distilling are associated with various types of harm (including lack of oversight and regulation regarding purity and safety), those making taxation policies must consider the potential increase in these activities. Finally, the costs are borne by all drinkers, rather than simply those who have problems with alcohol.

Despite these concerns, a recent review of taxation policies suggests that within the United States, a substantial increase in alcohol taxation would probably lead to an overall reduction in alcohol-related harm (Kenkel & Manning, 1996). It remains to be seen whether the U.S. public would support such an increase.

Local Control and Community Intervention

Many of the policies reviewed in this section have shown the potential for decreasing alcohol-related harm. However, enforcement of these alcohol policies has been shown to be a limiting factor in their efficacy. Several researchers have concluded that the U.S. public has or will have little interest in increased enforcement; even when enforcement is a priority, alcohol beverage control boards are generally woefully understaffed and underfunded to accomplish their stated aims (Wagenaar & Wolfson, 1994).

Several recent studies have examined community intervention as a means of increasing awareness and enforcement of the laws governing server liability, the minimum legal drinking age, and drunk driving. Researchers have also examined the use of local control measures (e.g., zoning ordinances and conditional use permits) for controlling alcohol availability without resorting to assistance from the alcohol beverage control boards. The results of these studies are encouraging: Community intervention trials have demonstrated significant reductions in various types of alcohol-related harm, including traffic accidents and fatalities, pedestrian injuries, drunk driving, and underage drinking (Holder & Wagenaar, 1994; Saltz, 1997; Wittman, 1997).

ENVIRONMENTAL HARM REDUCTION

In addition to clinical, pharmacological, and policy-level interventions to reduce harm, a number of environmental changes can reduce risks associated with drinking. Unlike most policy interventions, environmental changes are aimed primarily at reducing the consequences of drinking, rather than at reducing drinking per se. Perhaps the earliest examples of these include regulations regarding the cleanliness of licensed establishments (Musto, 1997); these regulations were not designed to reduce consumption, but rather to increase the safety of drinking patrons.

Recent environmental interventions include attempts to make bars and autos safer, and strategies making it easier to avoid drunk driving. For example, Graham and Homel (1997) describe changes in bar glasses in Scotland aimed at reducing injuries by making glasses crumble when broken, rather than shatter into sharp pieces. Programs providing free taxi rides home for intoxicated patrons aim to decrease the risk of drunk driving by making it easy to choose safer transportation home (Single, 1996). Designated-driver programs share this aim, although research suggests that these programs are not uniformly successful, because of frequent drinking (albeit at a more moderate level) by designated drivers (Shore, Gregory, & Tatlock, 1991).

Improvements in motor vehicle safety devices, as well as in highway safety, also contribute to decreases in alcohol-related injuries and accidents. For example, research indicates that drunk drivers are less likely to utilize seat belts, thereby increasing their risk for injuries in an accident (Hingson, 1996). Safety devices such as passive restraints and air bags help mitigate this risk. Research also indicates that alcohol-sensitive vehicle ignition locks, which require that drivers have a breath alcohol concentration below the legal limit in order to operate their vehicles, are associated with decreased recidivism among convicted drunk-driving offenders (Hingson, 1996). It is possible that expanded use of such devices may lead to significant reductions in drunk driving, at least among those already known to be at risk.

Finally, Geller, Kalsher, and Clarke (1991) have demonstrated that other aspects of the drinking environment (e.g., the alcohol content of beverages served, having alcohol served by bartenders vs. available *ad libitum,* and having food available) can all influence the intoxication level of those drinking in this setting. Harm can be reduced by careful attention to these factors. Thus, changes to the physical and social environment can affect the individual drinker in such a way as to minimize harm to both the individual and society.

CONCLUSION

This is an exciting time to be working in the alcohol field. The adoption of the IOM (1990) recommendations, and the culmination of more than 30 years of research on controlled drinking and alternatives to the disease model (Sobell & Sobell, 1995), have resulted in a much broader array of services available to clients seeking to change harmful drinking patterns. There is a movement away from dichotomous and moralistic views of alcohol problems, and toward conceptualizing alcohol problems as simply part of the continuum of physical and mental health issues confronting society today (McLellan et al., 1996; O'Brien, 1997). Whereas sometimes harsh, confrontational, coercive, and directive approaches once dominated the treatment field (Morgan & Cohen, 1993), it is now becoming increasingly common to see discussions of client choice, consumer-driven approaches, client–treatment matching, and the need to document treatment efficacy (O'Brien, 1997; McLellan et al., 1996). There is also a recognition that not all individuals with alcohol problems need, desire, or benefit from formal treatment (Dawson, 1996; Sobell et al., 1996); "one size" drinkers (IOM, 1990).

These advances in the alcohol field have benefited significantly from the development and explication of harm reduction philosophy in regard to illicit drug use (Single, 1996). The adoption of harm reduction as a broad public health goal helps place many of the earlier advances in alcohol treatment into a clearer context, and also helps to direct future research and intervention approaches.

It is important to recognize that harm reduction approaches for alcohol problems are not limited to clinical approaches or self-management training programs. Changes in the physical and social environment can also be implemented (Plant et al., 1997), along with public policy changes designed to minimize harm (Single, 1996). The best results may occur when all three methods are combined. For example, to reduce the harm of drunk driving, it is possible to combine programs mandated for drunk drivers (e.g., programs designed to modify drinking and prevent intoxicated driving) with physical and social environmental changes (e.g., use of car ignition systems that are designed to foil intoxicated drivers) and policy changes (e.g., reductions in the blood alcohol level used to define driver intoxication). Similarly, to reduce the risks of excessive drinking by youth, it is possible to combine alcohol prevention and education programs with laws restricting access to alcohol for minors, and with policies to shift enforcement and penalties to target providers of alcohol rather than youth. Social and environmental changes that focus on increasing the availability of nondrinking alternative activities for young adults may also help reduce harm for this population.

It is also important to realize that harm reduction approaches can be applied to both illicit and licit drugs, including alcohol. Even when abstinence is the goal in the treatment of alcohol dependence, harm reduction can be applied to reduce the frequency or intensity of relapse episodes; relapse prevention programs include tertiary prevention procedures to reduce harmful consequences (Marlatt & Gordon, 1985). Harm reduction can also be utilized as secondary prevention of alcohol problems through moderation goals. In sharp contrast to the insistence of disease model and Twelve-Step programs that abstinence be the "First Step" in dealing with all alcohol problems, harm reduction encourages a gradual, "step-down" approach to reduce the harmful consequences of alcohol or drugs. When the harm is reduced incrementally, drinkers can be encouraged and supported to pursue proximal subgoals along the way to either moderation or abstinence. Clearly, the "just say no" message no longer applies for people who have already said "yes." In these cases, harm reduction provides answers to the next question: "Just say how?" Harm reduction offers a realistic and compassionate alternative to the prevailing abstinence-only or zero-tolerance policies derived from the traditional disease model.

ACKNOWLEDGMENTS

Portions of this chapter have been adapted from G. Alan Marlatt's presidential address at the 1992 Association for Advancement of Behavior Therapy convention, entitled "Controlled Drinking: A Decade of Controversy." Some portions have also been adapted from Marlatt, Larimer, Baer, and Quigley (1993) (copyright 1993 by the Association for Advancement of Behavior Therapy; adapted by permission). The research described on prevention of binge drinking in college students was supported in part by a Research Scientist Award and a MERIT award (Grants No. AA00113 and No. AA05591) to G. Alan Marlatt, and by research grants awarded to Mary E. Larimer (Grant No. AA07702) and John S. Baer (Grant No. AA08632) by the National Institute on Alcohol Abuse and Alcoholism.

REFERENCES

Adrian, M., Ferguson, B. S., & Her, M. (1996). Does allowing the sale of wine in Quebec grocery stores increase consumption? *Journal of Studies on Alcohol, 57,* 434–448.

Alcohol and Drug Abuse Weekly. (1997, May 12). Researcher: Naltrexone minus drinking equals failure, pp. 1, 6.

Alden, L. E. (1988). Behavioral self-management controlled-drinking strategies in a context of secondary prevention. *Journal of Consulting and Clinical Psychology, 56,* 280–286.

Alterman, A. I., Bridges, K. R., & Tarter, R. E. (1986). Drinking behavior of high risk college men: Contradictory preliminary findings. *Alcoholism: Clinical and Experimental Research, 10,* 305–310.

American Psychiatric Association. (1980). *Diagnostic and statistical manual of mental disorders* (3rd ed.). Washington, DC: Author.

American Psychiatric Association. (1994). *Diagnostic and statistical manual of mental disorders* (4th ed.). Washington, DC: Author.

Anderson, P. (1995). Controlled drinking and a public health approach to alcohol. *Addiction, 90,* 1162–1164.

Anton, R. F., Kranzler, H. R., & Meyer, R. E. (1995). Neurobehavioral aspects of the pharmacotherapy of alcohol dependence. *Clinical Neuroscience, 3,* 145–154.

Armor, D. J., Polich, J. M., & Stambul, H. B. (1978). *Alcoholism and treatment.* New York: Wiley.

Babor, T. F., Grant, M., Acuda, W., Burns, F. H., Campillo, C., Del Boca, F. K., Hodgson, R., Ivanets, N. N., Lukomskya, M., & Machona, M. (1994). A randomized clinical trial of brief interventions in primary care: Summary of a WHO project. *Addiction, 89,* 657–678.

Baer, J. S., Kivlahan, D. R., & Marlatt, G. A. (1995). High-risk drinking across the transition from high school to college. *Alcoholism: Clinical and Experimental Research, 19,* 54–61.

Baer, J. S., Marlatt, G. A., Kivlahan, D. R., Fromme, K., Larimer, M. E., & Williams, E. (1992). An experimental test of three methods of alcohol risk reduction with young adults. *Journal of Consulting and Clinical Psychology, 60,* 974–979.

Baer, J. S., Marlatt, G. A., & McMahon, R. J. (Eds.). (1993). *Addictive behaviors across the life span: Prevention, treatment, and policy issues.* Newbury Park, CA: Sage.

Baker, T. (1989). An open letter to *Journal* readers. *Journal of Studies on Alcohol, 50,* 481–483.

Berkowitz, A. D., & Perkins, H. W. (1986). Problem drinking among college students: A review of recent research. *Journal of American College Health, 35,* 21–28.

Boffetta, P., & Garfinkel, L. (1990). Alcohol drinking and mortality among men enrolled in an American Cancer Society prospective study. *Epidemiology, 1,* 342–348.

Boffey, P. M. (1982, June 28). Alcoholism under new attack. *The New York Times,* p. A12.

Booth, P. G., Dale, B., & Ansari, J. (1984). Problem drinkers' goal choice and treatment outcome: A preliminary study. *Addictive Behaviors, 9,* 357–364.

Braucht, G. N., & Braucht, B. (1984). Prevention of problem drinking among youth: Evaluation of educational strategies. In P. M. Miller & T. D. Nirenberg (Eds.), *Prevention of alcohol abuse* (pp. 253–272). New York: Plenum Press.

Brennan, A. F., Walfish, S., & AuBuchon, P. (1986). Alcohol use and abuse in college students. *International Journal of the Addictions, 21,* 449–474.

Brickman, P., Rabinowitz, V. C., Karuza, J., Coates, D., Cohn, E., & Kidder, L. (1982). Models of helping and coping. *American Psychologist, 37,* 368–384.

Buhringer, G., & Kufner, H. (1995). Controlled drinking: A typical American debate. *Addiction, 90,* 1173–1174.

Caddy, G. R., Addington, H. J., & Perkins, D. (1978). Individualized behaviour therapy for alcoholics: A third year independent double-blind follow-up. *Behaviour Research and Therapy, 16,* 345–362.

Chassin, L., & DeLucia, C. (1996). Drinking during adolescence. *Alcohol Health and Research World, 20,* 175–180.

Chick, J., Ritson, B., Connaughton, J., Stewart, A., & Chick, J. (1988). Advice versus extended treatment of alcoholism: A controlled study. *British Journal of Addiction, 83,* 159–170.

Coate, D. (1993). Moderate drinking and coronary heart disease mortality: Evidence from NHANES I and the NHANES I follow-up. *American Journal of Public Health, 83,* 888–890.

Collins, J. J., & Messerschmidt, P. M. (1993). Epidemiology of alcohol-related violence. *Alcohol Health and Research World, 17,* 93–100.

Cook, D. R. (1985). Craftsman versus professional: Analysis of the controlled drinking controversy. *Journal of Studies on Alcohol, 46,* 433–442.

Cook, D. R. (1989). A reply to Maltzman. *Journal of Studies on Alcohol, 50,* 484–486.

Cornelius, J. R., Salloum, I. M., Cornelius, M. D., Perel, J. M., Thase, M. E., Ehler, J. G., Jarrett, P. J., Levin, R. L., Black, A., & Mann, J. J. (1995). Preliminary report: Double blind, placebo-controlled study of fluoxetine in depressed alcoholics. *Psychopharmacological Bulletin, 31,* 297–303.

Davidson, D., Swift, R., & Fitz, E. (1996). Naltrexone increases the latency to drink alcohol in social drinkers. *Alcoholism: Clinical and Experimental Research, 20,* 732–739.

Davies, D. L. (1962). Normal drinking in recovered alcoholics. *Quarterly Journal of Studies on Alcohol, 23,* 94–104.

Dawson, D. A. (1996). Correlates of past-year status among treated and untreated persons with former alcohol dependence: United States, 1992. *Alcoholism: Clinical and Experimental Research, 20,* 771–779.

Dickens, B. M., Doob, A. N., Warwick, O. H., & Winegard, W. C. (1982). *Report of the committee of inquiry into allegations concerning Drs. Linda and Mark Sobell.* Toronto: Addiction Research Foundation.

Dimeff, L. A., Baer, J. S., Kivlahan, D. R., & Marlatt, G. A. (1998). *Brief alcohol screening and intervention for college students (BASICS): A harm reduction approach.* New York: Guilford Press.

Duckert, F. (1995). The impact on the controlled drinking debate in Norway. *Addiction, 90,* 1167–1168.

Edwards, G., Arif, A., & Hodgson, R. (1981). Nomenclature and classification of drug- and alcohol-related problems: A WHO memorandum. *Bulletin of the World Health Organization, 59,* 225–242.

Edwards, G., Orford, J., Egert, S., Guthrie, S., Hawker, A., Hensman, C., Mitcheson, M., Oppenheimer, E., & Taylor, C. (1977). Alcoholism: A controlled trial of "treatment" and "advice." *Journal of Studies on Alcohol, 38,* 1004–1031.

Engelsman, E. L. (1989). Dutch policy on the management of drug-related problems. *British Journal of Addiction, 84,* 211–218.

Fillmore, K. M. (1987). Prevalence, incidence and chronicity of drinking patterns and problems among men as a function of age: A longitudinal and cohort analysis. *British Journal of Addiction, 82,* 77–83.

Fillmore, K. M., & Midanik, L. (1984). Chronicity of drinking problems among men: A longitudinal study. *Journal of Studies on Alcohol, 45,* 228–236.

Fingarette, H. (1988). *Heavy drinking: The myth of alcoholism as a disease.* Berkeley: University of California Press.

Finney, J. W., & Moos, R. H. (1981). Characteristics and prognoses of alcoholics who become moderate drinkers and abstainers after treatment. *Journal of Studies on Alcohol, 42,* 94–105.

Fleming, M. F., Lawton, B. K., Baer, M. L., Johnson, K., & London, R. (1997). Brief physician advice for problem drinkers: A randomized controlled trial in community-based primary care practices. *Journal of the American Medical Association, 277,* 1039–1045.

Foy, D. W., Nunn, L. B., & Rychtarik, R. G. (1984). Broad-spectrum behavioral treatment for chronic alcoholics: Effects of training controlled drinking skills. *Journal of Consulting and Clinical Psychology, 52,* 218–230.

Foy, D. W., Rychtarik, R. G., O'Brien, T. P., & Nunn, L. B. (1979). Goal choice of alcoholics: Effects of training controlled drinking skills. *Journal of Clinical Psychology, 34*(3), 781–783.

Fuller, R. K., Branchey, L., Brightwell, D. R., Derman, R. M., Emrick, C. D., Iber, F. L., James, K. E., Lacoursiere, R. B., Lee, K. K., & Lowenstein, I. (1986). Disulfiram treatment of alcoholism: A Veterans Administration cooperative study. *Journal of the American Medical Association, 256,* 1449–1455.

Gaziano, J. M., Buring, J. E., Breslow, J. L., Goldhaber, S. Z., Rosner, B., VanDenburgh, M., Willett, W., & Hennekens, C. H. (1993). Moderate alcohol intake, increased levels of high-density lipoprotein and its subfractions, and decreased risk of myocardial infarction. *New England Journal of Medicine, 329,* 1829–1834.

Geller, E. S., Kalsher, M. J., & Clarke, S. W. (1991). Beer versus mixed-drink consumption at fraternity parties: A time and place for low-alcohol alternatives. *Journal of Studies on Alcohol, 52,* 197–204.

George, W. H., Crowe, L. C., Abwender, D., & Skinner, J. B. (1989). Effects of raising the drinking age from 19 to 21 in New York State on self-reported consumption by college students. *Journal of Applied Social Psychology, 19,* 623–635.

Glatt, M. M. (1995). Controlled drinking after a third of a century. *Addiction, 90,* 1157–1159.

Godfrey, C. (1997). Can tax be used to minimise harm?: A health economist's perspective. In M. Plant, E. Single, & T. Stockwell (Eds.), *Alcohol: Minimising the harm—what works?* (pp. 29–42). London: Free Association Books.

Gonzalez, G. M. (1989). Early onset of drinking as a predictor of alcohol consumption and alcohol-related problems in college. *Journal of Drug Education, 19,* 225–230.

Goodstadt, M. S. (1986). School-based drug education in North America: What is wrong? What can be done? *Journal of School Health, 56,* 278–281.

Gordis, E. (1996). Alcohol research and social policy: An overview. *Alcohol Health and Research World, 20,* 208–212.

Graham, K., & Homel, R. (1997). Creating safer bars. In M. Plant, E. Single, & T. Stockwell (Eds.), *Alcohol: Minimizing the harm—what works?* (pp. 171–192). London: Free Association Books.

Grant, B. F., & Harford, T. C. (1995). Comorbidity between DSM-IV alcohol use disorders and major depression: Results of a national survey. *Drug and Alcohol Dependence, 39,* 197–206.

Gruenewald, P. J., Millar, A. B., & Roeper, P. (1996). Access to alcohol: Geography and prevention for local communities. *Alcohol Health and Research World, 20,* 244–251.

Hawkins, J. D., Graham, J. W., Maguin, E., Abbott, R., Hill, K. G., & Catalano, R. F. (1997). Exploring the effects of age of alcohol use initiation and psychosocial risk factors on subsequent alcohol misuse. *Journal of Studies on Alcohol, 58,* 280–290.

Heather, N. (1995). The great controlled drinking consensus: Is it premature? *Addiction, 90,* 1160–1162.

Heather, N., Robertson, I., MacPherson, B., Allsop, S., & Fulton, A. (1987). Effectiveness of a controlled drinking self-help manual: One-year follow-up results. *British Journal of Clinical Psychology, 26,* 279–287.

Helzer, J. E., Robins, L. N., Taylor, J. R., Carey, K., Miller, R. H., Combs-Orme, T., & Farmer, A. (1985). The extent of long-term moderate drinking among alcoholics discharged from medical and psychiatric treatment facilities. *New England Journal of Medicine, 312,* 1678–1682.

Hester, R. K., & Delaney, H. D. (1997). Behavioral self-control program for Windows: Results of a controlled clinical trial. *Journal of Consulting and Clinical Psychology, 65*(4), 686–693.

Hingson, R. (1996). Prevention of drinking and driving. *Alcohol Health and Research World, 20,* 219–229.

Hogan, C. M. (1993). *Substance abuse: The nation's number one health problem. Key indicators for policy.* Princeton, NJ: Robert Wood Johnson Foundation.

Holder, H. D., & Wagenaar, A. C. (1994). Mandated server training and reduced alcohol-involved traffic crashes: A time-series analysis of the Oregon experience. *Accident Analysis and Prevention, 26,* 89–98.

Holman, C. D., & English, D. R. (1996). Ought low alcohol intake be promoted for health reasons? *Journal of the Royal Society of Medicine, 89,* 123–129.

Hore, B. (1995). You can't just leave the goal choice to the patient. *Addiction, 90,* 1172.

Institute of Medicine (IOM). (1990). *Broadening the base of treatment for alcohol problems.* Washington, DC: National Academy Press.

Jellinek, E. M. (1960). *The disease concept in alcoholism.* New Brunswick, NJ: Hill House Press.

Johnston, L. D., O'Malley, P. M., & Bachman, J. G. (1995). *National survey results on drug use from Monitoring the Future study, 1975–1994: Vol. 1. Secondary school students.* Rockville, MD: U.S. Department of Health and Human Services.

Jones, N. E., Pieper, C. F., & Robertson, L. S. (1992). The effect of legal drinking age on fatal injuries of adolescents and young adults. *American Journal of Public Health, 82,* 112–115.

Kahan, M., Wilson, L., & Becker, L. (1995). Effectiveness of physician-based interventions with problem drinkers: A review. *Candian Medical Association, 152,* 851–859.

Kahler, C. W., Epstein, E. E., & McCrady, B. S. (1995). Loss of control and inability to abstain: The measurement of and the relationship between two constructs in male alcoholics. *Addiction, 90,* 1025–1036.

Kantor, G. K. (1993). Refining the brushstrokes in portraits of alcohol and wife assaults. In S. E. Martin (Ed.), *Alcohol and interpersonal violence: Fostering multidisciplinary perspectives* (NIAAA Research Monograph No. 24, pp. 280–290). Rockville, MD: U.S. Department of Health and Human Services.

Kenkel, D., & Manning, W. (1996). Perspectives on alcohol taxation. *Alcohol Health and Research World, 20*(4), 230–238.

Keso, L., & Salaspuro, M. (1990). Inpatient treatment of employed alcoholics: A randomized clinical trial of Hazelden-type and traditional treatment. *Alcoholism: Clinical and Experimental Research, 14,* 584–589.

Kilmer, J. R., Larimer, M. E., Baer, J. S., Parks, G. A., Dimeff, L. A., & Marlatt, G. A. (1998). *Correlates of fraternity and sorority members' opposition to constraints on drinking.* Manuscript submitted for publication.

Kishline, A. (1994). *Moderate drinking: The new option for problem drinkers.* New York: Sharp Press.

Kivlahan, D. R., Marlatt, G. A., Fromme, K., Coppel, D. B., & Williams, E. (1990). Secondary prevention with college drinkers: Evaluation of an alcohol skills training program. *Journal of Consulting and Clinical Psychology, 58,* 805–810.

Kranzler, H. R., Burleson, J. A., Del Boca, F. K., Babor, T. F., Korner, P., Brown, J., & Bohn, M. J. (1994). Buspirone treatment of anxious alcoholics: A placebo-controlled trial. *Archives of General Psychiatry, 51,* 720–731.

Kreitman, N. (1986). Alcohol consumption and the preventive paradox. *British Journal of Addiction, 88,* 591–595.

Lacey, J., Jones, R., & Fell, J. (1996, October 7–9). *The effectiveness of the Checkpoint Tennessee program.* Paper presented at the 40th Annual Meeting of the Association for the Advancement of Automotive Medicine, Vancouver, BC, Canada.

Levine, H. G. (1978). The discovery of addiction: Changing conceptions of habitual drunkenness in America. *Journal of Studies on Alcohol, 39,* 143–174.

Levy, D. T., & Miller, T. R. (1995). A cost–benefit analysis of enforcement efforts to reduce serving intoxicated patrons. *Journal of Studies on Alcohol, 56,* 240–247.

Linnoila, V. M., & Virkkunen, M. (1992). Aggression, suicidality, and serotonin. *Journal of Clinical Psychiatry, 53,* 46–51.

Litten, R. Z., & Allen, J. P. (1991). Pharmacotherapies for alcoholism: Promising agents and clinical issues. *Alcoholism: Clinical and Experimental Research, 15,* 620–633.

Litten, R. Z., Allen, J., & Fertig, J. (1996). Pharmacotherapies for alcohol problems: A review of research with focus on developments since 1991. *Alcoholism: Clinical and Experimental Research, 20,* 859–876.

Littleton, J. (1995). Acamprosate in alcohol dependence: How does it work? *Addiction, 90,* 1179–1188.

Lovibond, S. H., & Caddy, G. (1970). Discriminated aversive control in the moderation of alcoholics' drinking behavior. *Behavior Therapy, 1,* 437–444.

Maltzman, I. (1989). A reply to Cook, "Craftsman versus professional: Analysis of the controlled drinking controversy." *Journal of Studies on Alcohol, 50,* 466–472.

Mann, R. E., Vingilis, E. R., Gavin, D., Adlaf, E., & Anglin, L. (1991). Sentence severity and the drinking driver: Relationships with traffic safety outcome. *Accident Analysis and Prevention, 23,* 483–491.

Manning, W. G., Blumberg, L., & Moulton, L. H. (1995). The demand for alcohol: The differential response to price. *Journal of Health Economics, 14,* 123–148.

Marlatt, G. A. (1983). The controlled drinking controversy: A commentary. *American Psychologist, 38,* 1097–1110.

Marlatt, G. A., Baer, J. S., Kivlahan, D. R., Dimeff, L. A., Larimer, M. E., Quigley, L. A., Somers, J. M., & Williams, E. (1998). Screening and brief intervention for high-risk college student drinkers: Results from a two-year follow-up assessment. *Journal of Consulting and Clinical Psychology, 66*(4), 604–615.

Marlatt, G. A., Baer, J. S., & Larimer, M. E. (1995). Preventing alcohol abuse in college students: A harm reduction approach. In G. M. Boyd, J. Howard, & R. A. Zucker (Eds.), *Alcohol problems among adolescents: Current directions in prevention research* (pp. 147–172). Hillsdale, NJ: Erlbaum.

Marlatt, G. A., & Gordon, J. R. (Eds.). (1985). *Relapse prevention: Maintenance strategies in the treatment of addictive behaviors.* New York: Guilford Press.

Marlatt, G. A., Larimer, M. E., Baer, J. S., & Quigley, L. A. (1993). Harm reduction for alcohol problems: Moving beyond the controlled drinking controversy. *Behavior Therapy, 24,* 461–504.

Marlatt, G. A., Tucker, J. A., Donovan, D. M., & Vuchinich, R. E. (1997). Help-seeking by substance abusers: The role of harm reduction and behavioral–economic approaches to facilitate treatment entry and retention. In L. S. Onken, J. D. Blaine, & J. J. Boren (Eds.), *Beyond the therapeutic alliance: Keeping the drug-dependent individual in treatment* (NIDA Research Monograph No. 165, pp. 44–84). Rockville, MD: U.S. Department of Health and Human Services.

McKnight, A. J. (1993). Server intervention: Accomplishments and needs. *Alcohol Health and Research World, 17,* 76–83.

McKnight, A. J. (1996). Server intervention to reduce alcohol-involved traffic crashes. *Alcohol Health and Research World, 20,* 227–229.

McKnight, A. J., & Streff, F. M. (1994). The effect of enforcement upon service of alcohol to intoxicated patrons of bars and restaurants. *Accident Analysis and Prevention, 26,* 79–88.

McLellan, A. T., Woody, G. E., Metzger, D., McKay, J., Durell, J., Alterman, A. I., & O'Brian, C. P. (1996). Evalutating the effectiveness of addiction treatments: Reasonable expectations, appropriate comparisons. *Milbank Quarterly, 74,* 51–84.

Miller, P. M., & Nirenberg, T. D. (Eds.). (1984). *Prevention of alcohol abuse.* New York: Plenum Press.

Miller, W. R. (1983). Controlled drinking: A history and a critical review. *Journal of Studies on Alcohol, 44,* 68–83.

Miller, W. R. (1993). Alcoholism: Toward a better disease model. *Psychology of Addictive Behaviors, 7,* 129–136.

Miller, W. R., & Kurtz, E. (1994). Models of alcoholism used in treatment: Contrasting AA and other perspectives with which it is often confused. *Journal of Studies on Alcohol, 55,* 159–166.

Miller, W. R., Leckman, A. L., Delaney, H. D., & Tinkcom, M. (1992). Long-term follow-up of behavioral self-control training. *Journal of Studies on Alcohol, 53,* 249–261.

Miller, W. R., & Page, A. C. (1991). Warm turkey: Other routes to abstinence. *Journal of Substance Abuse Treatment, 8,* 227–232.

Miller, W. R., & Rollnick, S. (1991). *Motivational interviewing: Preparing people to change addictive behavior.* New York: Guilford Press.

Miller, W. R., & Sovereign, R. G. (1989). The check-up: A model for early intervention in addictive behaviors. In T. Loberg, W. R. Miller, P. E. Nathan, & G. A. Marlatt (Eds.), *Addictive behaviors: Prevention and early intervention* (pp. 219–231). Amsterdam: Swets & Zeitlinger.

Miller, W. R., Sovereign, R. G., & Krege, B. (1988). Motivational interviewing with problem drinkers: II. The Drinker's Check-Up as a preventative intervention. *Behavioural Psychotherapy, 16,* 251–268.

Moore, R. D., & Pearson, T. A. (1986). Moderate alcohol consumption and coronary artery disease: A review. *Medicine, 65,* 242–267.

Morgan, P., & Cohen, L. (1993). Controlled-drinking advocates challenge use of abstinence model in treatment of addiction. *Canadian Medical Association Journal, 149,* 706–713.

Morse, R. M., & Flavin, D. K. (1992). The definition of alcoholism: The Joint Committee of the National Council on Alcoholism and Drug Dependence and the American Society of Addiction Medicine to study the definition and criteria for the diagnosis of alcoholism. *Journal of the American Medical Association, 268,* 1012–1014.

Mosher, J. F. (1995). The merchants, not the customers: Resisting the alcohol and tobacco industries' strategy to blame young people for illegal alcohol and tobacco sales. *Journal of Public Health Policy, 16,* 412–432.

Moskowitz, J. M. (1989). The primary prevention of alcohol problems: A critical review of the research literature. *Journal of Studies on Alcohol, 50,* 54–88.

Musto, D. F. (1997). Alcohol control in historical perspective. In M. Plant, E. Single, & T. Stockwell (Eds.), *Alcohol: Minimising the harm—what works?* (pp. 10–25). London: Free Association Books.

National Clearinghouse for Alcohol and Drug Information (NCADI). (1995). *1993 National Household Survey on Drug Abuse* [On-line]. Available: http://www.health.org/mtf/index.htm

National Clearinghouse for Alcohol and Drug Information (NCADI). (1997). *1995 National Household Survey on Drug Abuse* [On-line]. Available: http://www.health.org/mtf/index.htm

National Highway Traffic Safety Administration (NHTSA). (1989). *The impact of minimum drinking age laws on fatal crash involvements: An update of the NHTSA analyses* (NHTSA Technical Report No. DOT-HS-807-349). Washington, DC: U.S. Department of Transportation.

National Highway Traffic Safety Administration (NHTSA). (1994). *FEARS.* Washington, DC: U.S. Department of Transportation.

National Highway Traffic Safety Administration (NHTSA) & National Institute on Alcohol Abuse and Alcoholism (NIAAA). (1996). *A guide to sentencing DUI offenders* (NHTSA & NIAAA Technical Report No. DOT-HS-808-365). Washington, DC: U.S. Department of Transportation.

National Institute on Alcohol Abuse and Alcoholism (NIAAA). (1993). *Eighth special report to the U.S. congress on alcohol and health.* Rockville, MD: U.S. Department of Health and Human Services.

National Institute on Alcohol Abuse and Alcoholism (NIAAA). (1997). *Ninth special report to the U.S. Congress on alcohol and health.* Rockville, MD: U.S. Department of Health and Human Services.

Nordstrom, G., & Berglund, M. (1987). Ageing and recovery from alcoholism. *British Journal of Psychiatry, 151,* 382–388.

O'Brien, C. P. (1993). Treatment of alcoholism as a chronic disorder. *Alcohol, 11*(6), 433–437.

O'Brien, C. P. (1996). Recent developments in the pharmacotherapy of substance abuse. *Journal of Consulting and Clinical Psychology, 64,* 677–686.

O'Brien, C. P. (1997). A range of research-based pharmacotherapies for addiction. *Science, 278,* 66–70.

Ogborne, A. C. (1987). A note on the characteristics of alcohol abusers with controlled drinking aspirations. *Drug and Alcohol Dependence, 19,* 159–164.

Ojehagen, A., & Berglund, M. (1989). Changes of drinking goals in a two-year out-patient alcoholic treatment program. *Addictive Behaviors, 14,* 1–9.

O'Malley, P. M., & Wagenaar, A. C. (1991). Effects of minimum drinking age laws on alcohol use, related behaviors and traffic crash involvement among American youth: 1976–1987. *Journal of Studies on Alcohol, 52,* 478–491.

O'Malley, S. S., Jaffe, A. J., Chang, G., Rode, S., Schottenfeld, R., Meyer, R., &

Rounsaville, B. (1992). Naltrexone and coping skills therapy for alcohol dependence: A controlled study. *Archives of General Psychiatry, 49,* 881–887.

O'Malley, S. S., Jaffe, A. J., Chang, G., Rode, S., Schottenfeld, R., Meyer, R., & Rounsaville, B. (1996). Six-month follow-up of naltrexone and psychotherapy for alcohol dependence. *Archives of General Psychiatry, 53,* 217–224.

Orford, J., & Keddie, A. (1986). Abstinence of controlled drinking in clinical practice: A test of the dependence and persuasion hypotheses. *British Journal of Addiction, 81,* 495–504.

Pachman, J. S., Foy, D. W., & Van Erd, M. (1978). Goal choice of alcoholics: A comparison of those who choose total abstinence vs. those who choose responsible, controlled drinking. *Journal of Clinical Psychology, 34,* 781–783.

Paille, F. M., Guelf, J. D., Perkins, A. C., Royer, R. J., Steru, L., & Parot, P. (1995). Double-blind randomized multicentre trial of acamprosate in maintaining abstinence from alcohol. *Alcohol and Alcoholism, 30,* 239–247.

Peele, S. (1992). Alcoholism, politics, and bureaucracy: The consensus against controlled-drinking therapy in America. *Addictive Behaviors, 17,* 49–62.

Peele, S. (1993). The conflict between public health goals and the temperance mentality. *American Journal of Public Health, 83,* 805–810.

Pendery, M. L., Maltzman, I. M., & West, L. J. (1982). Controlled drinking by alcoholics?: New findings and a reevaluation of a major affirmative study. *Science, 217,* 169–175.

Plant, M., Single, E., & Stockwell, T. (Eds.). (1997). *Alcohol: Minimising the harm—what works?* London: Free Association Books.

Polich, J. M., Armor, D. J., & Braiker, H. B. (Eds.). (1981). *The course of alcoholism: Four years after treatment.* New York: Wiley.

Prochaska, J. O., & DiClemente, C. C. (1983). Stages and processes of self-change of smoking: Toward an integrative model of change. *Journal of Consulting and Clinical Psychology, 51,* 390–395.

Project MATCH Research Group. (1997). Matching alcoholism treatments to client heterogeneity: Project MATCH posttreatment drinking outcomes. *Journal of Studies on Alcohol, 58,* 7–29.

Quigley, L. A., & Marlatt, G. A. (1996). Drinking among young adults: Prevalence, patterns, and consequences. *Alcohol Health and Research World, 20,* 185–191.

Razay, G., Heaton, K. W., Bolton, C. H., & Hughes, A. O. (1992). Alcohol consumption and its relation to cardiovascular risk factors in British women. *British Medical Journal, 304,* 80–83.

Rehm, J., & Fischer, B. (1997). Measuring harm: Implications for alcohol epidemiology. In M. Plant, E. Single, & T. Stockwell (Eds.), *Alcohol: Minimising the harm—what works?* (pp. 248–261). London: Free Association Books.

Rimm, E. B., Giovannucci, E. L., Willet, W. C., Colditz, G. A., Ascherio, A., Rosner, B., & Stampfer, M. J. (1991). Prospective study of alcohol consumption and risk of coronary disease in men. *Lancet, 338,* 464–468.

Rimm, E. B., Klatsky, A., Grobbee, D., & Stampfer, M. J. (1996). Review of moderate alcohol consumption and reduced risk of coronary heart disease: Is the effect due to beer, wine, or spirits? *British Medical Journal, 312,* 731–736.

Rosenberg, H. (1993). Prediction of controlled drinking by alcoholics and problem drinkers. *Psychological Bulletin, 113,* 129–139.

Rychtarik, R. G., Foy, D. W., Scott, T., Lokey, L., & Prue, D. M. (1987). 5–6 year follow-up of broad-spectrum behavioral treatment for alcoholism: Effects of training controlled drinking skills. *Journal of Consulting and Clinical Psychology, 55*, 106–108.

Ryder, D. (1996). Shades of gray: Some observations on Sobell & Sobell's "Controlled drinking after 25 years: How important was the great debate?" *Addiction, 91*, 603–604.

Saltz, R. F. (1997). Prevention where alcohol is sold and consumed: Server intervention and responsible beverage service. In M. Plant, E. Single, & T. Stockwell (Eds.), *Alcohol: Minimising the harm—what works?* (pp. 72–84). London: Free Association Books.

Sanchez-Craig, M., Annis, H. M., Bornet, A. R., & MacDonald, K. R. (1984). Random assignment to abstinence and controlled drinking: Evaluation of a cognitive-behavioral program for problem drinkers. *Journal of Consulting and Clinical Psychology, 52*, 390–403.

Sanchez-Craig, M., & Lei, H. (1986). Disadvantages to imposing the goal of abstinence on problem drinkers: An empirical study. *British Journal of Addiction, 81*, 505–512.

Sanchez-Craig, M., Spivak, K., & Davila, R. (1991). Superior outcome of females over males after brief treatment for the reduction of heavy drinking: Replication and report of therapist effects. *British Journal of Addiction, 86*, 867–876.

Sanchez-Craig, M., Wilkinson, D. A., & Davila, R. (1995). Empirically based guidelines for moderate drinking: 1-year results from three studies with problem drinkers. *American Journal of Public Health, 85*, 823–828.

Sandahl, C., & Ronnberg, S. (1990). Brief group psychotherapy in relapse prevention for alcohol dependent patients. *International Journal of Group Psychotherapy, 40*, 453–476.

Sass, H., Soyka, M., Mann, K., & Zieglgansberger, W. (1996). Relapse prevention by acamprosate. *Archives of General Psychiatry, 53*, 673–680.

Schuckit, M. A. (1996). Recent developments in the pharmacotherapy of alcohol dependence. *Journal of Consulting and Clinical Psychology, 64*, 669–676.

Scribner, R. A., MacKinnon, D. P., & Dwyer, J. H. (1994). Alcohol outlet density and motor vehicle crashes in Los Angeles County cities. *Journal of Studies on Alcohol, 55*, 447–453.

Shaper, A. G. (1993). Alcohol, the heart, and health. *American Journal of Public Health, 83*, 799–801.

Shore, E. R., Gregory, T., & Tatlock, L. (1991). College students' reactions to a designated driver program: An exploratory study. *Journal of Alcohol and Drug Education, 37*, 1–6.

Singh, M. (1991). Alcoholic pancreatitis. *International Journal of Pancreatology, 8*, 111–118.

Single, E. (1996). Harm reduction as an alcohol-prevention strategy. *Alcohol Health and Research World, 20*, 239–243.

Sitharthan, T., Kavanagh, D. J., & Sayer, G. (1996). Moderating drinking by correspondence: An evaluation of a new method of intervention. *Addiction, 91*, 345–355.

Skinner, H. A. (1988). *Executive summary: Spectrum of drinkers and intervention responses* (Report prepared for the Institute of Medicine Committee for the Study of Treatment and Rehabilitation Services for Alcohol and Alcohol Abuse). Washington, DC: National Academy of Sciences.

Skinner, H. A. (1994). *Computerized lifestyle assessment.* New York: Multi-Health Systems.

Skinner, H. A., & Horn, J. L. (1984). *Alcohol Dependence Scale: User's guide.* Toronto: Addiction Research Foundation.

Skutle, A., & Borg, G. (1987). Training in controlled drinking for early-stage problem drinkers. *British Journal of Addiction, 82,* 493–501.

Sobell, L. C., Cunningham, J. A., Sobell, M. B., Agrawal, S., Gavin, D. R., Leo, G. I., & Singh, K. N. (1996). Fostering self-change among problem drinkers: A proactive community intervention. *Addictive Behaviors, 21,* 817–833.

Sobell, M. B., & Sobell, L. C. (1973). Alcoholics treated by individualized behaviour therapy: One year treatment outcome. *Behaviour Research and Therapy, 11,* 599–618.

Sobell, M. B., & Sobell, L. C. (1976). Second year treatment outcome of alcoholics treated by individualized behavior therapy: Results. *Behaviour Research and Therapy, 14,* 195–215.

Sobell, M. B., & Sobell, L. C. (1978). Evaluating the external validity of Ewing and Rouse. *British Journal of Addiction, 73,* 343–345.

Sobell, M. B., & Sobell, L. C. (1989). Moratorium on Maltzman: An appeal to reason. *Journal of Studies on Alcohol, 50,* 473–480.

Sobell, M. B., & Sobell, L. C. (1993). *Problem drinkers: Guided self-change treatment.* New York: Guilford Press.

Sobell, M. B., & Sobell, L. C. (1995). Controlled drinking after 25 years: How important was the great debate? [Editorial]. *Addiction, 90,* 1149–1154.

Stampfer, M. J., Colditz, G. A., Willett, W. C., Speizer, F. E., & Hennekens, C. H. (1988). A prospective study of moderate alcohol consumption and the risk of coronary disease and stroke in women. *New England Journal of Medicine, 319,* 267–273.

Stampfer, M. J., Rimm, E. B., & Walsh, D. C. (1993). Commentary: Alcohol, the heart, and public policy. *American Journal of Public Health, 83,* 801–804.

Stockwell, T., Murphy, D., & Hodgson, R. (1983). The Severity of Alcohol Dependence Questionnaire: Its use, reliability, and validity. *British Journal of Addiction, 78*(2), 145–155.

Stockwell, T., Sitharthan, T., McGrath, D., & Lang, E. (1994). The measurement of alcohol dependence and impaired control in community samples. *Addiction, 89,* 167–174.

Tollefson, G. D., Montague-Clouse, J., & Tollefson, S. L. (1992). Treatment of comorbid generalized anxiety in a recently detoxified alcoholic population with a selective serotonergic drug (buspirone). *Journal of Clinical Psychopharmacology, 12,* 19–26.

Toomey, T. L., Rosenfeld, C., & Wagenaar, A. C. (1996). The minimum legal drinking age: History, effectiveness, and ongoing debate. *Alcohol Health and Research World, 20,* 213–218.

Trachtenberg, R. L. (1984). *Report of the steering group to the administrator, Alcohol, Drug Abuse and Mental Health Administration, regarding its attempts to investigate allegations of scientific misconduct concerning Drs. Mark and Linda Sobell.* Rockville, MD: Alcohol, Drug Abuse, and Mental Health Administration.

Tuyns, A. J. (1990). Alcohol and cancer. *Proceedings of the Nutrition Society, 49,* 145–151.

Vaillant, G. (1996). A long-term follow-up of male alcohol abuse. *Archives of General Psychiatry, 53,* 243–249.

Vaillant, G. E., & Milofsky, E. S. (1982). Natural history of male alcoholism: IV. Paths to recovery. *Archives of General Psychiatry, 39,* 127–133.

Voas, R. B., & Lacey, J. H. (1989). Issues in the enforcement of impaired driving laws in the United States. In *The Surgeon General's workshop on drunk driving* (pp. 136–156). Rockville, MD: U.S. Department of Health and Human Services.

Volpicelli, J. R., Alterman, A. I., Hayashida, M., & O'Brien, C. P. (1992). Naltrexone in the treatment of alcohol dependence. *Archives of General Psychiatry, 49,* 876–880.

Volpicelli, J. R., Clay, K. L., Watson, N. T., & Volpicelli, L. A. (1994). Naltrexone and the treatment of alcohol dependence. *Alcohol Health and Research World, 18,* 272–278.

Wagenaar, A. C. (1983). Drinking and driving: New directions. *Journal of Psychiatric Treatment and Evaluation, 5,* 539–544.

Wagenaar, A. C., & Holder, H. D. (1991). Effects of alcoholic beverage server liability on traffic crash injuries. *Alcoholism: Clinical and Experimental Research, 15,* 942–947.

Wagenaar, A. C., & Holder, H. D. (1995). Changes in alcohol consumption resulting from the elimination of retail wine monopolies: Results from five U.S. states. *Journal of Studies on Alcohol, 56,* 566–572.

Wagenaar, A. C., & Langley, J. D. (1995). Alcohol licensing system changes and alcohol consumption: Introduction of wine into New Zealand grocery stores. *Addiction, 90,* 773–783.

Wagenaar, A. C., Toomey, T. L., Murray, D. M., Short, B. J., Wolfson, M., & Jones, W. R. (1996). Sources of alcohol for underage drinkers. *Journal of Studies on Alcohol, 57,* 325–333.

Wagenaar, A. C., & Wolfson, M. (1994). Enforcement of the legal minimum drinking age in the United States. *Journal of Public Health Policy, 15,* 37–53.

Wechsler, H., & Isaac, N. (1992). "Binge" drinkers at Massachusetts colleges. Prevalence, drinking style, time trends, and associated problems. *Journal of the American Medical Association, 267,* 2929–2931.

Wells, P. E., Bangert, D. R., McMillen, R., & Williams, R. (1995). Final results from a meta-analysis of remedial interventions with drink/drive offenders. *Addiction, 90,* 907–926.

Wells, J. K., Greene, M. A., Foss, R. D., Ferguson, S. A., & Williams, A. F. (1997). Drinking drivers missed at sobriety checkpoints. *Journal of Studies on Alcohol, 58,* 513–517.

White, H. R., & Labouvie, E. W. (1989). Towards the assessment of adolescent drinking. *Journal of Studies on Alcohol, 50,* 30–37.

Wittman, F. D. (1997). Local control to prevent problems of alcohol availability: Experience in California communities. In M. Plant, E. Single, & T. Stockwell (Eds.), *Alcohol: Minimising the harm—what works?* (pp. 43–71). London: Free Association Books.

World Health Organization (WHO) Brief Intervention Study Group. (1996). A cross-national trial of brief interventions with heavy drinkers. *American Journal of Public Health, 86,* 948–955.

CHAPTER FIVE

Harm Reduction, Nicotine, and Smoking

JOHN S. BAER
HEATHER BRADY MURCH

OVERVIEW

A commonly used analogy still has dramatic effect. Imagine two jumbo jets colliding in midair, killing all aboard. One thousand people die in the disaster. Such an incident would no doubt result in bold headlines throughout the country, if not the world. Imagine further that the same accident occurs again the following day, and again the day after that. What would be the public and governmental response to such loss of life? How many days would this pattern continue before all flights were grounded? What kind of inquiries about the safety of innocent passengers would ensue? Would it make a difference if the individuals dying in these planes were not young, but rather in their sixth and seventh decades of life? The answer to this thought exercise is obvious: No society concerned about public health would ever allow such a pattern to continue. Yet these are the numbers of individuals who lose their lives prematurely each day, in the United States alone, because of the health consequences of smoking. Few question that the societal harm associated with nicotine addiction and smoking exceeds that of all other drugs of abuse combined.

Yet the public and governmental response to smoking in the United States has been almost as ambivalent as the response to alcohol. Tobacco is a legal commodity and an extremely profitable business as well. Tobacco farmers have received federal farm subsidies for decades, and tobacco companies spend enormous sums advertising their products. Tobacco companies argue that smoking is a lifestyle choice, that nicotine is not addicting,

122

and that there is little proof that smoking causes life-threatening disease. Tobacco companies invoke the U.S. Constitution's Bill of Rights to suggest that individuals have a right to choose to smoke. Yet other arms of the government, as well as essentially all of the scientific health community, acknowledge smoking as the single greatest cause of preventable death in the United States (U.S. Department of Health and Human Services [DHHS], 1994). Public health efforts to reduce the prevalence of smoking are extensive and date back over 30 years. The content of the public health message can be summarized fairly briefly: "If you smoke, stop. If you don't smoke, don't start."

Although literally millions of individuals have stopped smoking, efforts to prevent it and to treat its effects have been only partially successful. The profound harm associated with smoking and other tobacco use has prompted many to question whether there are ways in which this harm might be reduced. In this chapter, we explore selectively how harm reduction approaches can be applied to the addictive use of nicotine, with a primary focus on smoking. We do not attempt to review all possible interventions; rather, we discuss both the potential advantages and risks of harm reduction strategies.

A Brief History of Tobacco Use in the United States

Tobacco was first introduced to Western cultures in the 16th century as a medicinal herb. Reportedly, Columbus observed Indians smoking in the New World. Tobacco was cultivated in Portugal by 1558 (Vogt, 1982). Although the new substance was popular, until the 19th century tobacco was most frequently chewed or smoked in pipes or as cigars. In 1884 cigarettes were first mass-produced, and within 40 years (the 1920s), cigarette smoking had overtaken pipes, cigars, and chewing as the most common form of tobacco use (Ray, 1983). Cigarette smoking reached its peak popularity in the early 1960s, with over 40% of the U.S. adult population smoking regularly. Rates of smoking have declined, albeit unevenly, over the past 30 years. In the mid-1990s, roughly a quarter (25%) of the adult population smoked cigarettes regularly (U.S. DHHS, 1994). Other tobacco products have been popularized in recent years as well. For example, between 1970 and 1985, the percentage of the male U.S. population over age 12 using smokeless tobacco products (i.e., snuff and chewing tobacco) rose from 1% to 12% (Adams, Gfroerer, & Rouse, 1989; U.S. DHHS, 1986).

The use of tobacco products begins at a young age. Although it is illegal in the United States for persons under the age of 18 to purchase tobacco, nearly 90% of current smokers report that they began smoking as minors (U.S. DHHS, 1988, 1994), with the average age for having first tried a cigarette being 14.5 years. The average age for becoming a daily smoker is 17.7 years (Breslau, 1993; Elders, Perry, Eriksen, & Giovino,

). The pattern for smokeless tobacco initiation is similar to that for cigarettes (Elders et al., 1994). When the tobacco use rates (for both smoking and smokeless tobacco use) of high school seniors and high school dropouts are combined, the prevalence rate reaches about 25% (Boyd & Darby, 1989; Johnston, O'Malley, & Bachman, 1991; Pirie, Murray, & Luepker, 1988); this is roughly consistent with that of older adult populations (26%; U.S. DHHS, 1994).

Health Implications of Tobacco Use

The first scientific paper on the relationship between cigarette smoking and lung cancer was published in 1950 (Doll & Hill, 1950). The clear and convincing evidence accumulated until 1964, when the first U.S. Surgeon General's report on smoking and health was issued (U.S. Department of Health, Education and Welfare, 1964). At this time smoking was publicly linked to cancer and heart disease, and the U.S. population was encouraged to stop.

In the years following the 1964 report, evidence has continued to accumulate that smoking and the use of smokeless tobacco products cause a variety of negative, often deadly physical consequences. In the United States, about 400,000 people die each year from smoking-related ailments (Klesges & DeBon, 1994; Russell, 1993). These include lung, oral, and esophageal cancer; coronary heart disease, atherosclerotic peripheral vascular disease, and stroke; emphysema; and decreases in the effectiveness of the immune system (Fielding, 1985; U.S. DHHS, 1989). The use of smokeless tobacco is correlated with oral cancer, leukoplakia, gingival recession, destruction of periodontal bone and soft tissue, and tooth abrasion (Hatsukami, Nelson, & Jensen, 1991). In women, smoking increases the risk of infertility, ectopic pregnancy, and miscarriage (Campbell & Gray, 1987). Women who smoke have higher rates of abnormal Pap smears, cervical cancer, and pelvic inflammatory disease (Schols, Daling, & Stergachis, 1992). More recent data associate "passive" or "involuntary" smoking (i.e., inhaling secondhand smoke) with respiratory diseases in healthy nonsmokers (U.S. Environmental Protection Agency [EPA], 1992; U.S. DHHS, 1986), especially children of smokers (Burchfiel et al., 1986). Babies of smokers have a higher chance of having low birth weight (Hebel, Fox, & Sexton, 1988) and of dying from sudden infant death syndrome (Hoffman, Damus, Hillman, & Krongrad, 1988; Kleinman, Pierre, Madans, Lamd, & Schramm, 1988). It is estimated that an additional 4,000 people die each year from the effects of secondhand or passive smoke.

Nicotine as an Addictive Substance

It is commonly acknowledged that tobacco users have difficulty quitting once they have begun regular use. An extensive scientific literature indicates that nicotine is the drug in tobacco products that causes addiction (Henningfield, Cohen, & Slade, 1991; U.S. DHHS, 1988). Nicotine differs from most other drugs of abuse, in that its effects are subtle. Unlike alcohol and many other drugs, nicotine does not bring on violent or disruptive behavior, cause "blackouts" or memory loss, or physically or emotionally impair its users (Russell, 1993). Individuals can use this drug throughout the day, relatively wherever and whenever they so choose, without fear of directly diminishing their performance or facing legal consequences. Yet individuals also use nicotine systematically, feel poorly when nicotine is unavailable, develop tolerance, use the substance compulsively, and have considerable difficulty stopping its use. In short, any definition of "addictive behavior" applies quite well to the systematic use of nicotine (U.S. DHHS, 1988).

With the release of the U.S. Surgeon General's 1988 report on nicotine addiction, it has been more widely accepted that nicotine is a highly addictive substance (Henningfield, Cohen, & Slade, 1991; U.S. DHHS, 1988). The 1988 report concluded that "the pharmacologic and behavioral processes that determine tobacco addiction are similar to those that determine addiction to drugs such as heroin and cocaine" (U.S. DHHS, 1988, p. 9). Indeed, the proportion of individuals who go on from initial exposure to addictive use is higher for nicotine than for any other substance (Anthony, Warner, & Kessler, 1994). Although smoking is the most common pathway to nicotine addiction, most smokeless tobacco products contain nicotine amounts that far exceed those contained in cigarettes (Russell, Jarvis, Devitt, & Feyerabend, 1981; U.S. DHHS, 1988). Acquisition of addictive patterns of nicotine use can be rapid. About 90% of children who smoke more than three or four cigarettes go on to become regular smokers, and teenagers who smoke regularly report withdrawal symptoms similar to those of adults when they attempt to quit (McNeill, West, Jarvis, Jackson, & Bryant, 1986; Russell, 1990).

HARM REDUCTION AND SMOKING: CONCEPTUAL ISSUES

In spite of the efforts in the past several decades to reduce tobacco use in the United States, a decline of only about 16% has been achieved since 1965 (U.S. DHHS, 1994; U.S. Department of Health, Education and Welfare, 1964). There is disagreement among tobacco researchers and policy experts in the interpretation of this sobering reality. Some feel that efforts to motivate and assist individuals to stop smoking have not been sufficient; essentially, those taking this view feel that we need more money and more programs aimed at smoking cessation. Others feel that the current policies of supporting cessation have been successful with those individuals who are able and willing to quit; they contend that other policy approaches and clinical strategies are needed to minimize harm for those still smoking.

A national conference, "Smoking Cessation: Alternative Strategies," sponsored by the Johns Hopkins School of Medicine and the Society for Research on Nicotine and Tobacco, was convened in 1994 to consider "alternative" (i.e., harm-reductive) approaches to tobacco use. The conference challenged tobacco researchers and policy makers to consider harm reduction as one approach for the promotion of public health in the area of smoking and tobacco use. It is noteworthy that conference participants were by no means in uniform agreement on the utility of harm reduction approaches. Concerns and the need for future research are noted below. The application of harm reduction to nicotine addiction and tobacco use has been described in recent publications, most notably by Kozlowski (1989; Kozlowski & Herman, 1984), Russell (1990, 1993), Hughes (1995), and Benowitz (1995); the 1995 publications are from the national conference on treatment alternatives.

Because most nicotine use is legal, applications of harm reduction principles in this area differ somewhat from applications to illicit drug use. First, as described by Reuter and MacCoun (1995), the harm due to tobacco use is not the consequence of policy or prohibition (as with illicit drugs), but rather is a consequence of use of the substance itself. Second, the harm due to tobacco use develops for the users themselves, for the most part. Although secondhand smoke does result in health implications, such effects are relatively small. As a result, users of tobacco do not generally compromise the well-being of their families through addictive behavior. Third, there are few direct adverse behavioral effects of smoking or other tobacco use. In contrast to most illicit drugs, nicotine can be used in the course of normal human functioning. Harm accrues in the forms of economic hardship from treating disease and shortened lifespan. This state of affairs contrasts with that for illicit drugs, to be discussed in Chapter 6.

Any discussion of harm reduction and smoking in particular also necessitates an understanding of basic relationships between health, harm, and smoking behavior. Some would argue that smoking causes no harm, and hence there is nothing to reduce! We feel that the data presented above, many of which have now been available for the past 50 years, argue convincingly to the contrary. Yet an analysis of harm reduction and smoking requires understanding of mechanisms of how specific toxins create health problems, how substances are used, and whether changes in patterns of use of the substances or in the substances themselves will significantly alter harm for people.

For example, we have noted above that nicotine is the addictive agent in tobacco products. Yet it is not the nicotine in cigarettes that causes most of the health problems associated with smoking. Acute dosing of nicotine increases heart rate, blood pressure, and myocardial work, and is likely to aggravate preexisting coronary problems (Benowitz, 1995). Yet there are few data to date suggesting that long-term, low doses of nicotine (like those used in nicotine replacement therapy) lead to cardiovascular problems (Benowitz, 1995). In contrast, the majority of serious ailments experienced by smokers (and passive smokers) are caused by tars, carbon monoxide, and other additives and by-products of cigarettes. Thus, reductions in the use of cigarettes will only be harm-reducing to the extent that they are accompanied by reductions in the consumption of tars and carbon monoxide.

Dose–response relationships are also critical. For example, a 50% reduction in the consumption of tars may not be harm-reducing if a minimal threshold of tar exposure is responsible for health risks. It is the case, for example, that a near-linear dose–response relationship does exist between rates of smoking and lung cancer. Hence, reductions in the rate of cigarette smoking should produce health benefits on average. Compensatory processes must also be assessed, however, for any evaluation of harm reduction strategies. For example, reduced nicotine in cigarettes routinely produces deeper inhalation by smokers. Such deeper inhalation may actually increase exposure to tars, and hence may paradoxically increase health risks.

Below, we review several different strategies for harm reduction from the use of tobacco products, especially cigarettes. Some strategies, such as making cigarettes less available, are currently being utilized and are generally not controversial. Other strategies, such as providing cigarettes that deliver nicotine more safely, have not been accepted and are much more controversial. Still other approaches, such as nicotine replacement, are widely accepted but generally not appreciated as potential harm-reductive interventions. We feel encouraged that the harm due to smoking and other tobacco use can be reduced, but we have much left to learn. Ultimately, research can help us understand which strategies are most likely to benefit most individuals.

HARM REDUCTION STRATEGIES

Harm reduction strategies for smoking and other use of tobacco products can be categorized in several ways. From a quite general perspective, any strategy that reduces tobacco use, such as smoking prevention and cessation, is consistent with a harm reduction approach. This model is exemplified in the analysis of Russell (1993), where four general approaches to reduce smoking-related harm are proposed: reducing recruitment of new smokers, increasing cessation, reducing the risks of active smoking, and reducing secondhand smoke. Although we agree with Russell's assessment, we choose to emphasize and explore how a harm reduction approach results in new or overlooked behavioral and policy interventions.

Smoking cessation programs have a long history in behavioral science, and have been reviewed comprehensively (see Shiffman, 1993). Prevention programs similarly have received considerable attention from both researchers and policy advocates (Bruvold, 1993; Elder et al., 1993; Glynn, 1993). Both prevention and cessation programs have shown modest but nevertheless limited successes. A harm reduction approach, however, offers more unusual and creative strategies, particularly when one assumes that many individuals will use the substance, that not all are willing or ready to quit, and that the health and well-being of those who do use can be improved with behavioral or policy initiatives. In our discussion of nicotine use, we describe four general areas of potential change: (1) restricting access (including advertising and taxation), (2) altering how people use nicotine, (3) changing the nature of consumer products that contain nicotine, and (4) replacing nicotine. Although we discuss these areas of intervention separately, there is no reason why they cannot be combined in a multidimensional harm reduction effort.

Limiting Access

Access to tobacco products, as a general concept, includes issues of physical availability, cost, and marketing. In general, although the use of tobacco products follows an addictive pattern, it is quite elastic with respect to changes in access (Grossman, 1989). As reviewed briefly above, the initiation of smoking occurs almost exclusively among adolescents. Efforts to affect access to nicotine products tend to emphasize youth, although restricting access benefits individuals beyond adolescence.

First, making cigarettes more expensive reduces consumption. As an example, Hu, Sung, and Keeler (1995) recently estimated that a 25% state tax increase in California resulted in a 2-year reduction of 819 million packages of cigarettes sold. Thus taxation and other price controls seem to be likely targets for campaigns to promote public health (and to reduce harm; Cummings, Pechacek, & Shopland, 1994; Elders et al., 1994). It is noteworthy that excise taxes on cigarettes have not kept pace with inflation in the general U.S. economy (Lewit, 1989): Economic analyses indicate that cigarettes, relative to standard wages and prices, were in fact cheaper in the 1980s than they were in the 1950s. Effects of cost on rates of use seem to be greatest among younger smokers (Lewit, 1989).

A study in Canada found that a 10% increase in the price of cigarettes resulted in a 14% decline in the prevalence of smoking by 15- through 19-year-olds (Ferrence, Garcia, Sykora, Collishaw, & Farinon, 1992). Although increases in taxation have their greatest impact on initiation (hence the effects on adolescent rates of smoking), reductions in the rates of use among continuing smokers are also observed (Townsend, 1993). Given linear relationships between rates of consumption and health consequences, significant public harm reduction can be achieved through increased prices. Grossman (1989) has estimated that, for the cohort of Americans 12 years and older in 1984, over 800,000 premature deaths could have been averted in the United States if federal excise taxes on cigarettes had remained at the levels established in 1951.

Physical availability is another aspect of product access. Although tobacco products are only legally sold to those aged 18 or older, it is clear that minors do not have much difficulty obtaining them (Cummings et al., 1994). Studies have shown that when the laws pertaining to sales of tobacco products to minors are better enforced, the sales can be considerably reduced (Cummings & Coogan, 1992; Feighary, Altman, & Shaffer, 1991; U.S. DHHS, 1992). In addition, there is also evidence that enforced restrictions on the sales of tobacco products to minors can actually lower the prevalence of smoking among adolescents (DiFranza, Carlson, & Caisee, 1992; Jason, Ji, Anes, & Birkhead, 1991).

The United States has actually made some significant efforts in this regard during the 1990s. In 1992 the U.S. Congress passed an amendment to the Alcohol, Drug Abuse and Mental Health Administration Reorganization Act, intended to discourage the use of tobacco by adolescents. Called the Synar Amendment, it requires that as a condition of receiving grant funds for substance abuse prevention and treatment, states must enact and enforce a law prohibiting the sale or distribution of tobacco products to anyone under the age of 18 (Federal Register, 1996). The states are required to conduct random, unannounced inspections of places where tobacco is sold, and to submit a report each year detailing these activities. If a state fails to put forth a reasonable effort to enforce the restrictions, it will lose a percentage of the grant funds for the next year.

The use of nicotine can also be affected by limiting the contexts or environments where smoking is acceptable. The last several years have seen a host of restrictions on public smoking, most stemming from efforts to restrict secondhand smoke. Smoking is now commonly restricted in work sites, public buildings, and many businesses (e.g., restaurants). Studies of environmental restrictions suggest health benefits by way of rate reductions. Kinne, Kristal, White, and Hunt (1993) conducted a large survey of smokers concerning restrictions on smoking in work sites. About half (48% of men and 53% of women) reported reduced smoking rates on working days as a result of such restrictions. In fact, male survey respondents who worked in sites with smoking restrictions reported reduced smoking on nonworking days as well.

The advertising practices of the tobacco industry have been widely criticized. Although the industry argues that advertising efforts are intended solely to create brand loyalty, considerable data indicates the contrary. Pierce and Gilpin (1995), via a historical analysis, demonstrated increases in smoking rates among specific subgroups (women, youth) coincident with marketing campaigns directed at the same subgroups. Smoking increased only in young males prior to 1890, when marketing focused solely on males. Initiation of smoking by women increased markedly in the 1920s with the introduction of women's marketing campaigns. Similar patterns of increased consumption were observed when women were targeted by a new wave of advertisements in the late 1960s.

Considerable concern has been raised recently about the targeting of adolescents in marketing campaigns. The tobacco industry obviously realizes that adolescents make up the majority of its new consumers (Fischer, Schwartz, Richards, Goldstein, & Rojas, 1991; Pierce et al., 1991). For example, young people report familiarity with cigarette advertisements as early as age 6 (Fischer et al., 1991; George H. Gallup International Institute, 1992). Following the introduction of advertisements that appeal to young people, such as campaigns featuring cartoon characters, the prevalence of the use of those brands increases (DiFranza, Richards, & Paulman, 1991; Pierce et al., 1991; Tye, Warner, & Glantz, 1987). Efforts to restrict the amount and content of cigarette marketing are consistent with a harm reduction approach.

Despite much public attention to advertising and health education, it is worth emphasizing again that access to and availability of tobacco products are potent options for harm reduction. A comparative analysis of taxation and antismoking media message in California suggests a considerably larger impact of taxation (Hu et al., 1995). Most commentators advocate a multidimensional effort for greater regulation of tobacco products (Kessler, 1995; Kaplan, Orleans, Perkins, & Pierce, 1995). Limiting the advertising of tobacco products, aiming the focus of such advertising away from children, increasing prices, and restricting physical availability are likely to result in less smoking and thus in the promotion of public health (Madden & Grube, 1994; Kessler, 1995).

Changing Tobacco Use Practices to Reduce Harm

Tobacco use is often incorporated into many aspects of a user's daily life, and the thought of giving up the habit completely can be an overwhelming possibility. Many users find the thought of reducing the amount they use a more attainable goal; their eventual aim may be either cessation or permanent reduction. We are unaware of any evidence to support a "safe" level of tobacco use (Russell, 1993). The amount of tobacco one takes in is directly related to the amount of damage caused, even at very low levels (Hill, Weiss, Walker, & Jolley, 1988). Thus, any smoking or other tobacco use is dangerous, but reduced use may provide some health benefits.

Russell (1993) notes the long history of thought about reducing the harm associated with smoking as a function of methods or patterns of use. As early as 1962, the Royal College of Physicians (quoted in Russell, 1993, pp. 160–161) recommended "leaving longer butts, and switching to safer forms of smoking such as pipes and cigars." A second report in 1971 further recommended that individuals "[smoke] fewer cigarettes, inhale less, smoke less of each cigarette, take fewer puffs from each cigarette, take the cigarette out of the mouth between puffs and . . . smoke brands with low nicotine and tar content" (p. 161). Such efforts are typically assumed to be unsuccessful in the face of compensatory behaviors by smokers.

Studies on "controlled smoking" have revealed that there are generally two groups of individuals who smoke at low rates: those who have always smoked a small amount (fewer than 10 cigarettes a day), often referred to as "chippers" (Shiffman, 1989); and those who have cut down from a higher-risk level of smoking. Benowitz, Jacob, Kozlowski, and Yu (1986) found that physical dependence symptoms are generally not maintained with fewer than 10 cigarettes a day. Those individuals who have regularly used tobacco (a maximum of 5 cigarettes a day for at least 4 days a week) without developing dependence do inhale smoke and are exposed to nicotine, but show no signs of nicotine withdrawal when abstinent. They are less likely to smoke for affective or pharmacological reasons, and they report less stress, better coping, and more social support than dependent smokers (Shiffman, 1989). Unfortunately, current research suggests that these "chippers" are not necessarily consciously controlling smoking; rather, they may constitute a completely separate category of smokers who are somehow "protected" from dependence by a variety of lifestyle factors (Shiffman, 1989).

The success of controlled smoking in already dependent smokers who have chosen reduced smoking as their goal has been examined in only a few studies. Many smokers typically reach a "stuck point" of about 12–14 cigarettes a day (Levinson, Shapiro, Schwartz, & Tursky, 1971; Shapiro, Tursky, Schwartz, & Shnidman, 1971), which may be due to increasing difficulty in maintaining blood nicotine levels. Perhaps frustrated by high relapse rates in smoking cessation program, some researchers began to document significant rate reductions among those who do not achieve cessation, and questioned whether controlled smoking might be a beneficial option for those unwilling or unable to quit (Colletti, Supnick, & Rizzo, 1982). Controlled-smoking interventions, when tested, were quite success-ful in documenting that reductions in the rates of smoking, proportion of each cigarette smoked, and level of nicotine in cigarettes could be achieved with behavioral interventions (Glasgow, Klesges, Godding, & Gegelman, 1983; Glasgow, Klesges, & Vasey, 1983). In fact, at least one long-term follow-up indicated that rate and nicotine reductions were generally main-tained as long as 30 months after treatment (Glasgow, Klesges, Klesges, Vasey, & Gunnarson, 1985).

As noted by Glasgow, Morray, and Lichetenstein (1989), these con-trolled smoking interventions have been criticized on several fronts. The first criticism pertains to the questionable health benefits of smoking reduction in the face of compensatory behaviors. The health benefits achieved may be quite small. Rate reductions are also thought to be difficult to maintain. The most serious concern, of course, is that individuals who attempt controlled smoking will be unlikely to try to quit in the future, because they have "achieved their goals." Hence, the option with the most potent health benefits (quitting) may be undermined by a controlled-smoking intervention.

Glasgow et al. (1989) designed a study to examine these concerns directly. The study randomly assigned smokers to two different treatment programs—a traditional abstinence-based program and one that offered a controlled-smoking option. Results of this study are well stated in the title of the article, "Controlled Smoking versus Abstinence as a Treatment Goal: The Hopes and Fears May Be Unfounded." Essentially, there were no differences between these two treatment groups. There was no evidence that the controlled-smoking option caused fewer individuals to attempt cessation, thus allaying fears that controlled-smoking goals would undermine cessation attempts. On the other hand, there was no evidence that the controlled-smoking option led to greater reductions in smoking rates than those achieved in the traditional cessation-oriented program. The long-term reduction in smoking was no different at a 1-year follow-up for those with controlled smoking as their goal than for those with abstinence as the stated goal (see also Hill et al., 1988).

Glasgow's group's results are quite consistent with data from our own research, where we compared smoking cessation programs that were strongly abstinence-based with ones that were based on learning principles and relapse prevention (Curry, Marlatt, Gordon, & Baer, 1988). The learning-based program resulted in *lower* initial quit rates, but *more* quit attempts after relapses; a 1-year follow-up revealed few differences between the groups. What remains untested, of course, is whether harm reduction programs such as controlled-smoking programs create a lower threshold for involvement in services. That is, do such programs attract individuals who would otherwise avoid all services?

Changing the Nature of Products Containing Nicotine

Efforts to minimize smoking-related health harm via product changes have a long history. In fact, the introduction of filters and changes in tobacco pressing significantly reduced the delivery of tar in cigarettes in the 1950s (Russell, 1993). Peto (1986, cited in Russell, 1993) has suggested that these changes in the 1950s may have reduced lung cancer risk by half. As is typical in discussion of harm reduction efforts, however, Slade (1992) has expressed a contrary view—in this case, that the promotion of less toxic filtered cigarettes in the 1950s helped to sustain the prevalence of smoking and perpetuated public health problems. Of course, understanding the potential tradeoffs of product changes is essential for the evaluation of harm reduction programs (see "Summary and Limitations," below). The introduction of filters for cigarettes is but the first example of this basic conflict.

Reducing Tars and Nicotine in Cigarettes

In the past 30 years, efforts have been focused on reducing the tar and nicotine yield in cigarettes, primarily via ventilated filters. The notion seems fairly straightforward: If toxins in cigarettes create health hazards, reduce the toxins; if nicotine causes compulsive use, reduce the nicotine. Benowitz and Henningfield (1994), have suggested that the nicotine content of cigarettes be regulated to minimize addictiveness. They suggest that allowing 0.4 to 0.5 mg of nicotine per cigarette would be adequate to limit the development of addiction in most adolescents, while still providing enough nicotine for taste and sensory stimulation. Such limits are based on bioavailability of cigarettes, so that differences in style of smoking could not result in sufficient nicotine delivery for addictive patterns of use.

There are two common criticisms of this proposal. The first pertains to compensatory behaviors noted among smokers when they switch to lower-nicotine-yield cigarettes. Smokers using low-nicotine cigarettes have been shown to increase their rate of smoking, to take more puffs per cigarette, to inhale more deeply, and (most importantly) to block the filter vents in the cigarettes (Kozlowski, Rickert, Pope, Robinson, & Frecker, 1982). In a worst-case example, exposure to tars and carbon monoxide may actually be increased when smokers "oversmoke" in attempting to deliver nicotine from low-yield cigarettes. Hence, the health benefits of low-yield cigarettes are routinely questioned.

Some data exist to address this concern. The Benowitz and Henningfield (1994) proposal would make mandatory what is currently represented by a small portion of the cigarette market. Many different brands of cigarettes are available, and these brands vary widely in the amounts of nicotine (from 0.1 mg to 1.7 mg or more per cigarette) and other harmful substances that they contain. As reviewed by Hughes (1995), direct evidence of health benefits from the use of low-tar/low-nicotine cigarettes is limited. There are no data showing that those who smoke lower-yield brands are at less risk of illness. Hughes (1995) also notes, however, that compensatory behaviors are marked in the short term (laboratory studies) but have been studied in only a limited fashion across the long term (years). We simply do not have sufficient research data to evaluate any harm reduction that may accrue over the long term from the choice of particular cigarette brands.

Benowitz and Henningfield (1994) suggest that compensatory smoking or overcompensation for reduced nicotine exposes smokers to increased tars and carbon monoxide, but perhaps only for a few days or weeks. Several studies suggest that oversmoking does not negate benefits of brand switching (Hughes, 1995). Studies of brand switching suggest that although nicotine reductions are below what would be predicted from the yield of the cigarettes, significant reductions in cotinine and expired carbon monoxide levels are observed (Guyatt, Kirkham, Mariner, & Baldry, 1989; Lynch & Benowitz, 1987). In one study reviewed earlier, where brand switching was accomplished among those who did not wish to stop smoking, reductions in nicotine content were generally maintained at a 2½ year follow-up (Glasgow, Klesges, Klesges, et al., 1983).

A second and perhaps more general problem with low-tar/low-nicotine cigarettes is that they are generally unacceptable to many smokers. A strategy of providing a choice of such cigarettes may not benefit the public health. The market share for brands low in tar and nicotine has consistently remained below 20% (Russell, 1993). From a public health perspective, a safer product is of little help if people will not use it.

Maintaining Nicotine but Reducing Tar in Cigarettes

Russell (1993) is a critic of reducing the nicotine in cigarettes. He notes that "the obvious strategy is to identify those constituents that are harmful and to then eliminate or reduce them as far as possible without seriously impairing acceptability or giving rise to significant compensatory increases in inhalation" (p. 164). Thus, he has proposed reducing the tar (or possibly the carbon monoxide) in cigarettes, while maintaining or even increasing the nicotine so that people will use the product.

If the levels of tar can be significantly reduced, public health benefits seem likely. Such an approach is central to the concept of harm reduction, because addiction itself may not be the focus of a harm-reductive intervention. Although advocated for many years (see Russell, 1974), this approach has never been evaluated (Hughes, 1995). In fact, many efforts to produce a safer cigarette have been opposed by many health experts. Benowitz and Henningfield (1994), for example, argue against this strategy, suggesting that any smoking is highly toxic, and that maintaining nicotine in cigarettes will ensure that future generations will continue to become addicted. Safer cigarettes have historically been seen as a form of manipulation by the tobacco industry to diffuse concern about health hazards. It simply is not known, however, whether medium-nicotine/low-tar cigarettes would result in changes in smoking rates or addiction.

Resistance to a strategy of safer nicotine delivery has been exemplified with tobacco company efforts to develop nicotine delivery systems that do not involve the burning of tobacco (and hence result in little to no emission of tars). For example, RJR Nabisco (a major cigarette manufacturer) developed a cigarette that produced little smoke or odor, but still provided all of the nicotine of a regular cigarette. This cigarette did not burn tobacco directly, but instead used smoldering charcoal to extract the flavor. This method was designed to cut the ingestion of tars and other cancer-causing chemicals. This smoke-free cigarette might have also been successful in alleviating some of the problems of secondhand smoke, which have become issues for nonsmokers. However, the marketing of this product was opposed by the American Medical Association, the American Heart Association, the American Lung Association, and the American Cancer Society (U.S. House of Representatives, 1988, cited in Russell, 1993).

Curiously, the rationale behind maintaining nicotine in cigarettes but reducing the harm associated with other elements is similar to that for delivering nicotine independent of cigarettes altogether. Although it appears politically unacceptable for tobacco companies to pursue this line of product development, pharmaceutical companies have quite profitably taken this road for many years. In fact, nicotine replacement, reviewed next, has become one of the central strategies in smoking interventions in the last 10 years.

Nicotine Replacement

The logic for nicotine replacement treatment is both simple and essentially harm-reductive. Because nicotine is a physically addictive substance, withdrawal discomfort is an obstacle to quitting for many users (Hajek, 1991; Henningfield et al., 1991). Nicotine replacement allows a smoker to change habits with no (or much reduced) withdrawal symptoms, thus making cessation easier. Nicotine administered carefully under clinical supervision has few risks. Theoretically, once the smoking habit is extinguished, individuals can then be weaned from nicotine altogether.

Several different nicotine replacement techniques have been developed. Nicotine gum has been available in the United States since the mid-1980s at a 2-mg dose (per piece), and subsequently was approved by the FDA in a 4-mg dose as well. Nicotine gum became available over the counter in 1996. The gum, when used correctly, is capable of producing nicotine levels up to 64% of previous (smoking) levels (Fiore, Jorenby, Baker, & Kenford, 1992).

Success rates in treatment are greatly lowered if the nicotine gum is not used with some kind of counseling program (Russell, 1993; Cepeda-Benito, 1993). The gum tends to be somewhat difficult to use, has a larger number of minor but common side effects (such as hiccups and sore mouth, throat, and jaw), and patients often complain that the gum has an aversive or unpleasant taste (British Thoracic Society, 1983). Many also find the "parking" of the gum at the gumline difficult in actual use, and end up swallowing much of the nicotine through constant chewing of the gum. To complicate matters further, weaning users from the gum is not a simple process, and approximately 5% of users become dependent on the gum (Hajek, Jackson, & Belcher, 1988). Despite this host of difficulties, gum used within a comprehensive smoking cessation program improves quit rates (Fiore et al., 1992; Cepeda-Benito, 1993).

The nicotine transdermal delivery system ("the patch") was approved by the FDA in 1992 and became available over the counter in 1997. This nicotine cessation tool administers a fairly constant dose of nicotine through the user's skin, for either 24 or 16 hours a day. The patch is to be used for a period ranging from 2 weeks to about 2 months, depending on the severity of the addiction. Because of the potential simplicity and ease of use of this new product, many tobacco users, discouraged with failed attempts at cessation, have been motivated to give the patch a try.

In 1992 alone, there were more than 5 million users of the nicotine patch in the United States (Fiore et al., 1992). The patch is free of much of the difficulty found with nicotine gum, but a problem with it is that it administers nicotine slowly and gradually, and thus does not mimic the nicotine administration of cigarettes. Nevertheless, studies on the effectiveness of the nicotine patch have shown about a doubling of abstinence rates at a 12-month follow-up, compared with the rates of placebo-treated groups (Foulds, 1993). These rates are also influenced by the use of some kind of conjunctive smoking cessation counseling program (Fiore et al., 1992; Foulds, 1993; Russell, 1993).

Several new forms of nicotine replacement therapy are currently being developed, and these may widen the range of people who could potentially be reached by such therapy. These new methods concentrate on the drawbacks of the patch and gum choices available today—namely, convenience of use and rapidity of nicotine absorption in the blood. Three new methods currently being evaluated, with promising initial results, are the nicotine inhaler, the nicotine nasal spray, and nicotine lozenges (Foulds, 1993; Russell, 1991, 1993; Schneider, 1994; West, 1994). These are also attractive alternatives because the methods of delivery allow the smoker to reproduce the tactile, oral, and behavioral aspects of smoking to a certain extent (Glover, 1994).

Another possibility that has been less explored is that of combining nicotine replacement methods to match a tobacco user's particular needs, especially in the case of the heavier smoker, for whom one method may not be enough (Foulds, 1993; Glover, 1994). The nicotine vapor inhalers and nasal sprays that are being tested can potentially mimic the rapid high levels of nicotine that previously could only be achieved through smoking. These could be used in conjunction with the patch to provide both a constant, steady dose of nicotine and the instant "high" of the inhaler or the spray; this combination would virtually eliminate the need for tobacco use (Russell, 1991, 1993).

The wide acceptance of nicotine replacement is indeed fascinating, given that the theory behind the strategy is harm-reductive. It is frankly contradictory that nicotine delivered via a nasal spray gains public support while nicotine delivered via a cigarette does not. The difference, of course, is not so much in the products themselves as in the stated goals for use of the products. Nicotine replacement has been developed as a smoking cessation aid, rather than a harm reduction technique. In fact, smokers are usually instructed that they should not smoke and use nicotine replacement simultaneously. (Nicotine toxicity is one potential side effect from nicotine use.) In contrast, nicotine delivery systems sponsored by the tobacco industry are not meant as cessation aids, and, as documented above, have met with considerable opposition.

Of course, the stated goals for the use of nicotine replacement products may not reflect how the products are actually used by the public. To date, there have been few studies of patches or gum as methods of harm reduction. Yet one of the largest trials of nicotine patch use did find that individuals who did not quit smoking but did use nicotine patches exhibited significantly reduced smoking rates (Transdermal Nicotine Study Group, 1991). This trial evaluated three patch doses—21, 14, and 7 mg—as well as a placebo control. Patients who were given the 21- and 14-mg patches reduced their rates of use 66% and 67% more than the control group did, respectively. Reductions among the high-dose subjects were significantly better than those in the 7-mg and placebo control groups. It is noteworthy that persons who did not quit smoking represented over 25% of the patient group. These subjects, of course, reduced their smoking rates in the context of a cessation program. It simply is not clear how common it is for people to continue to use the patch when they have ceased trying to quit. It is likely, however, that this pattern is common.

Rennaurd et al. (1990) conducted a study in which harm reduction was both the treatment goal and the dependent measure in a research project involving nicotine replacement. In this study, 15 otherwise healthy chronic heavy smokers (consuming a minimum of two packs of cigarettes a day) who did not wish to quit smoking were enrolled. All were encouraged to reduce smoking by 50% and were instructed to use a minimum of 10 pieces of nicotine–polacrilex gum (2-mg dose per piece) daily. In addition to assessing smoking outcomes at baseline and a 2-month follow-up, the authors assessed expired carbon monoxide and conducted a bronchoscopy on each patient to assess lower-respiratory-tract inflammation.

Results indicated that smoking rates declined from an average of 50.7 cigarettes a day at baseline to 18.8 cigarettes a day after 2 months. Smoking reduction was associated with a reduction in expired carbon monoxide (48.5 to 27.3 parts per million). In addition, evidence of inflammation in the lungs significantly decreased. As one example, the visible evidence for bronchitis was significantly improved (the mean bronchitis index fell from 8.5 to 6.5), even among subjects who were selected to be asymptomatic and to have normal pulmonary function at baseline. The Rennaurd et al. (1990) study not only provides evidence that direct harm reduction can be achieved by using nicotine replacement with current smokers; it also provides an excellent example of the type of research that is necessary for the evaluation of nicotine delivery as a harm reduction strategy. The limited data available at present suggest that there is considerable potential for the improvement of public health through such strategies.

SUMMARY AND LIMITATIONS

A brief review of the harm reduction strategies applied to nicotine use suggests that such strategies have not received a great deal of research attention. Nevertheless, several behavioral, policy, and product alteration strategies have potential. In a general sense, we need to abandon the approach that labels those who attempt to quit smoking and do not as "treatment failures," and to begin studying processes of change that have the potential to lead to better health outcomes. The present review raises a number of questions and suggests some promising alternatives. Restricting access to nicotine products seems to be a consistently productive means to reduce smoking, even among heavy smokers. The long-term effects of smoking rate reductions ("controlled smoking") and brand switching need to be evaluated. It does appear that some long-standing changes may result from those strategies, but the potential health benefits of such behaviors have been largely dismissed without study. Two quite opposite proposals for altering the makeup of cigarettes have yet to be evaluated; each has both logical and practical benefits and limitations. Finally, nicotine replacement has been studied as a harm reduction strategy in only a very limited fashion, despite the fact that it may be used as such commonly.

There is clearly much we do not know about the application of harm reduction principles to smoking and tobacco use more generally. Each of the strategies reviewed above has some rationale for implementation, but there are also questions about the efficacy of each method. Furthermore, if reductions in harm can be associated with changing the makeup of cigarettes, with altering the pattern of their use, or with nicotine replacement, such health benefits need to be long-lasting to promote public health.

Several general and important questions about harm reduction and tobacco use remain. First, are smokers less likely to attempt cessation if harm reduction policies and strategies are given wide support? Clearly, cessation of smoking is the most harm-reductive strategy of all. Would the existence and support of harm reduction move fewer individuals toward quitting altogether? Policy makers are often concerned with presenting a single, simple, and coherent message; quitting smoking is such a message. Suggesting that individuals smoke differently or use different products might lessen the impact of the cessation message. This general concern (see Gritz, 1995) is common, but generally untested. One study (Glasgow et al., 1989) did not support this concern, but it tested the idea in only one context (that of a controlled-smoking option in a smoking cessation clinic).

Second, and relatedly, would pursuing harm reduction strategies at a policy level result in more young people beginning to smoke? On balance, would public health be improved or reduced? Recall the mixed opinions noted above about the introduction of filters for cigarettes in the 1950s. In another example, Henningfield and Heishman (1995) note that there seemed to be no appreciable reduction in smoking rates during the explosive rise in the use of smokeless tobacco in the United States. Thus, there seems to have been no benefit from smokeless tobacco as a form of nicotine substitution. Finally, would pursuing a policy of harm reduction spread resources for research, prevention, and treatment too thin? In an economy of limited funds for research and health promotion, resources should be targeted to the most efficacious strategies.

Of course, the answers to the questions above are empirical. Studies to examine the differential tradeoffs are well within the design capability of social science. At this time, it is not clear whether harm reduction policies would produce greater or lesser benefits to society than efforts focused solely on cessation would. It simply is not known whether harm reduction policies would undermine abstinence-based models of prevention and cessation.

The extent to which harm reduction programs can be integrated with cessation efforts is also not known. In stepped-care treatment models, as suggested by Abrams et al. (1993), treatments for smoking can be matched to clients as a function of client motivation, degree of dependence, and psychiatric and health comorbidities. Motivational interventions seem to make most sense for those who are not yet ready to quit, and brief and self-help interventions make sense for those who are less dependent and without comorbidities. Harm reduction approaches may prove to be another set of strategies that health care professionals can employ in their efforts to match programs to client needs, abilities, and motivation. As in harm reduction directed at alcohol use, failure in an initial harm reduction effort directed at tobacco use may be motivational for a subsequent cessation attempt. As stated above several times, such issues are easily subjected to controlled research, and only such investigations can ultimately answer these questions.

REFERENCES

Abrams, D., Orleans, C. T., Niaura, R., Goldstein, M., Velicer, W. F., & Prochaska, J. O. (1993). Treatment issues: Towards a stepped-care model. *Tobacco Control, 2,* 17–22.

Adams, E. H., Gfroerer, J. C., & Rouse, B. A. (1989). Epidemiology of substance abuse including alcohol and cigarette smoking. *Annals of the New York Academy of Sciences, 562,* 14–20.

Anthony, J. C., Warner, L. A., & Kessler, R. C. (1994). Comparative epidemiology of dependence on tobacco, alcohol, controlled substances, and inhalants: Basic findings from the National Comorbidity Survey. *Experimental and Clinical Psychopharmacology, 2*(3), 244–268.

Benowitz, N. L. (1995). Medical implications. *Tobacco Control: An International Journal, 4*(2), 44–48.

Benowitz, N. L., & Henningfield, J. E. (1994). Establishing a nicotine threshold for addiction: The implications for tobacco regulation. *New England Journal of Medicine, 331*(2), 123–125.

Benowitz, N. L., Jacob, P., Kozlowski, L. T., & Yu, L. (1986). Influence of smoking fewer cigarettes on exposure to tar, nicotine, and carbon monoxide. *New England Journal of Medicine, 315*(21), 1310–1313.

Boyd, G. M., & Darby, C. A. (1989). Smokeless tobacco use in the United States. *National Cancer Institute Monographs, 8,* 1–105.

Breslau, N. (1993). Daily cigarette consumption in early adulthood: Age of smoking initiation and duration of smoking. *Drug and Alcohol Dependence, 33,* 287–291.

British Thoracic Society. (1983). Comparison of four methods of smoking withdrawal in patients with smoking related diseases. *British Medical Journal, 286,* 595–597.

Bruvold, W. H. (1993). A meta-analysis of adolescent smoking prevention programs. *American Journal of Public Health, 83*(6), 872–880.

Burchfiel, C. M., Higgins, M. W., Keller, J. B., Howatt, W. F., Butler, W. J., & Higgins, I. T. (1986). Passive smoking in children: Respiratory conditions and pulmonary function in Tecumseh, MI. *American Review of Respiratory Diseases, 133,* 966–973.

Campbell, O. M., & Gray, R. H. (1987). Smoking and ectopic pregnancy: A multinational case–control study. In M. J. Rosenberg (Ed.), *Smoking and reproductive health.* Littleton, MA: PSG.

Cepeda-Benito, A. (1993). Meta-analytical review of the efficacy of nicotine chewing gum in smoking treatment programs. *Journal of Consulting and Clinical Psychology, 61*(5), 822–830.

Colletti, G., Supnick, J. A., & Rizzo, A. A. (1982). Long-term follow-up (3–4 years) of treatment for smoking reduction. *Addictive Behaviors, 7*(4), 429–433.

Cummings, K. M., & Coogan, K. (1992). Organizing communities to prevent the sale of tobacco to products to minors. *International Quarterly of Community Health Education, 13,* 77–86.

Cummings, K. M., Pechacek, T., & Shopland, D. (1994). The illegal sale of cigarettes to US minors: Estimates by state. *American Journal of Public Health, 84*(2), 300–304.

Curry, S. J., Marlatt, G. A., Gordon, J., & Baer, J. S. (1988). A comparison of alternative theoretical approaches to smoking cessation and relapse. *Health Psychology, 7*(6), 545–556.

DiFranza, J. R., Carlson, R. R., & Caisee, R. E. (1992). Reducing youth access to tobacco. *Tobacco Control, 1,* 58.

DiFranza, J. R., Richards, J. W., & Paulman, P. M., (1991). RJR Nabisco's cartoon camel promotes Camel cigarettes to children. *Journal of the American Medical Association, 266,* 3149–3153.

Doll, R., & Hill, A. B. (1950). Smoking and carcinoma of lung: Preliminary report. *British Medical Journal, ii,* 739–748.

Elder, J. P., Wildey, M. B., DeMoor, C., Sallis, J. F., Eckhardt, L., Edwards, C., Erickson, A., Golbeck, A., Hovell, M., Johnston, D., Levitz, M. D., Molgaard, C., Young, R., Vito, D., & Woodruff, S. I. (1993). The long-term prevention of tobacco use among junior high school students: Classroom and telephone interventions. *American Journal of Public Health, 83*(9), 1239–1244.

Elders, M. J., Perry, C. L., Eriksen, M. P., & Giovino, G. A. (1994). The report of the Surgeon General: Preventing tobacco use among young people. *American Journal of Public Health, 84*(4), 543–547.

Federal Register. (1996). Tobacco regulation for substance abuse prevention and treatment block grants. *Federal Register, 61*(13), 1492.

Feighary, E., Altman, D. G., & Shaffer, G. (1991). The effects of combining education and enforcement to reduce tobacco sales to minors. *Journal of the American Medical Association, 266,* 3168–3171.

Ferrence, R. G., Garcia, J. M., Sykora, K., Collishaw, N. E., & Farinon, L. (1992). The effects of pricing on cigarette use among teenagers and adults in Canada, 1980–1989. In *Health-oriented policy options on tobacco taxes in the 1992 Ontario budget.* Toronto: Council for a Tobacco-Free Ontario and the Non-smokers' Rights Association.

Fielding, J. E. (1985). Smoking: Health effects and control, Part 1. *New England Journal of Medicine, 313*(8), 491–498.

Fiore, M. C., Jorenby, D. C., Baker, T. B., & Kenford, S. L. (1992). Tobacco dependence and the nicotine patch. Clinical guidelines for effective use. *Journal of the American Medical Association, 268*(19), 2687–2694.

Fischer, P. M., Schwartz, M. P., Richards, J. W., Goldstein, A. O., & Rojas, T. H. (1991). Brand logo recognition by children aged 3 to 6 years: Mickey Mouse and Old Joe the Camel. *Journal of the American Medical Association, 266*(22), 3145–3148.

Foulds, J. (1993). Does nicotine replacement therapy work? *Addiction, 88,* 1473–1478.

George H. Gallup International Institute. (1992). *Teenage attitudes and behavior concerning tobacco.* Princeton, NJ: Author.

Glasgow, R. E., Klesges, R. C., Godding, P. R., & Gegelman, R. (1983). Controlled smoking, with or without carbon monoxide feedback, as an alternative for chronic smokers. *Behavior Therapy, 14*(3), 386–397.

Glasgow, R. E., Klesges, R. C., Klesges, L. M., Vasey, M. W., & Gunnarson, D. F. (1985). Long-term effects of a controlled smoking program: A 2½ year follow-up. *Behavior Therapy, 16*(3), 303–307.

Glasgow, R. E., Klesges, R. C., & Vasey, M. W. (1983). Controlled smoking for chronic smokers: An extension and replication. *Addictive Behaviors, 8,* 143–150.

Glasgow, R. E., Morray, K., & Lichtenstein, E. (1989). Controlled smoking versus abstinence as a treatment goal: The hopes and fears may be unfounded. *Behavior Therapy, 20,* 77–91.

Glover, E. D. (1994). The nicotine vaporizer, nicotine nasal spray, combination therapy, and the future of NRT: A discussion. *Health Values: The Journal of Health Behavior, Education, and Promotion, 18*(3), 22–28.

Glynn, T. J. (1993). Improving the health of U.S. children: The need for early interventions in tobacco use. *Preventive Medicine, 22,* 513–519.

Gritz, E. R. (1995). Panel discussion. *Tobacco Control: An International Journal, 4*(2), 74–75.

Grossman, M. (1989). Health benefits of increases in alcohol and cigarette taxes. *British Journal of Addiction, 84*(10), 1193–1204.

Guyatt, A. R., Kirkham, A. J., Mariner, D. C., & Baldry, A. G. (1989). Long-term effects of switching to cigarettes with lower tar and nicotine yields. *Pharmacology, 99*(1), 80–86.

Hajek, P. (1991). Individual differences in difficulty quitting smoking. *British Journal of Addiction, 86,* 555–558.

Hajek, P., Jackson, P., & Belcher, M. (1988). Long-term use of nicotine chewing gum. Occurrence, determinants, and effect on weight gain. *Journal of the American Medical Association, 260*(11), 1593–1596.

Hatsukami, D., Nelson, R., & Jensen, J. (1991). Smokeless tobacco: Current status and future directions. *British Journal of Addiction, 86*(5), 559–563.

Hebel, J. R., Fox, N. L., & Sexton, M. (1988). Dose–response of birth weight to various measures of maternal smoking during pregnancy. *Journal of Clinical Epidemiology, 41*, 483–489.

Henningfield, J. E., Cohen, C., & Slade, J. D. (1991). Is nicotine more addictive than cocaine? *British Journal of Addiction, 86*, 565–569.

Henningfield, J. E., & Heishman, S. J. (1995). The addictive role of nicotine in tobacco use. *Psychopharmacology, 117*(1), 11–13.

Hill, D., Weiss, D. J., Walker, D. L., & Jolley, D. (1988). Long-term evaluation of controlled smoking as a treatment outcome. *British Journal of Addiction, 83*(2), 203–207.

Hoffman, H. J., Damus, K., Hillman, L., & Krongrad, E. (1988). Risk factors for SIDS: Results of the National Institute of Child Health and Human Development SIDS Cooperative Epidemiological Study. *Annals of the New York Academy of Sciences, 533*, 13–29.

Hu, T. -W., Sung, H.-Y., & Keeler, T. E. (1995). Reducing cigarette consumption in California: Tobacco taxes vs. an anti-smoking media campaign. *American Journal of Public Health, 85*(9), 1218–1222.

Hughes, J. R. (1995). Applying harm reduction to smoking. *Tobacco Control: An International Journal, 4*(2), 33–38.

Jason, L. A., Ji, P. Y., Anes, M. D., & Birkhead, S. H. (1991). Active enforcement of cigarette control laws in the prevention of cigarette sales to minors. *Journal of the American Medical Association, 266*, 3149–3153.

Johnston, L. D., O'Malley, P. M., & Bachman, J. G. (1991). *Drug use, drinking, and smoking: National survey results from high school, college and young adult populations: 1975–1990* (Publication No. ADM 91-1638). Washington, DC: U.S. Government Printing Office.

Kaplan, R. M., Orleans, C. T., Perkins, K. A., & Pierce, J. P. (1995). Marshaling the evidence for greater regulation and control of tobacco products: A call for action. *Annals of Behavioral Medicine, 17*(1), 3–14.

Kessler, D. A. (1995). Nicotine addiction in young people. *New England Journal of Medicine, 333*(3), 186–189.

Kinne, S., Kristal, A. R., White, E., & Hunt, J. (1993). Work-site smoking policies: Their population impact in Washington State. *American Journal of Public Health, 83*(7), 1031–1033.

Kleinman, J. C., Pierre, M. B., Madans, J. H., Land, G. H., & Schramm, W. F. (1988). The effects of maternal smoking on fetal and infant mortality. *American Journal of Epidemiology, 126*, 274–282.

Klesges, R. C., & DeBon, M. (1994). *How women can finally stop smoking.* Alameda, CA: Hunter House.

Kozlowski, L. T. (1989). Reduction of tobacco health hazards in continuing users: Individual behavioral and public health approaches. *Journal of Substance Abuse, 1*(3), 345–357.

Kozlowski, L. T., & Herman, P. (1984). The interaction of psychosocial and biological determinants of tobacco use: More on the boundary model. *Journal of Applied Social Psychology, 14*(3), 244–256.

Kozlowski, L. T., Rickert, W. S., Pope, M. A., Robinson, J. C., & Frecker, R. C. (1982). Estimating the yield to smokers of tar, nicotine, and carbone monoxide from the "lowest yield" ventilated filter-cigarettes. *British Journal of Addiction, 77*(2), 159–165.

Levinson, B. L., Shapiro, D., Schwartz, G. E., & Tursky, B. (1971). Smoking elimination by gradual reduction. *Behavior Therapy, 2*(4), 477–487.

Lewit, E. M. (1989). U.S. tobacco taxes: Behavioural effects and policy implications. *Journal of Addiction, 84*(10), 1217–1235.

Lynch, C. J., & Benowitz, N. S. (1987). Spontaneous cigarette brand switching: Consequences for nicotine and carbon monoxide exposure. *American Journal of Public Health, 77*(9), 1191–1194.

Madden, P. A., & Grube, J. W. (1994). The frequency and nature of alcohol and tobacco advertising in televised sports, 1990 through 1992. *American Journal of Public Health, 84*(2), 297–299.

McNeill, A. D., West, R. J., Jarvis, M., Jackson, P., & Bryant, E. (1986). Cigarette withdrawal symptoms in adolescent smokers. *Psychopharmacology, 90*(4), 533–536.

Pierce, J. P., & Gilpin, E. A. (1995). A historical analysis of tobacco marketing and the uptake of smoking by youth in the United States: 1890–1977. *Health Psychology, 14*(6), 500–508.

Pierce, J. P., Gilpin, E. A., Burns, D. M., Whalen, E., Rosbrook, B., Shopland, D., & Johnson, M. (1991). Does tobacco advertising target young people to start smoking? *Journal of the American Medical Association, 266*(22), 3154–3158.

Pirie, P. L., Murray, D. M., & Luepker, R. V. (1988). Smoking prevalence in a cohort of adolescents, including absentees, dropouts, and transfers. *American Journal of Public Health, 78*, 176–178.

Ray, O. (1983). *Drugs, society, and human behavior* (3rd ed.). St. Louis, MO: C. V. Mosby.

Rennaurd, S. I., Daughton, D., Fujita, J., Oehlerking, M. B., Dobson, J. R., Stahl, M. G., Robbins, R. A., & Thompson, A. B. (1990). Short-term smoking reduction is associated with reduction in measures of lower respiratory tract inflammation in heavy smokers. *European Respiratory Journal, 3*, 752–759.

Reuter, P., & MacCoun, R. J. (1995). Lessons from the absence of harm reduction in American drug policy. *Tobacco Control: An International Journal, 4*(2), 28–32.

Russell, M. A. H. (1990). The nicotine addiction trap: A 40-year sentence for four cigarettes. *British Journal of Addiction, 85*(2), 293–300.

Russell, M. A. H. (1991). The future of nicotine replacement. *British Journal of Addiction, 86*(5), 653–658.

Russell, M. A. H. (1993). Reduction of smoking-related harm: The scope for nicotine replacement. In N. Heather, A. Wodak, E. A. Nadelmann, & P. O'Hare (Eds.), *Psychoactive drugs and harm reduction: From faith to science.* London: Whurr.

Russell, M. A. H., Jarvis, M. J., Devitt, G., & Feyerabend, C. (1981). Nicotine intake by snuff users. *British Medical Journal, 283*, 814–817.

Russell, R. D. (1974). Alcohol and other mood-modifying substances in ecological perspective: A framework for communicating and educating. *Quarterly Journal of Studies on Alcohol, 35*(2), 606–619.

Schneider, N. G., Olmstead, R., Mody, F. V., Doan, K., Franzon, M., Jarvik, M. E.,

& Steinberg, C. (1995). Efficacy of a nicotine nasal spray in smoking cessation: A placebo-controlled, double-blind trial. *Addiction, 90*(12), 1761–1682.

Schols, D., Daling, J. R., & Stergachis, A. S. (1992). Current cigarette smoking and risk of acute pelvic inflammatory disease. *American Journal of Public Health, 82*, 1352–1355.

Shapiro, D., Tursky, B., Schwartz, G. E., & Shnidman, S. R. (1971). Smoking on cue: A behavioral approach to smoking reduction. *Journal of Health and Social Behavior, 12*(2), 108–113.

Shiffman, S. (1989). Tobacco "chippers": Individual differences in tobacco dependence. *Psychopharmacology, 97*(4), 539–547.

Shiffman, S. (1993). Smoking cessation treatment: Any progress? *Journal of Consulting and Clinical Psychology, 61*(5), 718–722.

Slade, J. (1992). The tobacco epidemic: Lessons from history. *Journal of Psychoactive Drugs, 24*(2), 99–109.

Stitzer, M. L. (1995). Policy initiatives to enhance smoking cessation and harm reduction. *Tobacco Control: An International Journal, 4*(2), 67–73.

Townsend, J. (1993). Policies to halve smoking deaths. *Addiction, 88*(1), 37–46.

Transdermal Nicotine Study Group. (1991). Transdermal nicotine for smoking cessation. *Journal of the American Medical Association, 266*(22), 3133–3138.

Tye, J. B., Warner, K. E., & Glantz, S. A. (1987). Tobacco advertising and consumption: Evidence of a causal relationship. *Journal of Public Health Policy, 8*, 492–507.

U.S. Department of Health and Human Services (U.S. DHHS). (1986). *The health consequences of using smokeless tobacco: A report of the Advisory Committee to the Surgeon General* (NIH Publication No. 86-2874). Bethesda, MD: Author.

U.S. Department of Health and Human Services (U.S. DHHS). (1988). *The health consequences of smoking: Nicotine addiction. A report of the Surgeon General* (DHHS Publication No. CDC 880-8406). Washington, DC: U.S. Government Printing Office.

U.S. Department of Health and Human Services (U.S. DHHS). (1989). *Reducing the health consequences of smoking: 25 years of progress. A report of the Surgeon General* (DHHS Publication No. CDC 89-8411). Washington, DC: U.S. Government Printing Office.

U.S. Department of Health and Human Services (U.S. DHHS). (1992). *Youth access to tobacco.* Washington, DC: U.S. Government Printing Office.

U.S. Department of Health and Human Services (U.S. DHHS). (1994). *Preventing tobacco use among young people: A report of the Surgeon General.* Washington, DC: U.S. Government Printing Office.

U.S. Department of Health, Education and Welfare. (1964). *Smoking and health: Report of the Advisory Committee to the Surgeon General of the Public Health Service* (PHS Publication No. 1103). Bethesda, MD: Author.

U.S. Environmental Protection Agency. (1992). *Respiratory health effects of passive smoking: Lung cancer and other disorders.* Washington, DC: Author.

West, R. (1994). The future of nicotine replacement in smoking cessation? *Addiction, 89*(4), 438–439.

Vogt, T. M. (1982). Cigarette smoking: History, risks, and behavior change. *International Journal of Mental Health, 11*(3), 6–43.

CHAPTER SIX

Harm Reduction Strategies for Illicit Substance Use and Abuse

SUSAN F. TAPERT
JASON R. KILMER
LORI A. QUIGLEY
MARY E. LARIMER
LISA J. ROBERTS
ELIZABETH T. MILLER

OVERVIEW

The philosophy of harm reduction has been discussed in Part I of this book, and Chapters 4 and 5 have described its application to alcohol problems and to smoking, respectively. This chapter focuses on the reduction of harm from the use of illicit substances. When utilizing a harm reduction approach with illicit substances, one must consider a number of issues. Although a harm reduction goal of controlled or moderate use may be possible for some people, such a goal may not be appropriate for all cases. Some individuals' histories of using a particular substance may have been so problematic that avoiding *any* substance use may be the wisest option for them. Moreover, for some substances (e.g., crack cocaine), it is clear that any use at all can be both dangerous and illegal. Depending on an individual's problem history and the inherent dangers of a given substance, either a reduction in use may represent a favorable outcome, or moderation may be viewed as an intermediate step toward abstinence (the most valued outcome of a harm reduction program, because abstinence involves no risk for harm).

The "harm" that such an approach seeks to lessen manifests itself in many different ways with illicit drugs. The possible harm experienced on a personal level may include short- and long-term health risks; financial problems; potential legal consequences, including incarceration; and a decrease in efficacy across a number of different domains, including work and home. Harm with illicit drugs also becomes evident on interpersonal and societal levels. Interpersonal conflict can often surround illicit substance use, either because of problems that occur while a person is under the influence of the drug, or because of the fallout from earlier negative consequences of the substance use. Furthermore, drug dealing and crimes committed in order to acquire drugs detract from a community ethos of safety and nonviolence. Given the potential of illicit substances to cause harm at various levels, a comprehensive program designed to reduce such harm is needed.

In general, several different harm reduction strategies can be employed with illicit drug users. Aside from the potential danger of procuring illicit substances, often the primary risks to an individual are often more closely associated with the means in which the substance is consumed or administered than with the direct pharmacological effects of the substance itself. For example, needle sharing heightens risk for the transmission of HIV or AIDS. In addition, certain routes of administration can be more physiologically dangerous, and a change in how the drug is taken may reduce health risks. Thus, if abstinence is not an outcome that is immediately attainable, harm can be reduced by altering the individual's drug-taking practices.

Other attempts to reduce harm can be intermediate steps toward some other desired goal. For example, substance substitution allows one to reduce the addiction potential of a particular type of drug. Substitution of a less harmful substance or of the same substance in a less potent form can reduce the short-term dangers of the original substance of choice. On a long-term basis, a user who is hampered by severe withdrawal symptoms along the road to abstinence can substitute a less dangerous substance characterized by a less severe addiction potential for his or her drug of choice (e.g., methadone maintenance can be substituted for heroin use). Although substance substitution help• reduce the greater dangers associated with the initial drug being used, not all harm is eliminated, because there may still be risks associated with the alternative substance. Thus, the maintenance of abstinence remains the ideal method of reducing risk; however, with individuals for whom an immediate switch to a drug-free life is difficult to attain, intermediate or step-down approaches must take priority. Any steps toward the reduction of harm are steps in the right direction.

In 1996, just over a third of a representative sample of the U.S. adult population acknowledged the use of an illicit substance during their lifetimes and 6% acknowledged use in the past month (for more details about past-month use, see Table 6.1). The most commonly used illicit substance is cannabis. Although use of cocaine has remained stable, use of heroin has increased slightly, especially among young adults. In addi-

TABLE 6.1. Most Frequently Used Substances in the United States (Past-Month Use), 1996

Substance	Number of persons	Percent of population
Alcohol	109,149,000	51.0
Cigarettes	61,759,000	28.9
Any illicit drug use	13,035,000	6.1
Cannabis	10,095,000	4.7
Cocaine (including crack)	2,417,000	1.1
Hallucinogens	1,316,000	0.6
Heroin	216,000	0.1
Prescription drug misuse	3,082,000	1.4
Analgesics	1,884,000	0.9
Tranquilizers	952,000	0.4
Stimulants	763,000	0.4
Sedatives	232,000	0.1

Note. Data from SAMHSA (1997).

tion, use of hallucinogens and "designer drugs" has increased in certain populations (Substance Abuse and Mental Health Services Administration [SAMHSA], 1997). In the United States, the prevalence of illicit drug use is considered to be a primary indicator of drug abuse.[1] In a policy marked by "zero tolerance," any use of illicit substances is tantamount to abuse. From this absolute perspective, the "war on drugs" cannot be won until no one in the population uses illicit substances. Harm reduction strategies, on the other hand, focus on reducing the harm incurred by substance use, rather than on reducing the absolute number of substance users. Implicit in these strategies is the recognition that winning the so-called "war on drugs" is not a realistic goal and that some proportion of the population will continue to engage in illicit drug use. The success of harm reduction approaches is measured by reduction in heavy or problem use and attendant consequences, rather than (or in addition to) reduction in prevalence of use.

In this chapter, we discuss harm reduction strategies as they apply to illicit substance use. The chapter begins with an overview of strategies utilized to reduce the harm associated with opiate use. These strategies have been empirically evaluated more often than the approaches employed for other substances, perhaps because opiates have a longer history of abuse. Harm reduction treatment of problems with cocaine is addressed next, along with a discussion of the individual and societal issues that accompany these risk-reducing efforts. In addition, efforts to reduce the harm associated with problematic cannabis and hallucinogen use are reviewed, although such efforts are less fully described in the harm reduction literature. The misuse of prescription drugs is also briefly considered, though these drugs are not, strictly speaking, "illicit substances." Finally, other illicit substances such as amphetamines and steroids (for which there is a still less substantial body of literature regarding harm reduction approaches) are discussed.

OPIATES

The euphoria of opiate use and the suffering associated with opiate dependence have been topics of literature from Theophrastus in the 4th century B.C. to William S. Burroughs and Jim Carroll in the 20th century A.D. Although heroin is the most commonly abused opiate at present, other opiates can also lead to a pronounced and uncomfortable physiological withdrawal state. The opiate class of drugs includes heroin, morphine, and opium; methadone; analgesics (painkillers) such as oxycodone (Percodan), meperidine hydrochloride (Demerol), hydromorphone hydrochloride (Dilaudid), and codeine; and certain "designer drugs" synthesized to have chemical properties similar to those of opiates, such as fentanyl.

This section focuses on strategies with demonstrated success in reducing the harm associated with opiate use for both addicts and society. After a general discussion of opiates and their use, we discuss methadone maintenance and present suggestions for its optimal implementation. We then describe other forms of harm reduction for opiate addicts, including buprenorphine, L-alpha-acetylmethadol (LAAM), prescribed heroin, and ibogaine. These treatments all fall under the umbrella of harm reduction because they do not necessarily require abstinence from intoxicants for participation. Other treatments that do require abstinence, such as "cold turkey," rapid detoxification, and naltrexone, are not discussed here. These latter techniques have been used with varying degrees of success, but as a whole they have not been as effective in reducing the negative consequences of illicit opiate use as harm reduction methods have been (Gerstein & Harwood, 1990; Hubbard, Rachal, Craddock, & Cavanaugh, 1984; Hubbard, Marsden, Rachal, Valley, & Henrick, 1989; Institute of Medicine, 1995; Kreek, 1992; Ward, Mattick, & Hall, 1992). Other harm reduction strategies have been employed successfully in the reduction of risk of HIV seroconversion. The most notable of these strategies is needle or syringe exchange; this topic is covered in Chapter 7.

General Characteristics of Opiates and Their Use

Opiate addiction is less common than addiction to other drug types, but its effects are widespread. Approximately 2.4 million people in the United States reported having ever used heroin in 1996, and almost 12 million reported having used analgesic medications for nonmedicinal purposes at least once in their lifetimes (SAMHSA, 1997; see Table 6.2). Opiate use prevalence among young people remains low but is rising. In 1996, over 2% of U.S. eighth-grade students reported having used heroin at least once

TABLE 6.2. Prevalence of Nonmedical Opiate Use in the United
States

	Lifetime	Past-year use	Past-month use
Heroin	2,444,000	455,000	216,000
Analgesics	11,799,000	4,510,000	1,884,000
Total	14,243,000	4,965,000	2,100,000

Note. Data from SAMHSA (1997).

in their brief lifetimes, significantly more than in 1993 (Johnston, O'Malley, & Bachman, 1997). Approximately 141,000 people used heroin for the first time in 1996, and many were under age 26. Although injection was reported by about half of heroin users, those who reported ever smoking or snorting increased from 55% in 1994 to 82% in 1996. At least 216,000 Americans had used heroin in the past month in 1996 (SAMHSA, 1997). Over 1 million Americans are estimated to be opiate-dependent at some point in their lives. (American Psychiatric Association, 1994a).

The number of emergency room visits related to heroin use increased from 33,900 in 1990 to 76,000 in 1995 (Drug Abuse Warning Network, 1996). Opiate addiction has unfortunately been a prominent feature in news reports from the 1970s onward, due to the untimely deaths of numerous well-known young musicians. In addition to the deleterious effects of opiate dependence on addicts and their families, opiate dependence affects society in the form of criminal activity committed by addicts seeking funds for drugs. Related costs to the criminal justice system are conservatively estimated at $85 million per year in the United States (Deschenes, Anglin, & Speckart, 1991).

Opiates have been classified according to their analgesic properties by Jaffe and Martin (1990): (1) morphine-like agonists, including methadone, morphine, heroin, meperidine (Demerol), hydromorphone (Dilaudid), and fentanyl; (2) partial agonists, including codeine and oxycodone (Percodan); and (3) mixed agonist–antagonists, such as buprenorphine and pentazocine. The morphine-like agonists are strong analgesics. As the dose increases, pain relief effects increase and respiratory functioning decreases. In overdoses, the respiratory system fails. Partial agonists and mixed agonist–antagonists produce less analgesia and respiratory depression. Increasing the dose above a ceiling point does not increase analgesia (Zacny, 1995). Although heroin is the most commonly abused opiate, meperidine and fentanyl have been reported as frequent drugs of abuse among medical personnel (Ward, Ward, & Saidman, 1983).

Opiate intoxication involves pain relief and decreased pain sensation, euphoria, decreased sex drive, some sedation, nausea, constipation, respiratory depression, and suppression of the cough reflex. These effects are caused by opiates' binding to different opioid receptors, mostly in the central nervous system. The mu receptors affect pain and respiration. Kappa and sigma receptors affect sedation, hormones, mood, and hallucination. Delta receptors appear to respond preferentially to endogenous or natural brain opiates. An excess of opiates, or opiate overdose, can cause death by respiratory depression and failure. The effects of opiates have been put to use in medical settings. Opiate drugs such as morphine and heroin were once used as cough suppressants and diarrhea cures. Methadone and other opiate drugs are now commonly prescribed to cancer patients for pain relief (Bushnell & Justins, 1993; Jaffe & Martin, 1990).

Opiates are also often discussed in terms of their duration of action (see Table 6.3). Heroin and morphine are short-acting opiates. The effects of heroin are perceived by the user very soon after administration. Individuals addicted to these drugs report withdrawal symptoms after several hours of abstinence and report maximum severity of withdrawal symptoms between 24 and 72 hours after the most recent administration. Methadone is a longer-acting opiate with a slower, gentler slope of psychoactive onset. Its longer half-life allows opiate-dependent individuals to administer the drug less frequently. Initial withdrawal symptoms are not noted until after 24–48 hours of abstinence, and peak severity is usually reported up to 5–8 days after abstinence. In general, the severity and duration of withdrawal symptoms from opiates are proportional to the rate at which the opiates are removed from opioid receptors (Jaffe, 1995).

When an individual ceases opiate administration, opioid receptors are soon depleted of exogenous opiates. If the individual is addicted to opiates, the central nervous system develops tolerance to the increased presence of exogenous opiate by diminishing production of endogenous opiates, such as endorphins and enkephalins. With the absence of both endogenous and exogenous opiates, the individual typically experiences unpleasant abstinence symptoms, sometimes termed "opiate withdrawal syndrome" or "dependence syndrome." This involves flu-like symptoms such as chills,

TABLE 6.3. Comparison of Selected Opiates

	Heroin	Methadone	LAAM	Buprenorphine
Frequency of administration	2–5x/day	1x/day	3ö/week	1ö/day
Recommended dose	N/A	60–120 mg	50–120 mg	8–16 mg
Drug half-life	6 hours	24 hours	48–72 hours	24–36 hours
Peak withdrawal	24–72 hours	5–8 days	Up to 15 days	3–5 days
Route of administration	Injection	Oral	Oral	Sublingual
Legal status	Illegal	Legal in clinics	Legal in clinics	Under FDA investigation

shakes, sweating, nausea, vomiting, diarrhea, increased heart rate, restlessness, and increased physical sensitivity and pain. The severity of symptoms is related to the degree of tolerance an individual has developed and to his or her health status. Some individuals in poor health may risk heart problems and pneumonia. Many opiate-dependent individuals relapse to illicit opiates when faced with these unpleasant symptoms, as administration of an opiate immediately alleviates symptoms (Gold, 1993).

Alpha-adrenergic agonists, such as clonidine (Catapres), are commonly prescribed as antihypertensives. These drugs have also demonstrated utility in ameliorating certain opiate withdrawal symptoms: Because the drugs reduce excess activity in the locus coeruleus and other noradrenergic nuclei, withdrawal symptoms of increased heart rate and restlessness are reduced. Clonidine is not a controlled substance, nor is it intoxicating. However, because it is not an opiate, it does not delay withdrawal. The utility of clonidine is somewhat limited because it does not affect craving, insomnia, or muscle aches. A major side affect of clonidine is hypotension, so it should not be used with hypotensive individuals or pregnant women (Gold & Kleber, 1979; Jaffe, 1995).

Cross-tolerance develops among opiate drugs. For example, an individual with a developed tolerance to heroin will also have an immediate tolerance to methadone, and thus will require a higher dose of it. This is an important concern regarding treatment of pain in opiate-dependent individuals. Because they already have a high tolerance to opiates, they require a higher dose of analgesic opiates to curb medical pain successfully than most patients do. Also noteworthy is the relatively rapid loss of tolerance, so that an opiate addict, once abstinent over a period of time, cannot tolerate a dose of opiate previously tolerated and may risk overdose unless the dose is appropriately reduced. Relapses following reduction in tolerance often result in heroin overdoses. In its 1994 sample of emergency room incidents, the Drug Abuse Warning Network (1995) found 251 deaths directly attributable to heroin and morphine use, compared to 15 deaths attributed to methadone (including illicitly obtained methadone) and 13 aspirin-related deaths. Environmental cues also appear to play a role in physiological adaptation to the presence of opiates. Heroin injection in novel surroundings (i.e., those different from where the user typically injects), have been associated with an increased risk of heroin overdose (Gutierrez-Cebollada, de la Torre, Ortuno, Garces, & Cami, 1994).

Methadone Maintenance

What Is Methadone and How Does It Work?

Methadone is a synthetic opiate that prevents opiate abstinence symptoms (withdrawal), decreases craving for opiates, and blocks euphoric effects of other opiates by creating cross-tolerance. Methadone is typically administered orally and has a longer half-life than heroin. It is most often administered once per day. In contrast, heroin addicts usually administer heroin two to five times daily; thus, heroin attainment and administration become the focus of daily activities. Moreover, to continue experiencing opiate euphoria, users must administer larger and larger doses of heroin to surpass tolerance. Methadone is less intoxicating than heroin and most other opiates, and users experience less euphoria and impairment (Weddington, 1992), enabling them to proceed with life goals. Since tolerance develops to a consistent dose level, very little euphoria results from a consistent maintenance dose. Finally, a methadone dose can be controlled to the nearest milliliter; in contrast, the purity level and content of street heroin are unknown to the user.

Although methadone is cheaper than street drugs, participants in a methadone maintenance program in the United States are usually required to pay a fee for services. Methadone treatment is sometimes free or reduced for participants on public assistance or with health insurance. However, it should be noted that the average annual cost to society is $43,000 for each untreated abuser and $40,000 for each incarcerated abuser, whereas each individual in methadone maintenance treatment costs approximately $3,500 annually (Gerstein & Harwood, 1990; Swan, 1994). Residential drug treatment programs cost between $13,000 and $20,000 per addict annually, and have lower retention and success rates than methadone maintenance programs do (Gerstein & Harwood, 1990).

History of Methadone Maintenance Treatment

Methadone was developed by German chemists during World War II for use as an analgesic (Gerstein & Harwood, 1990), although others claim it was first synthesized by German chemists at I. G. Farben who were researching spasmolytica (Lap, 1995). It was first used with opiate addicts at the U.S. Public Health Hospital/Prison in Lexington, Kentucky, as a detoxification agent. Methadone was found to be preferable to morphine for clinical use because it was (and is) cheap, orally active, and longer-lasting than morphine.

Dr. Vincent Dole, an endocrinology researcher, and Dr. Marie Nyswander, a psychiatrist trained at the Lexington facility, began experiments with maintenance treatment for chronic heroin addicts in the mid-1960s at Rockefeller University in New York. Dole and Nyswander found that the opiate addicts maintained on methadone no longer experienced opiate euphoria or withdrawal (Dole, Nyswander, & Warner, 1968; Dole et al., 1969). They proposed that heroin induces a metabolic disorder that places patients in need of continued use of heroin or other opiates. Methadone was thought to correct this disorder and to block the euphoric opiate effects, allowing participants to function normally (Lap, 1995). Addicts were able to redirect their time away from obtaining and using drugs.

Supplementing methadone maintenance with therapeutic assistance, many were able to pursue life goals (Institute of Medicine, 1995).

The social and political climate demanded a solution to the increasing drug problem. By the late 1960s, heroin was the leading cause of death for 15- to 35-year-olds in New York City. Arrests for drug-related crimes were at an all-time high, and the incidence of hepatitis was on the rise (Institute of Medicine, 1995). U.S. President Richard Nixon's war on street crime was at the core of his domestic policy. Nixon and the U.S. Congress saw methadone as a potential strategy for reducing crimes committed by addicts (Nadelmann & McNeely, 1996; Renner, 1984). Federal officials rapidly expanded methadone programs. In 1968, fewer than 400 addicts were enrolled in U.S. methadone programs; by 1973, participants numbered 73,000 (U.S. Department of Health and Human Services, 1993). As more opiate addicts enrolled in New York's methadone programs, drug arrests dropped from 40,000 to 15,100. Complaints to the police for crimes associated with drug abuse, such as robbery, burglary, and larceny, dropped from 350,000 to 273,000. Drug dependence deaths and hepatitis cases among drug injectors also dropped during the period between 1971 and 1973 (Joseph, 1988).

Methadone found success in other countries as well. In Hong Kong, all addicts were given immediate access to methadone, starting in the 1970s. Hong Kong experienced a 70% decrease in the number of addicts arrested for drug or other criminal offenses during the first 5 years of its methadone maintenance program (Newman & Peyser, 1991). Reports of reduced criminality and enhanced health status soon emerged from Australia (Reynolds & Magro, 1976), Sweden (Gunne & Gronbladh, 1981), and Thailand (Vanichseni et al., 1991) following implementation of methadone programs.

When the U.S. Congress instituted methadone clinics in 1972, the Food and Drug Administration (FDA) began regulation of methadone distribution. Regulations were strict and often in opposition to Dole and Nyswander's guidelines for proper methadone prescribing (Gerstein & Harwood, 1990). Regulatory guidelines, imposed by both federal and state agencies, attempted to prevent diversion of methadone from program participants to street markets. Regulations also tended to limit methadone dose and the amount of time opiate-dependent individuals could continue on methadone. As a result of prohibitive regulations and the rapid expansion of treatment, the quality of methadone maintenance treatment began to suffer. Insufficient lengths of treatment stays and low doses of methadone resulted in many addicts' relapsing to street opiates (Nadelmann & McNeely, 1996). Treatment guidelines were not influenced by input from addicts, but by public policy and misinformed clinic staffs.

When injection drug use was recognized as a major transmission route for HIV, methadone maintenance received a resurgence of support as a means to curb the rise in HIV among injection drug users, many of whom were addicted to heroin and other opiates. Methadone has since been associated with significant reductions in HIV and hepatitis transmission (see Chaisson et al., 1989; McLachlan, Crofts, Wodak, & Crowe, 1993; Metzger et al., 1993; Serpelloni et al., 1994; Siddiqui, Brown, Meyer, & Gonzalez, 1993). In addition, clinics provide a useful outlet for condoms (Calsyn, Meinecke, Saxon, & Stanton, 1992).

As of 1994, approximately 115,000 opiate-dependent individuals were participating in methadone maintenance programs in the United States; of these participants, 40,000 were in New York State and about 20,000 in California (Institute of Medicine, 1995). Methadone is used worldwide in the treatment of opiate addiction. It is the most rigorously studied and the most effective treatment for opiate addiction to date (Ball & Ross, 1991; Hubbard et al., 1984, 1989; Gerstein & Harwood, 1990, 1995; Kreek, 1992; Ward et al., 1992).

Participant Demographics

Methadone maintenance participants vary widely on many dimensions. A 1985 sample of 617 male participants provides some information on sociodemographic characteristics; these participants were selected for representativeness as addicts in U.S. East Coast cities (Ball & Ross, 1991). In another sample of 309 methadone clients (Calsyn, Fleming, Wells, & Saxon, 1996), the participants were consecutive admissions to a Seattle methadone clinic from 1990 to 1991 (see Table 6.4).

Across studies, many methadone maintenance participants have medical problems (e.g., hepatitis, HIV, tuberculosis), and 25–35% of participants in some studies have psychiatric disorders (Rounsaville, Weissman, Kleber, & Wilber, 1982). Methadone may assist these addicts in coping with or stabilizing psychiatric symptoms (Zweben & Sorenson, 1988).

Criticisms of Methadone Maintenance

Despite the demonstrated effectiveness of methadone maintenance in reducing crime, improving the physical and psychological health of participants, and assisting participants in attaining life goals, methadone maintenance is not without controversy. Some sources of controversy pertain to genuine flaws, but others stem from lack of information.

"Not in My Backyard." Neighborhood-based controversies often arise regarding geographic placement of methadone clinics. The first methadone clinics in the 1960s and 1970s acquired reputations for being part of the drug problem rather than part of the solution. Neighbors of methadone clinics complained of participants' loitering. These "not in my backyard" complaints continue to block new methadone clinics (Nadelmann & McNeely, 1996). In Washington State, for example, methadone clinics are

TABLE 6.4. Methadone Patient Characteristics

	East Coast, 1985 (n = 617) (Ball & Ross, 1991)	Seattle, 1990–1991 (n = 309) (Calsyn et al., 1996)
% male	100%	67%
Age	72% between 25 and 39	38 (SD = 7.5)
Ethnicity		
European American	41%	60%
African American	51%	37%
Other	8%	3%
Occupation	71% previously employed 25% no work in 3 years	65% past-month illegal occupation
Marital status	28% ever married	—[a]
Drug use history	66% daily opiate use by 19	13 years of heroin injection 4 years of cocaine injection
Arrest history	85% one or more	—
Incarceration history	35% ever	—
Prior treatment	94%	—
Psychopathology[b]	—	32% affective disturbance 17% psychotic symptoms 90% some Axis II psychopathology

[a]Not reported.
[b]As assessed via Millon Clinical Multiaxial Inventory.

approved on a county-by-county basis, and only counties with large metropolitan areas have received approval, forcing many rural opiate-dependent individuals to commute long distances for treatment. In urban areas, local businesses and residents often fight to keep methadone clinics out of their neighborhoods for fear of increased crime. Use of mobile methadone-dispensing units may alleviate some of this controversy, because mobile programs are not fixed to sites (Besteman & Brady, 1994).

"Replacing One Addiction with Another." Some politicians as well as opiate addicts have argued that methadone maintenance is merely "replacing one addiction with another" (Gerstein & Harwood, 1990). The notion of maintaining a methadone dose level indefinitely is unappealing to some people, because participants are not truly "drug-free." It is useful to note that several other major medical and psychological problems are remedied by implementation of lifelong pharmacological treatments, including insulin for diabetes, lithium for bipolar disorders, and antihypertensives for high blood pressure.

Addicts are often ambivalent about methadone, and many do not seek methadone treatment until their drug use has reached a crisis level (Bell, Caplehorn, & McNeil, 1994). Other opiate-dependent individuals want to get off drugs altogether and do not consider methadone an appealing option. However, methadone has been used successfully as an intermediate step between heroin use and abstinence. In one study (Sorensen, Acampora, Trier, & Gold, 1987), treatment outcomes were assessed in opiate-dependent individuals enrolled in a therapeutic community to taper off from methadone. Over half (17 of 32) were successful in detoxification, and most addicts rated their living situation as improved since starting treatment and retained improved global functioning ratings at follow-up. However, some addicts did test positive for heroin at follow-up. Milby (1988) reviewed rates of detoxification completion by methadone program participants in the 1970s and found that psychotherapy-assisted detoxification showed greater completion rates. Detoxification is not easy, but methadone can ease the transition.

"Not Quite a Junkie, Not Quite Straight." Because of stigmatization, methadone maintenance participants often maintain secrecy regarding their addict status in many life contexts, because disclosure of personal histories and methadone use could eliminate them from social and occupational opportunities (Murphy & Irwin, 1992). A person receiving methadone also often reports problems with conceptualizing personal identity, as he or she is "not quite a junkie, not quite straight" (Murphy & Irwin, 1992, p. 259). Moreover, because methadone clients are not drug-free, sending them to Twelve-Step meetings was unacceptable until recently (Zweben & Sorensen, 1988). Now some cities offer special support group meetings for methadone maintenance participants.

Concomitant Use of Other Drugs. Some methadone maintenance participants continue to use other substances during treatment such as cocaine (Kosten, Rounsaville, & Kleber, 1987), benzodiazepines (Caplehorn, 1994), and other intoxicants. This is a major problem, as reducing illicit substance use is a primary goal of methadone maintenance. Sufficient methadone dosing attenuates illicit opiate use because of the pharmacological properties of methadone, as discussed previously; however, the pharmacological properties of methadone do not alter cravings for other substances. Overall, use of illicit opiates as well as other substances tends to decrease among methadone maintenance participants, compared to addicts not in methadone maintenance (Fairbank, Dunteman, & Condelli, 1993; Newman, 1995). Nonetheless, reduction of illicit drug and alcohol use among methadone clients has been the focus of much research activity. Contingency contracting, regular urinalysis screens, and take-home dose incentives reduce concomitant drug use among methadone maintenance participants, and are discussed later in this section.

Significant proportions of clients in methadone maintenance may be alcohol-dependent. El-Bassel, Schilling, Turnbull, and Su (1993) reported that 20% of methadone clients in the Bronx and Harlem met Michigan Alcoholism Screening Test criteria for alcohol dependence. Alcohol-dependent clients reported more psychopathology, needle sharing, and experience with detox programs. Alcohol use is particularly risky for opiate addicts who have had hepatitis, because of the added harm to the liver. Although most addicts with alcohol problems developed the alcohol problems prior to enrolling in methadone maintenance, few have received specific treatment for these problems. This may be due to the tendency of alcohol treatment programs to insist on methadone detoxification. Methadone as a medication is not effective in reducing alcohol use. Therefore, clinics need to provide additional psychosocial interventions and support for alcohol-dependent addicts.

Interestingly, continued cannabis use while in methadone maintenance does not appear to compromise medical status or treatment outcome. A high prevalence of methadone clients use marijuana. Saxon, Calsyn, Greenberg, et al. (1993) evaluated correlates of marijuana use during methadone maintenance treatment. Participants who used marijuana did not differ from those who did not use marijuana on neuropsychological testing, methadone dose, time in treatment, employment, or marital status. Furthermore, marijuana use was not associated with use of other, more harmful drugs. The results of this study call into question the need to spend additional clinic funds to screen for marijuana use.

Side Effects. Some opiate-dependent individuals avoid taking methadone for fear of negative side effects. For example, among a sample of incarcerated injection drug users, most expressed ambivalence regarding participation in methadone maintenance. Users reported fears of bone decalcification and overdose, even though these are highly unlikely to occur as results of methadone maintenance participation (Rosenblum, Magura, & Joseph, 1991). In general, methadone produces physical side effects similar to those of other opiates, and these tend to abate with tolerance. However, methadone has fewer side effects than street drugs, because street drugs are often cut with unknown substances. Methadone maintenance may coincide with physical changes emerging after a history of poor diet and hygiene, including sedentary weight gain and dental problems; these changes are usually simultaneous with, but not caused by, methadone maintenance. In women, methadone maintenance usually leads to stabilized hormonal functioning and regular menses, compared to those of women on heroin. Overall, medical evaluations of methadone maintenance participants have reported that even long-term methadone maintenance is not associated with negative medical sequelae (Novick et al., 1993). In a study of 111 male participants who had been maintained on methadone for 11 to 18 years, Kreek et al. (1993) reported no unexpected adverse effects, and general improvements in nutrition.

Withdrawal. Some addicts report that withdrawal from methadone is more protracted and uncomfortable than withdrawal from heroin. Gossop and Strang (1991) compared withdrawal symptoms among 83 opiate addicts in detoxification. Those detoxifying from methadone reported more severe withdrawal symptoms than those detoxifying from heroin, although the onset and duration of withdrawal symptoms were similar between groups. The authors suggest that methadone withdrawal may be more severe than heroin withdrawal, and that detoxification from methadone should involve tapered doses over a period of time.

Cognitive and Psychomotor Effects. Although the euphoric qualities of methadone are markedly less than those of heroin, some people fear that methadone-maintained individuals may not be capable of performing in the workplace or driving on the highways. In fact, most methadone maintenance participants can maintain jobs and operate vehicles safely.

The effects of methadone and other opiates on cognitive and psychomotor functioning have been extensively evaluated and reviewed (Zacny, 1995). Information processing and sustained attention do not appear to be negatively affected in methadone maintenance participants (Appel & Gordon, 1976; Appel, 1982; Kelley, Welch, & McKnelley, 1978; Rothenberg, Schottenfeld, Meyer, Krauss, & Gross, 1977; Walsh, Preston, Stitzer, Cone, & Bigelow, 1994). Similarly, learning and memory have not been shown to be impaired among methadone clients (Kelley et al., 1978). One study (Gritz et al., 1975) found that methadone-maintained individuals performed more poorly on tasks of learning nonsense words than abstinent, formerly opiate-dependent individuals. However, when stimuli were presented within a verbal context, group differences disappeared. Methadone-maintained individuals also perform normally on tests of overall intellectual functioning (Lombardo, Lombardo, & Goldstein, 1976).

Methadone-maintained individuals and nonusers perform similarly on tests of simple motor performance and reaction time (Gordon, 1970; Kelley et al., 1978; Rothenberg et al., 1977). Methadone causes impairments in oculomotor functioning among nondependent individuals, but does not produce these effects in methadone clients who have developed tolerance to opiates (Rothenberg, Schottenfeld, Gross, & Selkoe, 1980a, 1980b). Although methadone did not impair auditory threshold and time perception among methadone-maintained participants in one study, it was associated with overestimation of distances (Kelley et al., 1978).

To further assess the possible influence of opiates on driving, Tennessee Medicaid participants' automobile accidents were examined. Use of benzodiazepines and antidepressants was associated with an increased risk of automobile accidents, but use of oral opiates was not (Ray, Fought, & Decker, 1992). Examinations of Los Angeles traffic fatalities found that only 1 out of 594 drivers had opiates in biological samples (Budd, Muto, & Wong, 1989). Compared with 1,059 nonusers, 152 methadone maintenance participants were not involved in more traffic accidents (Blomberg

& Preusser, 1974). Opiates are safer than barbiturates and alcohol in terms of motor impairments related to driving ability (Stapleton, Guthrie, & Linnoila, 1986). Overall, use of opiates such as methadone does not appear to be associated with increases in intellectual deficits, psychomotor impairments, or automobile accidents (Zacny, 1995).

Outcome Evaluations of Methadone Maintenance

Methadone reduces crime, improves health status, and helps opiate-dependent individuals attain productive lifestyles. Ideally, health and legal risks are drastically reduced or eliminated completely, but society and opiate-dependent individuals experience significant benefits even if negative consequences associated with opiate addiction are only partially reduced. The risks methadone can reduce are clear. Because it is a legally obtained drug, users can remove themselves from the world of illicit drugs and crime; this results in significant societal benefits (reduced property crimes, prostitution, drug pushing, and demands on the criminal justice system), as well as individual benefits (fewer legal and social problems). The successes of methadone in reducing crime, death, disease, and drug use are well documented (Anglin & McGlothlin, 1984; Ball & Ross, 1991; Dole et al., 1968, 1969; Gerstein & Harwood, 1990; Gunne & Gronbladh, 1981; Hubbard et al., 1984; Institute of Medicine, 1995; Newman & Whitehill, 1979).

As described earlier, the first trials of methadone maintenance outcome were performed in New York by Dole and Nyswander (see Dole et al., 1968). They noted that most clients remained in treatment as long as it was available. They also found that participants used some illicit drugs in the first few weeks, but that this usually fell off gradually, in contrast to the rapid return to drugs observed in detoxified participants. Dole et al. also reported a steady increase in employment and a dramatic reduction in criminal behavior. Those randomly assigned to methadone maintenance rather than to a nonmaintenance treatment modality made statistically significant improvements in drug use, criminal involvement, employment, education, and child rearing.

The Treatment Outcome Prospective Study examined the outcomes of over 11,000 drug users and found that treatment retention was the single best predictor of treatment success, and that methadone programs had better retention rates than therapeutic communities, drug-free outpatient treatment, and chemical dependency treatment (Hubbard et al., 1984). Anglin and McGlothlin (1984) studied the sociological sequelae of the initiation of methadone maintenance in California in 1971. They examined the criminal involvement of heroin-dependent individuals under supervision by the state Civil Addict Program for prior criminal convictions. After the state supervision ended, those who enrolled in methadone maintenance remained significantly less involved in crime than those who did not enroll throughout the 3-year follow-up period. Ball and Ross (1991) also demonstrated substantial reductions in crime for 617 men in methadone maintenance. Participants reduced criminal activity by 79% after starting the methadone program; the reduction was greater for those who were in treatment longer. Although crime was not eliminated altogether, the reduction is very impressive.

Health risks have been found to be significantly reduced for methadone maintenance participants. Because methadone is administered orally, risks associated with injection are reduced, including HIV, hepatitis B, endocarditis, skin infections, vein deterioration, and abscesses (see Chaisson et al., 1989; McLachlan et al., 1993; Metzger et al., 1993; Serpelloni et al., 1994; Siddiqui et al., 1993). HIV risk associated with sexual behavior is also reduced, because methadone participants report lower numbers of past-year sex partners than do addicts not in methadone programs, even after adjustments for demographic factors are made. This reduction in sexual risk is positively related to length of time in treatment (Longshore, Hsieh, & Anglin, 1994). HIV-positive methadone maintenance participants have a substantially delayed onset of AIDS-related illnesses (Sorensen, Batki, Good, & Wilkinson, 1989). Finally, methadone reduces the health risks resulting from the unknown composition of street drugs, as well as the health risks associated with opiate withdrawal syndrome (Umbricht-Schneiter, Ginn, Pabst, & Bigelow, 1994).

Pregnant opiate-dependent women who participate in methadone treatment programs have reduced risks to their fetuses (Chang, Carroll, Behr, & Kosten, 1992; Dawe, Gerada, & Strang, 1992; Doberczak, Kandall, & Friedmann, 1993; Jarvis & Schnoll, 1994). Neonates born to methadone-maintained mothers tend to have lower birth weights overall, but no remarkable developmental abnormalities. If methadone programs take the opportunity to provide good prenatal care, nutritional counseling, and parenting skill classes, the incidence of low birth weight, prematurity, and morbidity is significantly reduced (Zweben & Sorensen, 1988).

Carroll, Chang, Behr, and Clinton (1995) randomly assigned 20 pregnant woman addicted to opiates to standard or enhanced methadone maintenance programs. Standard treatment consisted of daily methadone administration, weekly group counseling sessions, and urinalysis screening three times per week. Enhanced treatment added weekly prenatal care, relapse prevention groups, awards for abstinence, and child care availability during treatment visits. No group differences in concomitant use of other drugs were reported; however, women in the enhanced program had fewer premature births and heavier, healthier babies. These findings supported those of previous studies (Chang et al., 1992) which indicated that enhanced methadone treatment is safe and reduces risks for pregnant women. It should be noted that withdrawal from opiates stimulates uterine contractions, and that even gradual detoxification causes stress to the fetus (American Psychiatric Association, 1994b). In summary, methadone maintenance is safe for pregnant women and is associated with substantial improvements in the health of both mothers and babies.

Recommendations for Optimal Methadone Maintenance Programming

Methadone is dispensed under widely varying systems worldwide. Methadone may be dispensed through hospitals, general drug treatment facilities, private physicians, and free-standing methadone clinics. Units may be for-profit, nonprofit, or state-operated. In most European nations and Australia, methadone delivery is linked to public health programs. Differences in delivery influence addict retention rates and success. In a 1994 statement, the American Psychiatric Association recommended expanding public support for methadone treatment programs that offer counseling, occupational rehabilitation, and primary medical care. However, the statement condemned programs that abuse this treatment modality, particularly programs that offer take-home dosages primarily to reduce costs and skimp on adjunct services that are crucial to successful treatment outcome (American Psychiatric Association, 1994b).

In a recent survey of U.S. methadone programs, D'Aunno and Vaughn (1992) reported that these programs differ with regard to profit-making status, staff backgrounds, abstinence versus maintenance goals, dosage levels, take-home dosage privileges, client influence on program policies, and client awareness of dosage level. Many programs have practices that are not consonant with recommendations from methadone researchers. In particular, many programs provide methadone at dosages that are much lower than those recommended for client retention. In a 3-year outcome study of six methadone maintenance clinics, Ball and Ross (1991) reported that clinic factors contributed significantly to treatment outcome. Director and staff competence, a low staff turnover rate, and close staff–participant relationships were associated with effective treatment.

Although methadone programs in the United States operate under a wide array of practices, an exemplary program is described here to illustrate how effective methadone delivery can be designed. Evergreen Treatment Services, one of several methadone clinics in Seattle, Washington, is a nonprofit methadone delivery service. Addicts seeking methadone treatment must complete a two-step intake process. First, prospective clients undergo a psychological and social intake. Next, they must abstain from all opiates for a period of 24 hours, so that withdrawal symptoms can be demonstrated and documented in a medical intake evaluation. If sufficient withdrawal symptoms are noted, admission to methadone treatment proceeds. Most clients report histories of opiate addiction lasting 1 year or longer, as well as current addiction. Pregnant women are exempted from the "sick intake" requirement, due to the possibility of adverse fetal consequences of opiate withdrawal.

Prospective clients are typically placed on a 2-week or longer waiting list until a treatment slot becomes available. Once admitted, clients have access to limited on-site primary medical care, tuberculosis testing and treatment, HIV testing, psychiatric care, and disulfiram (Antabuse) for alcohol problems. Participation requires clinic visits 6 days per week for the first 90 days. After that, take-home dose privileges are available for clients with drug-free urinalyses who are involved in productive activities, such as employment or school. All methadone clinic records are subject to stringent Drug Enforcement Agency, FDA, and state regulatory authority and inspection. Detected use of cocaine, amphetamines, tranquilizers, or marijuana may be grounds for dismissal.

Low-Threshold Programs. Methadone maintenance can only be as effective as the number of opiate-dependent individuals who enroll. As discussed in Chapter 2 (see also Engelsman, 1989), the Dutch have employed a strategy of low-threshold drug treatment programs to allow any addict interested in behavior change into the treatment system. Treatment providers perform fieldwork in the streets, hospitals, and jails; provide programs that offer material support and social rehabilitation opportunities; and deliver services in a respectful manner. Brief courses or seminars in changing addictive behaviors are available, as are outpatient and intensive inpatient treatment facilities. Low-threshold programs have no admission requirement for commitment to abstinence or drug testing.

The Jellinekcentre in Amsterdam utilizes a mobile methadone clinic (the "methadone bus") to reach addicts in their own neighborhoods. Individuals can obtain methadone from the methadone bus only if they are in contact with a doctor and are enrolled in the program. Needle exchange, condoms, and first-aid materials are available upon request. Additional help and family assistance can be arranged if needed. Once in contact with an addict, outreach workers can lead the individual to seek further help and take steps toward a healthier lifestyle (Marlatt & Tapert, 1993). Participants can be reached with counseling, motivational enhancement strategies, and possibly referrals to therapeutic communities and vocational/educational resources. Mobile methadone delivery and health services may make methadone services more readily accessible to participants in the United States as well (Besteman & Brady, 1994).

The requirements of methadone maintenance participation contribute greatly to variance in treatment outcome, client satisfaction, and local controversy. Methadone may be dispensed with or without counseling, with or without urinalysis testing for illicit drug use, and with or without clients' contracting not to use illicit drugs while enrolled in the program. Varying federal, state, and local policies dictate how methadone distribution is handled. The following discussion gives further suggestions for optimal methadone service delivery, based on findings from researchers in this field.

Improving Treatment Access: Rapid Intake and Alternative Maintenance Formats. Briefer assessment procedures are believed to foster client motivation, to lead to less illicit drug use during treatment, and to enhance client retention (Bell et al., 1994). Prolonged intake evaluations to discourage undecided addicts from treatment may result in missed opportunities to demonstrate the benefits of methadone to opiate addicts. Budgetary constraints, as well as recent requirements to expand treatment slots rapidly to prevent the spread of HIV, are resulting in "interim" methadone maintenance clinics. Such clinics provide a very brief intake with a single physical examination, followed by nurse-administered methadone, AIDS education, and condoms. Interim clinics do not provide counseling or other services, just referrals. Clients may be on waiting lists for comprehensive treatment programs while participating in interim clinics. This service system has been criticized for not providing enough treatment for participants. However, minimal services may be better than none, especially in HIV-affected communities.

Yancovitz et al. (1991) randomly assigned 301 opiate-dependent individuals to interim methadone clinics or a waiting-list condition. Interim clinic participants reduced their heroin use by 50% in 1 month, as confirmed by urinalysis. Many interim clinic participants also enrolled in comprehensive treatment programs. Cocaine use, however, did not decrease. The authors conclude that interim services should not be viewed as a substitute for comprehensive methadone delivery, but they strongly recommend implementation of interim services instead of placing addicts on waiting lists.

Another recommendation for making methadone maintenance treatment available to a broader range of opiate-dependent individuals is to permit physicians to prescribe methadone. This format presents advantages over methadone clinics for some participants. Methadone clinics can be geographically distant; clinic procedures may entail long waits; and participants may come into contact with active drug users at or en route to the clinic. Receiving methadone from physicians' offices or health maintenance organizations may be more convenient and less costly than participation in methadone clinics for some individuals.

Senay et al. (1993) randomly assigned successful methadone maintenance participants to different methadone maintenance formats. They found that the reduced frequency of physician office visits was not associated with differential participant benefit, but with cost-effectiveness. Furthermore, participants reported preferring the physician office format because visits were less frequent and more convenient than prior methadone clinic experiences. Novick et al. (1994) supported these findings by transferring successful, long-term methadone participants to internists and family practitioners. They reported good retention and the possibility of broader methadone availability, requiring only brief physician training. This allows opiate-dependent individuals to receive a designated supply of methadone from a private local setting. Medical maintenance is recommended for participants who have been successfully stabilized on methadone for a period of time. Methadone is available by physician prescription in the United Kingdom and Australia (Gaughwin et al., 1993).

Long-Term Methadone Maintenance. Long-term methadone maintenance programs offer advantages over abstinence-based or tapering methadone programs (Caplehorn, 1994). Long-term maintenance participants have lower rates of illicit heroin use and are less likely to seek other methadone maintenance programs following discharge—findings suggesting lower rates of relapse.

Many methadone programs require clients to take urinalyses on a regular or random schedule, and if results indicate use of illicit drugs beyond what program regulations allow, the user is often refused further methadone and is forced to detoxify. This requires the client to experience the full effects of withdrawal, and most relapse to using street drugs, with their associated risks (Ball & Ross, 1991; McLellan, Arndt, Metzger, Woody, & O'Brien, 1993; Powell, Gray, & Bradley, 1993). Decisions regarding termination of drug-abusing clients present a clinical dilemma. Even if a client is still using drugs or alcohol regularly, is he or she benefiting from treatment? If the client was injecting heroin daily before methadone maintenance and now injects heroin every other day, are the reductions in risk clinically significant? On the other hand, will the threat of detoxification motivate some clients to cease illicit drug use? If the clinic has a long waiting list, which individual should get a treatment slot—a client who is still using, or someone on the waiting list? Discharging HIV-positive clients presents a further ethical dilemma, because they may relapse to injection drug use and become involved in needle sharing, which spreads HIV.

The American Psychiatric Association states, "Many patients need methadone maintenance for 5–10 years, and some patients may need a lifetime of treatment. Two years appears to be the minimum duration before detoxification is attempted" (1994b, p. 793). Although this may seem lengthy, retention is the best predictor of long-term positive outcome (Hubbard et al., 1984). In addition, time-limited methadone programs may not be as effective in reducing the use of other drugs (Bell, Chan, & Kuk, 1995).

Adequate Dosing. Programs differ in terms of philosophies of treatment duration, and dosing policies tend to differ likewise. Both variables have major implications for treatment effectiveness. For optimal relapse prevention, the American Psychiatric Association (1994a) recommends daily methadone dosages at 60–120 mg/day for at least 2 years before detoxification is attempted. However, only 9% of respondents to a nationwide survey of methadone programs waited beyond 2 years to encourage clients to detoxify, and only 3% of programs reported average dose levels above the recommended 60 mg/day (D'Aunno & Vaughn, 1992). A strong association has been reported between methadone dose and illicit heroin use. Participants on doses of 40 mg/day are more likely to test positive for heroin use than participants on doses of 80 mg/day (Bell et al., 1995). Another study found that when methadone maintenance participants were permitted to regulate personal methadone dose, increases in dosing did not occur (Maddux, Desmond, & Vogtsberger, 1995).

Contingency Contracting and Positive versus Negative Reinforcers. Strategies to reduce substance use among methadone participants have focused on implementing positive or negative consequences to participants for "clean" or "dirty" urine screens. Some programs ask clients to sign a contract promising not to use illicit drugs while in the program. Toxicology screens confirm subsequent behavior. Negative consequences, such as dose reduction, methadone detoxification, and program discharge, often follow "dirty" screens. Contracting and aversive reinforcers yield mixed results. Contingent dose reduction does not appear to enhance program efficacy (Iguchi, Stitzer, Bigelow, & Liebson, 1988); however, methadone clients who contract to discharge if substance use is detected appear to use illicit drugs less than clients who do not sign such contracts. Nonstimulant abusers who have been in treatment for long periods of time appear to respond particularly well (Saxon, Calsyn, Kivlahan, & Roszell, 1993). However, participants who are discharged are more likely to return to a drug-using, high-risk lifestyle, because they cannot or will not live up to their contracts (Calsyn et al., 1994; Dolan, Black, Penk, Robinowitz, & DeFord, 1985). In light of the high rate of HIV among injection drug users and lack of treatment on demand, this strategy is not recommended for all methadone clients.

In contrast, positive reinforcers, such as increased or supplemental dose levels (Higgins, Stitzer, Bigelow, & Liebson, 1986), money (McCaul, Stitzer, Bigelow, & Liebson, 1984), take-home dose privileges (Pani, Pirastu, Ricci, & Gessa, 1996), and retail vouchers, may be preferable because they do not lead to program discharge. Higgins, Budney, Bickel, Foerg, et al. (1994) reported that treatment retention rates in their program at the University of Vermont were improved significantly by offering voucher incentives to cocaine-dependent participants. The vouchers were redeemable for merchandise, and were awarded to participants for submission of drug-free urine specimens. Whereas only 40% of participants in the no-voucher group completed 24 weeks of treatment, 75% of those in the voucher group completed 24 weeks of treatment. In addition, those in the voucher group demonstrated greater success in maintaining abstinence goals, and greater improvement on the Drug and Psychiatric scales of the Addiction Severity Index. Although these participants were in treatment for cocaine addiction, similar strategies may prove useful in methadone programs.

Some participants travel great distances to their nearest methadone clinic, and this daily visit can be burdensome. Take-home doses of methadone allow participants flexibility in daily schedules by allowing them to skip visits to the clinic. Providing take-home dose incentives contingent on clean urinalyses has been associated with clinically mean-ingful improvements in urine test rates (Stitzer, Iguchi, & Felch, 1992).

Pani et al. (1996) recently examined the influence of a take-home dose policy to reinforce drug-free urine screens. Participants were rewarded with take-home doses when drug-free screens were submitted, and take-home privileges were removed when drug-positive screens were submitted. Among participants who had positive screens before the take-home policy, a 25% reduction in rates of positive screens was evidenced. Some studies have not found decreases in illicit drug use, but instead have found improvements in attendance at adjunctive therapy sessions, which increased in proportion to the number of days take-home doses were awarded (Kidorf, Stitzer, Brooner, & Goldberg, 1994; Stitzer et al., 1977). The possibility that take-home dosages may result in diversionary sale of methadone on the street can be controlled for by random recalls of take-home supplies, at which the client is asked to display the expected level of methadone remaining in the container. Convergence of empirical findings supports use of contingent take-home dose incentives to encourage abstinence.

Counseling Services. It seems intuitive that psychosocial counseling and occupational rehabilitation administered in concert with methadone maintenance should enhance participant adjustment to a new lifestyle. However, counseling is not always effective for all participants. One source of variability is the counselor. McLellan, Woody, Luborsky, and Goehl (1988) compared the patients of four different methadone clinic counselors. They found the most improvement among patients of a counselor who demonstrated a high level of organization, took thorough notes, accurately anticipated problems, and possessed good psychotherapy skills. Patients who were seen by a disorganized counselor who did not document cases well actually worsened. A second source of variability is participant characteristics. In particular, counseling helps methadone participants with significant psychiatric problems, which are relatively common. This benefit is most marked when psychotherapists are fully integrated into the methadone program (Woody et al., 1983). A third source of variability is participant interest in receiving counseling. For example, participants report that more counseling services are needed during tapering from methadone, to provide support through the physical discomfort experienced during tapering (Gold, Sorensen, McCanlies, Trier, & Dlugosch, 1988). Some studies report that counseling is less critical to outcome than other factors, such as use of contingency contracting (Calsyn et al., 1994) and participant involvement in decisions regarding methadone dose (Maddux et al., 1995). Overall, research suggests that counseling may be a useful adjunct to methadone maintenance treatment for some individuals and should be readily available, but it should not be a mandatory component of all methadone maintenance programs.

Methadone-maintained individuals with comorbid depression respond well to ancillary antidepressant therapy. Most antidepressants do not necessarily improve substance use patterns, but result in improvements on measures of mood state, and no interactive side effects have been reported (Nunes, Quitkin, Brady, & Post-Koenig, 1994; Titievsky, Seco, Barranco, & Kyle, 1982). A study by Margolin, Kosten, Petrakis, Avants, and Kosten (1991) demonstrated reductions in cocaine use when the antidepressant bupropion was administered to five methadone maintenance participants. An early study by Spensley (1974) demonstrated that tricyclic antidepressants reduced withdrawal symptoms in 25 of 27 methadone-maintained individuals.

Emphasis on Client Satisfaction. An emphasis on client satisfaction with a program contributes greatly to lower-dropout rates and improved treatment outcome (Joe, Simpson, & Hubbard, 1991). Because methadone programs remove the menace of withdrawal, they have the potential for bringing opiate-dependent individuals into treatment who otherwise might avoid it, and thus for bringing these addicts into contact with other services. Clinics need to be flexible enough to accommodate the wide range of lifestyles of the clients they serve. Clinic hours and location need to be convenient. Clinic staffs need to be respectful of clients, helpful, and aware of the problems they face. Methadone should be used as a tool to work with the clients to facilitate behavior change. Client input may also facilitate retention and appropriate program policies. The National Alliance of Methadone Advocates puts out a guide for participants who wish to start their own methadone program (Gilmore & Bowers, 1995). A useful study would compare an "expert"-operated program to one developed by the individuals it serves.

Summary of Recommendations. At this time, methadone is the most thoroughly studied and most effective method for reducing the harm caused to addicts and society by opiates. Based on existing research, several methods are recommended for methadone maintenance programs to yield maximum harm reduction:

- Foster an environment conducive to low staff turnover.
- Make treatment available to opiate-dependent individuals who haven't achieved abstinence yet.
- Expand the availability of services through mobile or physician office methadone delivery.
- When treatment slots are not available, provide rapid intake and interim services instead of putting people on waiting lists.
- Allow long or indefinite durations of maintenance treatment.
- Provide sufficient doses of methadone (e.g., 80–120 mg/day).
- Employ contingency contracting with take-home doses and vouchers as incentives.
- Offer (but don't require) counseling and vocational training, and strongly encourage counseling for participants with psychiatric needs.

- Finally, maximize participant input to program operations and policies.

L-Alpha-Acetylmethadol (LAAM)

Although the benefits of LAAM (also known as acetylmethadol) have been indicated by research since the 1970s, this drug has not been widely used in the treatment of human opiate dependence. Research diminished until LAAM was approved by the FDA as a maintenance treatment agent for opiate dependence in 1993. LAAM is a compound that is metabolized in the liver into two long-acting metabolites with potent opioid (mu agonist) activity (Jaffe, 1995). Like methadone, LAAM produces marked cross-tolerance to opiates. Animal models suggest that withdrawal from LAAM is less severe than withdrawal from morphine or methadone in opiate-dependent rats (Young, Moreton, Meltzer, & Khazan, 1977). In humans, withdrawal symptoms are similar to those experienced during methadone withdrawal (Jaffe, 1995).

LAAM is administered orally, like methadone; however, it prevents withdrawal symptoms for 72 hours, compared to just 24 hours with methadone. Opiate-dependent individuals using LAAM as a maintenance treatment need to visit a clinic only three times per week for dosing. Peak effects are experienced 4 hours following administration—a more delayed onset than methadone. LAAM is typically dispensed on Monday–Wednesday–Friday schedules, at 50–90 mg/day with a 40% increase in the Friday dose (Ling, Rawson, & Compton, 1994).

Results of LAAM trials with humans were first reported in 1970 (Jaffe, Schuster, Smith, & Blachly, 1970), and it was found to be an effective alternative to methadone in treating opiate dependence. In a later study (Wilson, Spannagel, & Thomson, 1976), LAAM was administered to heroin-addicted individuals three times per week; heroin-dependent individuals receiving daily doses of methadone served as the comparison group. Overall, no significant differences were found in terms of social adjustment or drug abuse patterns for heroin addicts treated with LAAM versus methadone. However, participants who received LAAM had increased motor activity, irritability, and restlessness, which suggested a mild stimulant effect of LAAM. These effects were most prominent in the early stages of treatment and appeared to abate with tolerance. Interestingly, LAAM is more active when administered orally than by injection (Ling et al., 1994).

Overall, LAAM is as effective as methadone in reducing heroin use and associated behaviors. For reasons that remain unclear, participants are somewhat more likely to drop out of LAAM treatment or to request transfer to methadone (Jaffe et al., 1970). This may be due to a perception that the drug is not taking effect. FDA regulations do not permit take-home doses of LAAM or use of this drug with pregnant women. Use of LAAM appears particularly beneficial for opiate-dependent individuals (1) who have transportation or scheduling problems that make daily clinic visits burdensome; or (2) who have developed a negative impression of methadone from either personal experiences or hearsay.

Buprenorphine

Although not approved for general use, buprenorphine (Bruprenex) is under investigation as a maintenance strategy for opiate addiction. It was first proposed as a pharmacotherapeutic agent for treating drug dependence in 1978 (Jasinski, Pevnick, & Griffith, 1978). Buprenorphine is an analgesic with properties of both an opiate agonist and an opiate antagonist. This means that it satiates addicted opioid receptors, offsetting withdrawal symptoms, and that it also blocks effects of subsequently administered opiates.

Opiate-dependent and nondependent participants report subjective experiences after buprenorphine use similar to those following methadone and heroin use (Jasinski et al., 1978). Side effects are also similar, with the exception that buprenorphine does not appear to depress respiratory functioning as much as other opiates do (Cowan, Doxey, & Harry, 1977). This improves the safety profile of buprenorphine and permits administration of higher doses. Buprenorphine has a ceiling for drug effects, so that higher doses simply stretch the duration of the effects instead of raising their intensity. Agonist activity appears to last for 24 hours, but may last longer with increased doses near 16 mg (Walsh et al., 1994), suggesting that buprenorphine could be therapeutically administered every other day or possibly every third day. Antagonist activity does not appear to extend beyond 24 hours without readministration (Bickel et al., 1988a). A further advantage of buprenorphine is that the withdrawal symptoms are somewhat milder than withdrawal from full opiate agonists such as morphine and methadone (Fudala, Jaffe, Dax, & Johnson, 1990; Kosten, Morgan, & Kleber, 1991).

Several studies have examined the efficacy of buprenorphine maintenance in reducing illicit drug use. A randomized trial comparing buprenorphine to methadone reported that both medications were equally effective in minimizing illicit opiate use and suppressing withdrawal (Bickel, Johnson, Stitzer, & Bigelow, 1987). However, another study (Kosten, Schottenfeld, Ziedonis, & Falcioni, 1993) compared buprenorphine and methadone in 125 opiate addicts, and reported that buprenorphine was less successful than methadone in reducing number of days of illicit opiate use and money spent on illicit opiates. Retention rates of buprenorphine maintenance programs appear comparable to those of methadone programs (Johnson, Jaffe, & Fudala, 1992; Kosten et al., 1991; Strain, Stitzer, Liebson, & Bigelow, 1994). Buprenorphine also shows promise in reducing use of cocaine and "speedballs" (heroin and cocaine combined) (Kosten, Kleber, & Morgan, 1989).

Overall, buprenorphine appears comparable to methadone in terms of client satisfaction, and as effective or almost as effective in reducing illicit drug use (Bickel et al., 1988b; Rosen & Kosten, 1991). This medication provides another alternative to opiate-dependent individuals seeking to reduce drug-related harm.

Prescribed Heroin

As described in Chapter 2, the Merseyside Drug Dependency Service in Liverpool, England, provides legal prescriptions for cocaine or heroin to addicts for personal use. The idea is to keep opiate-dependent individuals off the street and away from illicit drugs. A primary goal is to prevent injection, but some addicts whose preferred route is injection are permitted to do so in a physician's office with a clean syringe. Drugs are also made available in smokable form ("reefer" cigarettes) and in oral forms. The results of this highly controversial program appeared promising in one evaluation (O'Hare et al., 1992): The HIV rate was held to 5% among opiate addicts in Liverpool (much lower than in other U.K. cities), and drug-related crime in Liverpool decreased. The rigorous evaluation of prescribed heroin maintenance in Switzerland is discussed in Chapter 2.

Some researchers report that snorting and smoking heroin ("chasing the dragon") may be growing in popularity as alternatives to injecting the drug (Jenkins, Keenan, Henningfield, & Cone, 1994; Schuckit, 1995). Although "dragon chasers" may experience the same opiate dependence symptoms as heroin injectors do, these individuals do not appear particularly likely to move on to opiate injection (Gossop, Griffiths & Strang, 1988). By smoking heroin instead of injecting, these individuals place themselves at risk for fewer health problems. If heroin injectors are unable or unwilling to attempt existing forms of treatment, changing the route of drug administration may reduce some risks. Prescribing heroin in noninjection formats may reduce criminal involvement and serious health risks such as HIV.

Not all heroin users are heroin-dependent, although heroin-dependent individuals clearly capture the bulk of attention in the mass media and the scientific literature. Zinberg (1979) reviewed the scant literature of the 1970s on nonaddictive opiate use and described factors related to controlled use. In his study of 90 controlled opiate users, Zinberg reported that most of these "chippers" did not go on to addictive opiate use. Most evidenced consistent use patterns over time. Although some reported past episodes of compulsive opiate use, these periods were significantly briefer than periods of controlled use. The majority of the study participants were gainfully employed or in college. Although no distinct personality patterns were noted, similarities in the management of drug use emerged. Controlled users placed limits on their heroin use, such as only using on weekends. Social sanctions and rituals limited the diversity of contexts in which heroin was used and created peer norms for avoiding harmful drug risks. These social sanctions were articulated explicitly by participants; they included using heroin only in safe situations that did not interfere with work and "testing" the drug before taking more to avoid overdose. These chippers also reported refusing to share injection equipment—a notable finding, as this research was completed before HIV emerged as a major public health problem.

Ibogaine

Ibogaine is a rainforest indole alkaloid derived from the root of *Tabernanthe iboga,* a shrub that grows in west central Africa. Ibogaine has long been used by native peoples in low doses to treat illnesses and to combat fatigue. It is used in higher doses for hallucinogenic properties in religious rituals. The use of *iboga* (ibogaine and associated alkaloids) in Bwiti initiation ceremonies has been studied by ethnologists in Gabon (Goutarel, Gollnhofer, & Sillans, 1993). Unlike methadone, LAAM, and buprenorphine, ibogaine is not a substitute for narcotics, and it is not addicting (Mash, 1995).

Physiological responses to ibogaine have been examined since the early 1900s. In the 1950s, Ciba-Geigy Pharmaceuticals investigated the antihypertensive properties of ibogaine, but discontinued research because of skepticism over its commercial value (Mash, 1995). Ibogaine was reported as a beneficial adjunct to psychotherapy by Claudio Naranjo (1973), a Chilean psychotherapist and physician. Howard Lotsof, an American filmmaker and political activist, found that ibogaine was particularly useful in treating opiate addiction, based on his own experience and that of his friends since the early 1960s. Over a period from 1985 to 1992, Lotsof received patent rights for use of ibogaine in the treatment of narcotic, stimulant, alcohol, nicotine, and polydrug dependence. Investigations of ibogaine's physiological properties, toxicity, and mechanisms of action for treating drug dependence were prompted by activists' reports that a single dose could virtually eliminate opiate withdrawal and cravings for cocaine and heroin. Lotsof (1995) and others describe the effect of ibogaine as "interrupting" the addiction.

Laboratory studies have determined that ibogaine indeed attenuates opiate withdrawal (Dzoljic, Kaplan, & Dzoljic, 1988; Glick, Rossman, Rao, Maisonneuve, & Carlson, 1992) and reduces morphine self-administration in rats (Glick, Rossman, Steindorf, Maisonneuve, & Carlson, 1992). Using radioligand binding assays, Sweetnam et al. (1995) found that ibogaine interacts at a wide variety of neurotransmitter receptors. These include the mu, delta, kappa, and sigma opioid receptors, as well as dopamine, norepinephrine, and serotonin uptake sites. A possible mechanism for reduced drug craving following ibogaine ingestion relates to its action at opioid receptors. Ibogaine binds weakly to the NMDA receptor, acting as a competitive inhibitor of MK-801 (Mash et al., 1995; Popik, Layer, & Skolnick, 1994). MK-801 is an excitatory amino acid antagonist that has been associated with attenuation of opiate tolerance (Marek, Ben-Eliyahu, Gold, & Liebeskind, 1991; Trujillo & Akil, 1991).

Cocaine self-administration in rodents is also reduced by ibogaine (Cappendijk & Dzoljic, 1993; Sershen, Hashim, & Lajtha, 1993). Animal models show that ibogaine reverses cocaine-induced changes in dopamine levels (Broderick, Phelan, & Berger, 1992; Maisonneuve, Keller, & Glick, 1991; Maisonneuve, Rossman, Keller, & Glick, 1991; Sershen, Hashim, Harsing, & Lajtha, 1992) and reduces motor activity and side effects related to cocaine administration (Broderick, Phelan, Eng, & Wechsler, 1994; Sershen et al., 1992). Multiple administrations over time appear to yield greater reductions in morphine and cocaine self-administration (Cappendijk & Dzoljic, 1993; Glick, Rossman, Steindorf, et al., 1992).

The results of preclinical animal studies thus indicate great promise for the use of ibogaine in treatment of addiction, but official enthusiasm has been tempered by studies indicating selective loss of Purkinje cells in the cerebellar vermis of rats (O'Hearn & Molliver, 1993). However, these findings have not been replicated in primates, and the rodents in O'Hearn and Molliver's research received higher doses than are required for therapeutic effects. The authors propose that the toxicity observed in rats may be caused by release of excitatory amino acids in the inferior medullary olive, rather than by the direct effect of ibogaine itself. This hypothesis is under investigation at Johns Hopkins University. In addition, three deaths among human subjects worldwide have been associated with ibogaine treatment, although the causes of death in these cases appear to have been preexisting health problems and simultaneous use of other drugs. Nonetheless, these reports have added to the concerns of government officials who are skeptical about funding research for a Schedule I hallucinogenic drug to treat drug addiction.

Further studies on the potential neurotoxic properties of ibogaine are warranted. However, the risks of damage must be considered in the context of risks to untreated addicts. Significant numbers of drug addicts die every year from overdose, violence, injection-related health problems, and other risks associated with hard drug use (10 deaths per 1,000 per year among untreated opiate addicts; American Psychiatric Association, 1994a). Other addicts experience physiological damage as a direct result of substance abuse. Although "as little harm as possible" is the goal in treatment development, what is an acceptable level of risk?

Addict self-help groups from the Netherlands, U.S. activists, and physicians who have observed ibogaine treatment sessions have continued to push for research funding and investigation of ibogaine in humans. These activists have seen addicts who received ibogaine treatment and did not experience withdrawal (Lotsof, Della Sera, & Kaplan, 1995), were no longer interested in using intoxicating substances and also were not chained to maintenance treatment (Lotsof, 1995). In fact, some individuals who underwent ibogaine treatment dramatically changed their lifestyle: They were observed to resume healthy weight, eat better, reduce alcohol consumption, and quit smoking!

Preclinical and clinical trials have begun to establish the safety of ibogaine in human volunteers. The FDA has approved the use of limited doses of ibogaine in research, which may increase if results are encouraging. Mash and colleagues at the University of Miami are investigating the neurological and neuropsychological effects of ibogaine on drug-dependent male volunteers who received ibogaine treatments in Panama. Preliminary results for six subjects were reported at the Symposium on Maturational Issues in Behavioral Disorders in Maastricht, the Netherlands (Mash, 1995). Participant behavior was assessed before, during, and after treatment on a wide variety of addiction and withdrawal symptom checklists, psychiatric screenings, mood profiles, and neuropsychological tests. Participants were evaluated for cerebellar and extrapyramidal signs by neurological exam.

Ibogaine was not associated with neurobehavioral impairments for the dose range tested. While under the direct influence of ibogaine, participants first exhibited mild tremor and transient ataxia. Next, participants reported vivid visual images that some described as repressed memories. The content of the visual images produced fearful emotions in some participants. Tremors, ataxia, and vivid visual imagery lasted up to 8 hours. Most participants reported a relaxation period 24 hours after ibogaine ingestion, by which time most of the ibogaine was eliminated, as confirmed by blood and urine samples. However, some participants reported mild insomnia for several days. Participants maintained orientation to time and place and showed no amnesia throughout the ibogaine treatment session. Postibogaine neuropsychological testing did not reveal impairments compared to baseline performance. The chronology of participants' experiences correlated with ibogaine blood levels (Mash, 1995).

A specific clinical procedure for ibogaine treatment has been developed by Lotsof (1995). He describes key elements in the treatment setting to minimize participant discomfort, including building trust and maintaining safety. Some participants may feel more comfortable in the presence of former addicts who are experienced with the treatment procedure (Frenken & Nodelman, 1996). An informal self-help network has been providing ibogaine treatments to addicts in Europe since 1987 (Lotsof, 1995).

Ibogaine is particularly appealing to some opiate-dependent individuals because the ibogaine is administered only one to three times. In contrast, methadone, LAAM, and buprenorphine are designed for use as maintenance or tapering drugs, requiring regular administrations. From the limited data available to date, ibogaine appears to show promise for interrupting addiction in healthy, relatively high-functioning individuals (Lotsof, 1995; Lotsof et al., 1995; Sheppard, 1994).

If the results of toxicity studies allow research to continue in humans, treatment-matching methodology will be appropriate to determine participant factors most strongly associated with improvement. For example, are age, socioeconomic status, psychiatric symptoms, motivation, history of drug abuse, and past experience with hallucinogens related to outcome? Are there risks that participants should be aware of? Controlled clinical studies are required to support reports that either single or repeated ibogaine administrations are effective in treating substance use disorders. Deciding upon an appropriate control drug to use in double-blind studies presents significant challenges to researchers. If subjects and attending physicians are aware of the withdrawal attenuation, hallucinogenic effects, and 24- to 36-hour duration of ibogaine, group assignment can easily be ascertained if effects are not comparable to expectations, and the results will thus be rendered invalid. Furthermore, the criteria for success must be assessed in relation to the outcomes that are possible with existing treatments.

Like other pharmacological agents, ibogaine will probably be most successful if its use is coupled with therapy and appropriate psychosocial support. The interruption of addiction that is proposed to result from ibogaine treatment provides an excellent opportunity to introduce psychotherapy, social skills training, occupational guidance, and medical intervention to treat sequelae of drug abuse.

Ibogaine continues to be controversial, despite numerous documented successes. It is unclear why this promising treatment is not slated for more funding when opiate and cocaine addiction are clearly not going away. Perhaps ibogaine's classification as a hallucinogen conjures up images of Timothy Leary's "Tune in, turn on, and drop out" message of the 1960s in the minds of those who oppose its use. Certainly, reports of toxicity in animals are relevant, but if follow-ups of humans treated with ibogaine do not indicate clinically relevant damage, then the benefits seem to outweigh the risks. Although ibogaine probably will not end opiate addiction, it appears that it can provide another much-needed treatment option for opiate-dependent individuals who do not want to become involved in maintenance treatment.

Summary of Harm Reduction Strategies for Opiate Addiction

Methadone maintenance treatment is the best-studied and most successful treatment available to date for opiate addiction. Its success in reducing crime is well documented, which has helped public officials overcome its controversial aspects. LAAM operates similarly to methadone. Although it has been less thoroughly studied, it appears to have comparable treatment efficacy, and provides participants with a less cumbersome clinic visit schedule because of its longer duration of action. Buprenorphine provides yet another alternative to maintenance and tapering forms of opiate treatment. It is not quite as effective in reducing illicit drug use as methadone, but buprenorphine withdrawal appears to be less daunting than methadone withdrawal for addicts.

Although relatively well studied, all the maintenance drugs remain somewhat controversial, largely because of public discomfort with "replacing one drug with another." In addition, some opiate-dependent individuals feel trapped by their continued physical dependence on the maintenance drug. Treatments that facilitate interruption of addiction by single administrations are appealing to these individuals. Ibogaine has been reported to interrupt the addiction process by attenuating withdrawal and significantly reducing cravings for opiates. However, ibogaine is also very controversial, not only because of possible side effects, but due to its hallucinogenic properties.

Opiate addicts come from many walks of life and cannot all be treated by the same method. A wide variety of strategies must be made available to attract opiate-dependent individuals to treatment, including maintenance, tapering, interruption, and nonpharmacological treatments. Determination of treatment efficacy must be compared to risks incurred without treatment. If a treatment appears to reduce the risks associated with opiate use without introducing serious new risks, that treatment should be made available.

COCAINE

Historically, cocaine has been perceived both as relatively safe and as deadly (Gawin & Ellinwood, 1988; Morgan & Zimmer, 1997). The potential for harm associated with cocaine is confounded by such factors as dose, route of administration, patterns of use, and cocaine production (Gold, 1997). Although these variables make understanding the phenomenon of cocaine use more complicated, they are also the variables that are most conducive to harm reduction strategies. This section first briefly describes the history of cocaine use, from the chewing of coca leaves to the smoking of crack cocaine. Subsequently, a summary of the negative consequences associated with cocaine use is provided. Interventions aimed at reducing cocaine use are then summarized, and suggestions for intervening within a harm reduction framework are provided.

History

Cocaine is one of several alkaloids found in the *Erythroxylon coca* plant. The chewing of coca leaves by the Incas and other tribes of the Andes mountains of Peru dates back to before 500 A.D. According to Gold (1997), the amount of cocaine ingested by the Incas was probably low (about 200–300 mg over a 24-hour period). Despite the reports of the stimulating effects of the coca leaf, Europeans were initially unimpressed until a process for extracting cocaine from the coca leaves was developed (Diaz, 1997). Cocaine hydrochloride is the salt or powder form and is water-soluble, so it can be used either intranasally or intravenously. By 1860, the perceived virtues of cocaine led to its addition to wines and tonics, and eventually to a snuff that was advertised as a remedy for asthma and hay fever (Gold, 1997). In 1880 the anesthetic properties of cocaine were described and applied (as cited in Diaz, 1997), and by 1906 both procaine hydrochloride (Novocain) and lidocaine had been synthesized (Diaz, 1997). John Pemberton developed a product that contained two naturally occurring stimulants, cocaine and caffeine, which eventually became known as Coca-Cola; in 1903, cocaine was removed from the formulation in response to public pressure and news reports on the dangers of cocaine (as described by Gold, 1997). The Harrison Narcotic Act of 1914 levied taxes on certain drugs and also increased the amount of paperwork necessary to obtain drugs. It mistakenly listed cocaine as a narcotic and tightened the restrictions on the manufacture and distributions of products that contained coca (Gold, 1997). According to Diaz (1997), there were reports in the early 1900s that cocaine use was reaching epidemic levels among Southern blacks and that it was responsible for a crime wave in the South. In 1914, records in Georgia were examined, and this alleged high use among blacks was not found.

It was not until the 1970s that cocaine use escalated in the United States, especially among middle- and upper-class populations. By 1986, another epidemic of cocaine use had developed. It was estimated that 3 million people abused cocaine regularly, more than five times the number of people addicted to heroin (Gawin & Ellinwood, 1988). Between 1978 and 1982 the routes of administration also changed. "Free-basing" (smoking cocaine in which the adulterants have been removed by boiling with alkali and ether) provides a method of rapid self-administration without intravenous injection. Smoking cocaine provides a more intense euphoria, followed by an intense "crash" that leads to a cycle of use until the user is physically or financially exhausted (Wallace, 1991). Although first reported in the literature in the early 1970s, widespread use of "crack" cocaine in large U.S. cities began in the early 1980s. Media attention began to focus on crack in 1985 (Smith, Wesson, Sees, & Morgan, 1988). Crack is produced by mixing cocaine powder (cocaine hydrochloride) with ammonia or water and baking soda, then heating the mixture to remove the hydrochloride. The remaining substance forms into pebble-sized chunks, which readily burn at moderate temperatures (Smart, 1991). Packaging and marketing techniques include the selling of crack at low prices (ranging from $2 to $20), and instant availability through dealers who often wear beepers to alert them to a need for their goods (Wallace, 1991). Recent reports have suggested that crack smoking is predominant among blacks. It is unclear, however, whether this distribution reflects socioeconomic status or other factors associated with race or ethnic groups (Lillie-Blanton, Anthony, & Schuster, 1993).

Smoking free-base or crack is the most efficient way to get cocaine to the brain, because the drug is absorbed from the lungs to the heart and then to the brain. Because it is smoked, the user feels the effects in less than 10 seconds. Researchers are studying the "rate hypothesis," which posits that the faster a drug occupies enough brain receptors to produce a psychoactive effect, the greater the euphoria it produces and the addiction potential it has. In addition, the "duration of action," or length of time a drug occupies a receptor once it gets there, may also play an important role in the potential for abuse. Smoked cocaine has a fast rate of action and a short duration of action, both of which promote its frequent reuse and abuse (Mathias, 1997). Crack is sometimes confused with free-base cocaine; however, free-base is cocaine in which the adulterants have been removed, whereas crack is a smokable form of cocaine in which the adulterants are still present (Smart, 1991).

Approximately 9% of the U.S. population over age 12 have used cocaine at least once in their lifetimes. In 1996, the National Household Survey on Drug Abuse (NHSDA) estimated that approximately 608,000 (0.3% of the population) were frequent cocaine users (i.e., use on 51 or more days during the past year), and that 668,000 had smoked crack in the past month. The highest rates of cocaine use were found among persons aged 18–25 and 26–34, at 2.0% and 1.5%, respectively (SAMHSA, 1997). Cocaine-related crimes and lost productivity cost U.S. society approximately $10 billion per year (Rand Corporation, 1995).

Cocaine-related consequences are reported more frequently than marijuana-related consequences. When assessed in NHSDA, the most commonly reported consequence was "felt very nervous or anxious" (14%), followed by "became depressed and lost interest in things" (10%). Nineteen percent of past-year cocaine users indicated at least one cocaine-related consequence within that year (National Institute on Drug Abuse [NIDA], 1991). Two or more consequences were reported by 14% of the sample, and almost 10% acknowledged three or more cocaine-related concerns.

Negative Consequences of Cocaine Use

Entire books have been devoted to describing the medical and psychiatric complications associated with cocaine use. Some of the potential harmful consequences associated with cocaine use are described below, with additional recommended readings.

Cardiovascular Consequences

Cocaine blocks the reuptake of the neurotransmitter norepinephrine, producing an excess of norepinephrine in both the central and peripheral nervous system. The resulting cardiovascular effects are tachycardia, vasoconstriction, hypertension, cardiomyopathy, and ventricular arrhythmia

(Chakko & Myerburg, 1995). Complications associated with cocaine use include myocardial ischemia, infarction, coronary spasm, cardiac arrhythmia, myocarditis, dilated cardiomyopathy, acute pulmonary edema, and sudden death (Chakko & Myerburg, 1995; Cregler & Mark, 1986; Cregler, 1991; Isner & Choksi, 1991).

Respiratory Consequences

Recent evidence suggests that smoking crack cocaine can cause acute respiratory symptoms, abnormalities in lung function, and (in some instances) life-threatening acute lung injury.(Tashkin, Gorelick, Khalsa, Simmons, & Chang, 1992).

Neurotoxicity

The euphoria of cocaine has been hypothesized to result from its effect on reward pathways of the brain. Cocaine blocks the reuptake of dopamine into the presynaptic neuron, which leaves greater dopamine in the synaptic cleft, and at the postsynaptic site for stimulation of receptors. Cocaine also blocks the reuptake of other neurotransmitters, including serotonin and (as noted above) norepinephrine. The reinforcing properties of cocaine are hypothesized to be associated with enhanced dopamine transmission in mesocortical pathways (Diaz, 1997). It has been hypothesized that drug-induced changes in the brain may last for many months or even years after abstinence, and one area in which these deficits have been investigated is neurotoxicity (Gold & Miller, 1997). Interested readers should review the monograph edited by Majewska (1996).

One aspect of neurotoxicity that is pertinent to harm reduction and substance abuse treatment is the effect of combinations of cocaine and other drugs. For example, cocaethylene is a metabolic by-product of cocaine ingested in combination with ethyl alcohol (Gorelick, 1992; Landry, 1992). What is interesting about this by-product is that it "represents the only known example of the body producing a third psychoactive drug that is produced exclusively during the co-administration of two drugs of abuse" (Landry, 1992, p. 275). Thus, the coadministration of cocaine and alcohol involves the interaction of three drugs, all of which are psychoactive and toxic (Landry, 1992). This is particularly important, because there is a high prevalence of alcohol dependence among individuals with cocaine dependence (Higgins, Budney, Bickel, Hughes, et al., 1994).

Prenatal Effects

In the late 1980s, the escalation of crack use in inner cities spawned a largely media-driven concern about the offspring of crack-addicted women. "Crack babies" were described as a scourge of inner-city hospitals and a harbinger of the bleak future of urban America. Case studies reported infants with low birth weight and significant developmental delays. However, subsequent research that included examination of other maternal factors, such as alcohol use, cigarette smoking, prenatal nutrition, and infant caretaking, have concluded that the prenatal effects of cocaine are relatively modest in comparison to those produced by alcohol and tobacco (Lester, LaGasse, Freier, & Brunner, 1996; Riley & LaFiette, 1996).

Cocaine use during pregnancy can produce an increased probability of preterm labor, congenital abnormalities, intrauterine growth retardation, low birth weight, neonatal death, and sudden infant death syndrome (Fox, 1994; Miller & Hyatt, 1992; Zuckerman et al., 1989). A 2-year follow-up study found that intrauterine drug exposure could place infants at risk for poor developmental outcome and that cocaine exposure was the single best predictor of head circumference. By 18 months of age, the relative impact of cocaine on head growth had declined, probably as a result of postnatal nutrition and other environmental factors. The authors caution that long-term effects cannot be explained by cocaine exposure alone. Other factors, such as poverty, multigenerational drug use, and the impact of growing up in a drug-seeking environment, may also predict developmental outcomes for children (Chasnoff, Griffith, Freier, & Murray, 1992).

Consequences Related to HIV

Three mechanisms have been proposed to describe the "entangled epidemics" of cocaine use and HIV infection: (1) Cocaine users are at increased risk for HIV exposure; (2) cocaine increases the susceptibility to HIV infection; and (3) cocaine use facilitates the progression of HIV (Edlin et al., 1994; Larrat & Zierler, 1993).

Mitchell Ratner (1993) describes the results of a study funded by NIDA, in which interviews were conducted in "crack houses," in apartments, and on the street with prostitutes, drug dealers, and homeless individuals about trading sex for crack cocaine. In addition, the study explored the increased risk of spreading HIV through "sex-for-crack" exchanges. A NIDA research monograph reviews the HIV risks associated with drug use (Battjes, Sloboda, & Grace, 1994).

Cohen, Navaline, and Metzger (1994) compared crack-abusing women to opioid-abusing women in terms of their involvement in high-risk behaviors and other background variables. These authors concluded that both groups are at elevated risk for HIV because of the behaviors associated with their lifestyles. The crack-abusing group is at risk because of frequent unprotected sexual behavior, particularly when sex is exchanged for crack. In addition, a smaller subgroup is placed at risk by the combination of crack cocaine and injection drug use, because these behaviors frequently include unprotected sex with multiple partners and needle sharing (see Chapter 7).

Psychiatric Consequences

The lifetime prevalence rate of mental disorder diagnoses associated with cocaine abuse is approximately 76% (Regier et al., 1990). Individuals who suffer from DSM-IV Axis I disorders appear to be particularly susceptible to the effects produced by cocaine (Gold, 1997). Approximately 50% of individuals receiving treatment for cocaine abuse meet diagnostic criteria for mood disorders (Gawin & Kleber, 1986). In the past, it was hypothesized that individuals suffering from depression might be self-medicating symptoms through use of cocaine. However, it now appears that one of the changing trends associated with cocaine is that as its use has become more widespread, premorbid psychopathology is less of a risk factor for the development of chronic cocaine abuse (Weiss, Mirin, Griffin, & Michael, 1988).

Although estimates of cocaine abuse among clinical samples may seem elevated because of sampling procedures (due to a phenomenon called "Berckson's fallacy"; see Mueser, Bellack, & Blanchard, 1992), it is also possible for cocaine use to go unrecognized (Shaner et al., 1993). There is a growing interest in the development of procedures that will increase the reliability and validity of diagnosing comorbid substance use and psychiatric disorders (Bryant, Rounsaville, Spitzer, & Williams, 1992; Drake, Rosenberg, & Mueser, 1996).

Treatments for Cocaine Dependence

Pharmacotherapy

According to a report from the U.S. General Accounting Office (U.S. GAO, 1996), 20 medications have been studied for the treatment of cocaine addiction by NIDA's Medications Development Division. Of these, 14 medications have been tested with humans, 5 with animals, and 1 with both humans and animals. According to the report, 6 of the medications studied (buprenorphine, carbamazepine, desipramine, imipramine, mazindol, and nifedipine) were "disappointing," and the remainder had equivocal findings. Although some of these pharmacotherapies may have yielded positive results in one or more clinical trials, "no medication has demonstrated effectiveness" in treating cocaine addicts (U.S. GAO, 1996, p. 3).

Investigators are attempting to use the "rate hypothesis" to guide the development of medications for the treatment of cocaine dependence. Specifically, the goal is to understand and develop a compound that "achieves the precise rate of action and degree of receptor occupancy that is needed to produce a milder effect and longer duration of action than cocaine" (Mathias, 1997, p. 11). Montoya, Hess, Preston, and Gorelick (1994) suggested that part of the difficulty in synthesizing the literature on the pharmacotherapy for cocaine dependence is due to lack of comparability of results from different treatment programs and to poor reliability and validity of research findings. They have proposed a model to standardize data collection across studies, which would allow for comparisons between studies. In addition, it will be important to design studies that have adequate follow-up periods, to assess whether there is a delayed emergence of treatment effects (Carroll et al., 1994).

Goldstein (1994, p. 167) presents another authority's summary of the situation:

> In 1991, a leading expert, Herbert D. Kleber, offered the following assessment: One can sum up the status of the pharmacotherapy of cocaine abuse by noting that a number of positive clinical reports exist, but most reports are anecdotal and uncontrolled ... the nature of addiction requires that pharmacotherapy be combined with appropriate psychological and behavioral therapy. It is unlikely that any "magic bullet" will stop drug addiction in and of itself.

Behavioral Treatment

A number of behavioral therapies have been developed for the treatment of cocaine dependence (see Liese & Najavits, 1997; Onken, Blaine, & Boren, 1993). These include relapse prevention (Carroll, Rounsaville, & Keller, 1991; Wallace, 1991), neurobehavioral therapy (Rawson et al., 1995), community reinforcement/contingency management (Higgins et al., 1993; Higgins, Budney, Bickel, Foerg, et al., 1994), cognitive therapy (Beck, Wright, Newman, & Liese, 1993), cue exposure (Childress et al., 1993), and intensive outpatient treatment (Washton, 1989). One commonality among these interventions is that they all have abstinence as the outcome goal.

The 1996 U.S. GAO report reviewed various types of federally funded treatment approaches evaluated from 1991 to 1995. Overall, the GAO's findings suggested that three cognitive-behavioral approaches have shown early promise for the treatment of cocaine dependence: relapse prevention, community reinforcement/contingency management, and neurobehavioral therapy.

Cost-Effectiveness of Treatment

As described by O'Brien (1996), a recent Rand Corporation study (Everingham & Rydell, 1994) modeled the cost of reducing cocaine use in the United States by 1%. The analysis found that "increasing treatment facilities would accomplish the reduction at a cost 23 times less than reducing the supply in countries where cocaine is grown and 7.3 times less than increasing domestic law enforcement" (O'Brien, 1996, p. 678).

Although increasing treatment may be an important step at reducing cocaine use, it does not necessarily imply that the mode of treatment must be inpatient. Alterman et al. (1994) have found little evidence of differential improvement for individuals who received inpatient as opposed to day treatment. In addition, the costs for day treatment were 40–60% of the costs of inpatient treatment, depending on the measure used.

Harm Reduction Implications

1. *Consider the continuum of harmful use for treatment and research.* In a report by the World Health Organization (1995), cocaine use is described as existing along a continuum. The behaviors along the continuum range from experimental use to occasional use to situation-specific use to intensive use and compulsive/dysfunctional use. The associated negative consequences increase along the continuum. For example, experimental use is associated with low doses of cocaine on one or two occasions, without the relationship, work, legal, or health problems that are associated with compulsive/dysfunctional use.

In addition, it is important to consider that many individuals who use cocaine may also use other drugs. A harm reduction approach will seek to reduce the number of substances used, particularly combinations such as alcohol and cocaine, which produce a third and potentially dangerous psychoactive agent (Gorelick, 1992; Higgins, Budney, Bickel, Hughes, et al., 1994; Landry, 1992).

2. *Increase the probability of sustained success.* Data from 20 years of substance abuse research have shed light on several factors that can enhance treatment success. In particular, effective treatment services need to address more than just the substance abuse, and treatments need to occur for a sufficient duration to allow major life changes to occur. In his recent review of substance abuse treatments, O'Brien (1996) commented: "Unfortunately, the general public often confuses the treatment of withdrawal with the treatment of addiction. Effective treatment of addiction requires a long term approach at reducing the risk of relapse and improving the ability of participants to function in society" (p. 677).

Successful long-term treatment necessitates good treatment retention. Attrition is a challenge in substance abuse treatment, especially with cocaine abusers (Hoffman et al., 1994). Treatment retention is a challenge in drug treatment in general and with cocaine abusers in particular (Hoffman et al., 1994). Increasing the frequency, intensity, and range of treatment services enhances the success of psychosocial treatments. In addition to program variables, it has been suggested that therapist variables should be considered to improve retention (Kleinman et al., 1992).

The provision of psychosocial services (such as employment counseling, psychotherapy, or family therapy) significantly predicted psychosocial adjustment after substance abuse treatment in one study (McLellan et al., 1994). Although the provision of these services was not strongly related to posttreatment alcohol and drug use, it was concluded that "psychosocial sessions and services may be essential to the reduction of psychosocial problems that are so important in the post-treatment environment of a patient and that have such a profound effect on sustained recovery" (p. 1156).

3. *Make it as easy to get services as it is to get drugs.* Most cocaine abusers have not received substance abuse treatment. One assumption is that untreated cocaine abusers have less severe drug use and therefore have a reduced need for treatment. This assumption is challenged by the findings of Carroll and Rounsaville (1992), who compared cocaine abusers seeking treatment to untreated cocaine abusers. The two groups were similar in terms of the severity of cocaine use, use of self-control strategies to restrict cocaine use, and rates of current and lifetime psychiatric disorders. However, the untreated cocaine abusers had higher levels of polysubstance abuse, had greater involvement with the legal system, had longer histories of prison time, spent more days involved in illegal activities, and perceived fewer negative consequences from cocaine use. In addition, the untreated cocaine abusers had less participation in social roles (e.g., employment, stable relationships, and religious affiliations).

Wallace (1991) provides an excellent description of how drug dealers are entrepreneurs and maximize their ability to meet the needs of their clients. Drug dealers are smart and accessible—often more so than treatment providers. Dealers deliver fast-acting, incredibly rewarding, short-duration drugs by car or in person (users can just page them when the supply is low) and will even provide drugs on loan, particularly if a buyer is perceived as a good credit risk (Shaner et al., 1995). Meanwhile, treatment services are often hard to access, inflexible, and absolute in terms of treatment goals (abstinence only).

CANNABIS

Substances in the cannabis class (i.e., marijuana, hashish, and sinsemilla) are the most widely used illicit drugs in the United States (Zimmer & Morgan, 1997). Approximately one-third of the U.S. adult population in 1996 acknowledged having used cannabis products, and approximately 9% had used marijuana within the past year. Marijuana use was most prevalent among young adults (age 18 to 25), with approximately 44% acknowledging lifetime use and 13% acknowledging past-month use (SAMHSA, 1997). From the 1970s until 1992, Americans reduced past-month use of cannabis products, and the rate has leveled off since. Almost 5% in 1996 had used within the past month and 3% were frequent users, defined as use of cannabis on at least 51 days during the past year (SAMHSA, 1997). This section describes the acute and chronic harmful effects of marijuana use, the therapeutic effects and medicinal usage of cannabis products, and treatment approaches to minimize harm associated with cannabis dependence.

A previous National Household Survey on Drug Abuse (NIDA, 1991) assessed consequences related to substance use across three primary domains: social (e.g., "had arguments and fights with family or friends"), health (e.g., "had health problems"), and psychological concerns (e.g., "became depressed or lost interest in things"). Fifteen percent of respondents who had used marijuana in the past year reported at least one marijuana-related consequence, 8% reported two or more, and 4% reported three or more consequences. Clearly, therefore, the majority of users did not report problems related to their cannabis use.

The assessment of cannabis dependence is a diagnostic challenge, for several reasons: lack of physical evidence of excessive use, possible distortions in subjective appraisal of related consequences, and difficulties in determining a standard marijuana dose because of variable potency (Roffman & George, 1988; Roffman & Stephens, 1993). However, 9% of regular users are estimated to become marijuana-dependent, defined as experiencing problems in at least three of four domains: (1) physiological effects, (2) control problems, (3) personal–social problems, and (4) adverse opinions from others (Roffman & Stephens, 1993; Weller & Halikas, 1980).

Harmful Effects of Cannabis

In the early 1980s, the Secretary of Health and Human Services and the Director of the National Institute of Health commissioned a 22-member Institute of Medicine committee to conduct a comprehensive review of the effects of marijuana on health (Institute of Medicine, 1982). The goals of this 15-month study were to analyze possible health hazards, benefits, and therapeutic potential of marijuana; to identify new directions for basic and applied research; and to provide an empirical basis for the development public policy. The committee concluded that there are definite acute effects of marijuana—that is, changes evident during cannabis intoxication. The acute effects primarily involve the central nervous system, including impaired motor coordination, sensory and perceptual functioning, short-term memory, and learning. Marijuana-induced affect may include feelings of euphoria, anxiety, or paranoia. Marijuana also exerts acute effects on the cardiovascular system by temporarily increasing heart rate and blood pressure, and on the respiratory system through bronchodilation and clearing of pulmonary airways (Institute of Medicine, 1982; National Institutes of Health, 1997).

Longer-term negative effects of marijuana may include lower levels of gonadotropins or pituitary reproductive hormones, and a small but reversible decrease in sperm production in men (Institute of Medicine, 1982). At high levels marijuana is also likely to induce chromosome aberrations, as demonstrated in cytogenetic studies (Zimmerman & Zimmerman, 1990); however, there are no clinical studies to suggest that such alterations are apparent in the offspring of marijuana users. Although there is evidence that the psychoactive ingredient in marijuana, tetrahydrocannabinol (THC), crosses the placenta, it has not been documented to be a cause of birth defects (Institute of Medicine, 1982; National Institutes of Health, 1997).

Although acute low doses of marijuana may lead to bronchodilation, higher doses or chronic use may lead to the constriction of bronchial airways. Marijuana smoke is chemically similar to tobacco smoke (Huber, First, & Gruber, 1991); therefore, it is likely that prolonged heavy smoking of marijuana may lead to a number of lung diseases, including cancer, emphysema, and bronchitis. Regular marijuana users may be at lower risk for cancer than regular tobacco smokers, however, because marijuana users are unlikely to inhale the same volume over time (Zimmer & Morgan, 1997).

The Institute of Medicine (1982) report documented no clear evidence for changes in immune functioning as a result of marijuana use. A later study has suggested that reduced immunosuppression may occur, but only at extremely high drug concentrations (Hollister, 1992). Although chronic marijuana use has been associated with behavioral and mental disorders, the causal direction of this relationship remains unclear (Institute of Medicine, 1982; Zimmer & Morgan, 1997).

Therapeutic Effects of Cannabis

Although the demonstrated negative effects of marijuana use have been minimal, substantial beneficial effects have been shown (Cohen, 1976; Hollister, 1986; Institute of Medicine, 1982; Nahas, 1977; National Institutes of Health, 1997; Ungerleider & Andrysiak, 1985; Vincent, McQuiston, Einhorn, Nagy, & Brames, 1983; Zimmer & Morgan, 1997). Medicinal use of cannabis has been traced back to 2737 B.C. in China (Ray & Ksir, 1993). Another Chinese physician reportedly recommended that a mixture of cannabis resin and wine could serve as a surgical anesthetic in 200 A.D. (Ray & Ksir, 1993). It has also been suggested that cannabis was utilized during the last stages of pregnancy or during labor for an adolescent girl in about 315 A.D. (Zias et al., 1993).

In recent years, marijuana and other cannabis products have been shown to have therapeutic effects as antiemetic agents for cancer patients with chemotherapy-induced nausea and vomiting (Lane et al., 1991; Plasse et al., 1991; Vincent et al., 1983). Effective antiemetics are needed for treatment not only of the nausea induced by cancer chemotherapy, but of that caused by HIV antiviral regimens. Ineffective antiemetics may affect patient compliance, which may compromise treatment efficacy. Dronabinol, a THC product taken orally, has been shown to reduce chemotherapy-induced nausea and vomiting; this effect is enhanced by treatment with another antiemetic agent, prochlorperazine (Lane et al., 1991; Plasse et al., 1991).

Although numerous anecdotal reports suggest the utility of smoked marijuana for the relief of nausea and vomiting, few controlled clinical trials have been conducted to test the effectiveness of smoked marijuana versus other THC products. Those that have been conducted have shown smoked marijuana to be effective in reducing these symptoms (Levitt, Faiman, Hawks, & Wilson, 1984; Vinciguerra, Moore, & Brennan, 1988). Vinciguerra et al. (1988) demonstrated the effectiveness of marijuana in treating nausea and vomiting in cancer chemotherapy patients who were refractory to other available antiemetic agents. A "Group of Experts" committee assembled by the National Institutes of Health for the purpose of evaluating areas for future research on marijuana's therapeutic effects has recommended that controlled double-blind randomized trials determine the therapeutic utility of smoked marijuana for patients, both as compared to standard antiemetics and as a pharmacotherapy adjunct (National Institutes of Health, 1997).

Two surveys of oncologists' opinions of marijuana as an antiemetic agent have shown support for its palliative benefits (Doblin & Kleiman, 1991; Schwartz & Beveridge, 1994). In the first of these studies, Doblin and Kleiman (1991) found that 44% of oncologists who were assessed under conditions of anonymity supported the use of marijuana in decreasing chemotherapy-induced nausea. Similar efficacy ratings were found for oral THC. However, this sample may not have been representative, due to a low response rate (43%) of members of the American Society of Clinical Oncology (Doblin & Kleiman, 1991). In 1997, the American Medical Association passed a resolution affirming the rights of physicians to discuss the potential medical benefits of marijuana use for their patients (although it did not explicitly endorse marijuana as a recommended medicine).

Schwartz and Beveridge (1994) also assessed oncologists' preference for antiemetic agents following cancer chemotherapy. This study also utilized an anonymous, randomly selected sample of clinical oncologists, and it had a 78% response rate. In this study, marijuana was ranked ninth in order of preference for the treatment of mild to moderate nausea and vomiting, and sixth for treatment of severe postchemotherapy nausea and vomiting. Only 18% of respondents had never prescribed or recommended cannabinoids. Over 75% of responding oncologists had either prescribed oral THC or recommended natural marijuana for the treatment of postchemotherapy nausea, and they estimated that natural marijuana or oral THC was effective in reducing nausea or vomiting in 50% of their patients with "bothersome" side effects. Surprisingly, Schwartz and Beveridge concluded that natural marijuana and oral THC products may be beneficial but are not necessary for the treatment of chemotherapy-induced nausea; their conclusion was presumably based on the presence of higher-ranked antiemetic agents. Although other antiemetic agents are available, smoked marijuana may be an important part of an oncologist's medicinal arsenal for countering chemotherapy side effects, particularly for those patients who are not aided by other available medications (Vinciguerra et al., 1988). Although the surveys described above did not assess patients' perceptions of efficacy in alleviating side effects of chemotherapy, the results are still useful in summarizing physicians' attitudes toward cannabinoids for oncology patients.

In studies involving healthy subjects, smokers of cannabis cigarettes showed greater caloric intake than smokers of placebo cigarettes did, but the variability was so large that the authors were uncertain whether this finding was clinically significant (for a review, see Institute of Medicine, 1982). Because of this effect, cannabis products may serve as an appetite stimulant in late-stage cancer patients and individuals with AIDS or HIV infection (Plasse et al., 1991). Dronabinol has been shown to reduce the rate of AIDS-related weight loss. Because substantial weight loss is generally associated with shorter survival times for HIV-positive individuals (Kotler, 1989), use of cannabis may increase survival time. Research is warranted to determine the extent to which marijuana use may be related to caloric intake, weight gain, immune status, and clinical outcome for HIV-positive individuals (National Institutes of Health, 1997).

Cannabis also has demonstrated medicinal value in the treatment of glaucoma (Institute of Medicine, 1982; National Institutes of Health, 1997). Glaucoma is the leading cause of blindness in the United States, involving increased pressure within the eye and eventual damage to the optic nerve. Conventional antiglaucoma medications regulate intraocular pressure, but generally have unpleasant side effects and are not effective with all patients. THC and cannabis in high doses have been demonstrated to reduce intraocular pressure when administered intravenously, orally, or by inhalation (Institute of Medicine, 1982; National Institutes of Health, 1997). Because high doses of these products have systemic side effects and are not well tolerated by the elderly, a topical cannabinoid was developed for the treatment of glaucoma. Unfortunately, this product was not effective in reducing intraocular pressure. The National Institutes of Health (1997) Group of Experts has recommended outcome studies of longer duration, as well as studies that evaluate the mechanism of action leading to therapeutic effects.

Anticonvulsant properties of marijuana have been demonstrated as well. In research conducted on mice and rats, cannabis derivatives have been shown to have a dose–response protective effect against seizures induced by electrical shock (Institute of Medicine, 1982). Evidence of tolerance to this effect occurred with repeated exposure to THC. In epileptic individuals, cannabis derivatives in conjunction with typical anti-convulsant medications have been shown to offer some additional improvement over standard medications alone (Institute of Medicine, 1982). Anecdotal reports also suggest that smoked and oral THC may reduce the spasticity experienced by individuals with multiple sclerosis (MS) or spinal cord injuries (SCI) (Hollister, 1986; National Institutes of Health, 1997).

THC has also been shown to exert antiasthmatic effects approaching those of a commonly prescribed drug, isoproterenol (Institute of Medicine, 1982). Mixed findings have been reported for THC's therapeutic potential as a tumor retardant, anxiolytic, and antidepressant agent (Institute of Medicine, 1982). Cannabis products may provide analgesic effects (Institute of Medicine, 1982; Noyes, Brunk, Baram, & Canter, 1975), particularly for those with neuropathic pain (National Institutes of Health, 1997).

Despite the status of marijuana as an illegal drug, and some dissension among those in the medical and scientific establishments, use of medicinal marijuana continues to receive wide support from the community of individuals who have found relief from their medical conditions through the use of cannabis products. A San Francisco organization, the San Francisco Cannabis Buyers Club, has been established to improve access to marijuana for individuals who have a doctor's letter documenting the existence of a condition that may be alleviated by marijuana, along with the physician's agreement to supervise its use. In 1995, there were reportedly 3,200 members of this club. At first, this organization did not experience legal disruption, due to a 1992 decision by city supervisors and the mayor to make medicinal marijuana law enforcement their lowest priority ("Pot Smoking," 1995). Recent court orders, however, have threatened to close down the club. In December 1997, the First District Court of Appeals in California ordered the reinstatement of an injunction that shut down the Cannabis Buyers Club after a raid by state agents in August 1996. Similar organizations have been established in other cities with varying degrees of public support. The use of marijuana by medical patients is likely to continue despite the legal difficulties involved, because of these patients' perceptions of the need for and efficacy of cannabis products.

In November 1996, California and Arizona passed voter initiatives to decriminalize the possession and use of marijuana for medicinal purposes. The Clinton administration responded to the passage of these initiatives by threatening to prosecute and revoke the prescription privileges of physicians who recommended marijuana to their patients.

In summary, cannabis-derived products show the most promise in the treatment of glaucoma, asthma, epileptic seizures, chemotherapy-induced nausea, neuropathic pain, MS- or SCI-related spasticity, and cancer- and AIDS-related wasting. This evidence of therapeutic potential warrants further clinical trials. However, marijuana is classified as a Schedule I narcotic (a category reserved for substances thought to have no medicinal benefits), and this is preventing further evaluation of its therapeutic potential at this time.

Treatment for Cannabis Dependence

Cannabis use commonly occurs within the context of other substance use. As a result, treatment for marijuana dependence has traditionally been conducted within the general rubric of addiction treatment, without special attention to the unique issues faced by marijuana-dependent individuals.

Rainone, Deren, Kleinman, and Wish (1987) identified a group of individuals who used marijuana heavily but did not use other illicit substances. Through anonymous phone interviews targeting heavy marijuana users, they identified 13% of a sample of 99 respondents who met the criteria for a "pure" marijuana user, defined as a person using marijuana at least three times a week over the past month but not engaging in the use of other illicit substances. Forty-seven percent of this sample regarded their use of marijuana as having some problems associated with it.

Also using an anonymous telephone interview, Roffman and Barnhart (1987) identified individuals who were concerned about their marijuana use. Almost three-quarters (74% of their 225 respondents) reported adverse consequences resulting solely from use of marijuana. In this study, multiple-drug use was distinguished from polysubstance abuse; respondents who used other substances without adverse consequences were classified as multiple-drug users. In addition, 92% of this sample expressed interest in participating in a treatment program for marijuana users (Roffman & Barnhardt, 1987). The results of this study support the utility of designing treatment programs tailored to the specific challenges faced by marijuana users (Roffman, Stephens, Simpson, & Whitaker, 1988; Zweben & O'Connell, 1988).

Roffman et al. (1988) recruited respondents from the telephone interview study who had expressed interest in treatment. A total of 212 individuals without other drug abuse, other ongoing treatment, or severe psychopathology agreed to participate in a 12-week treatment outcome study. Participants were randomly assigned to either a relapse-prevention-oriented cognitive-behavioral program or a social support and group discussion condition. Both treatments focused on abstinence as a goal. Treatment groups met for 10 2-hour sessions over a 12-week period, with posttreatment booster sessions at 3 and 6 months (Stephens, Roffman, & Simpson, 1993, 1994). Participants' posttreatment marijuana use was verified by collateral informants. The two treatment conditions resulted in comparable abstinence rates (15% in the relapse prevention treatment and 14% in the social support treatment), and both resulted in significant reductions in amount of marijuana used and problems related to use. These reductions were maintained throughout the 12-month follow-up (Stephens et al., 1994). Men in this sample were more likely than women to maintain abstinence, but men were less likely to successfully maintain a level of nonproblematic use of marijuana.

Overall, for the relatively small proportion of marijuana users who develop substantial interpersonal, occupational, or legal problems stemming from their cannabis use, treatments specifically designed to move the individuals toward cessation are the optimal starting point. A harm reduction approach to the management of cannabis-related harm will educate users about potential risks in a context of individual responsibility for use decisions.

HALLUCINOGENS

The use of hallucinogens in religious practices can be traced to the Aztec Indians who used *ololiuqui* (morning-glory seeds), psilocybin-containing *teonanacatl* (also called "flesh of the gods"), and peyote (described as the indirect catalyst of the psychedelic revolution; Hoffer, 1965). As far back as 1890 and up until the 1960s, clinical research protocols were developed to study the therapeutic effects of hallucinogens (Mitchell, 1896). Humans have long searched for ways to alter consciousness (Weil & Rosen, 1993), and the popularity of using hallucinogens recreationally peaked in the late 1960s.

The hallucinogenic class of drugs, also called psychedelics, includes lysergic acid diethylamide (LSD), mescaline (found in the peyote cactus), psilocybin (found in certain mushrooms), 2C-B ("Nexus"), 2,5-dimethoxy-4-methylamphetamine (DOM, also called STP), ibotenic acid, and muscimol. Dissociative anesthetics, such as phencyclidine (PCP) and ketamine ("special K"), are sometimes also classified as hallucinogens. The present discussion of hallucinogens is limited to harm reduction strategies associated with the use of LSD and peyote, since LSD is the most commonly used psychedelic agent, and peyote is the one traditionally used in religious and spiritual ceremonies.

Between 20 and 21 million individuals in the United States have used a hallucinogen at least once. Of those, 80% used have used LSD and 20% have used peyote. Psychedelics appear to be gaining resurgence in popularity among youth. Past-month use of hallucinogens among Americans aged 12 to 17 increased from 1% in 1994 to 2% in 1996 (SAMHSA, 1997). According to Johnston et al. (1997), approximately 46% of U.S. high school students reported that obtaining hallucinogens was "fairly easy" or "very easy."

Lysergic Acid Diethylamide (LSD)

The mechanisms by which LSD alters sensory and thought processes are still unknown. LSD is hypothesized to act in the brain as a serotonin inhibitor. This results in disinhibition of sensory and higher cortical function neurons, for which serotonin is an inhibitory neurotransmitter. The increase in electrical firing of the neurons in the brain causes distortions of perception and thought (Strassman, 1984). However, evidence for this theory is based on the positive clinical response of an LSD-induced psychosis when L-5l hydroxytryptophan, a serotonin precursor, is administered (Freedman, 1986).

Routes of administration include swallowing, smoking, snorting, injecting, and conjunctival instillation of liquid LSD. Doses vary from 25 µg to 500 µg, and the drug has a half-life of 8–12 hours. Tolerance develops after 3 or 4 days of continuous use, and there are no withdrawal symptoms with cessation of use. The negative consequences of hallucinogen use are rare, particularly in comparison to those associated with cocaine, heroin, and alcohol use. However, the number of LSD-related emergency room visits increased by 74% (from 3,400 to 6,000) from 1993 to 1995; these visits typically concerned dangerous behaviors or undesirable emotional reactions during hallucinogen intoxication (Drug Abuse Warning Network, 1996).

Initial objective symptoms of LSD intoxication include nausea, flushing, chills, tachycardia, hypertension, piloerection, pupillary dilation, and tremor (Strassman, 1984). The characteristic effects that follow include affective lability, a distortion of time and space, increases in eidetic imagery, heightened perception of colors, distorted visual perception, and occasional synesthesia (subjective report of feeling colors or seeing sounds; Abraham, Aldridge, & Aldridge, 1993). The subjective LSD intoxication involves feelings of "being one with the universe" and philosophical ideas regarding nature or space, which combine to give the perception of a religious or mystical experience (Strassman, 1984). Dangers associated with use of LSD include panic attacks, LSD-induced psychosis, exhaustion, depression, mood lability, operating motorized vehicles during a "high," risk taking, and suicide attempts. As with any other drug, the resultant behavior is mediated by several factors, including quantity ingested, concomitant other substance use, previous experience with hallucinogens, and set and setting (expectations for the drug-induced state and the environment in which the drug is used, respectively).

Acute intoxication may include anxiety, paranoia, and suspiciousness, or changes in cognition and judgment, which may lead to physical self-endangerment. Reports by Schick and Smith (1970) indicate that most psychedelic "bad trips" are best treated in a supportive, nonpharmacological fashion by restoring a positive, nonthreatening environment. Volunteers and outreach workers from the Haight-Ashbury Free Clinic in San Francisco set up a quiet space at large rock concerts in order to perform emergency "talk-down" procedures for those users who experienced distressing psychedelic experiences. Individuals were reassured that the effects they were feeling were the normal and expected results of psychedelic drug ingestion, and these strategies were usually sufficient.

The long-term adverse consequences of hallucinogen drug use may include prolonged psychotic symptoms, depression, flashbacks, exacerbation of preexisting psychiatric illness, or the relatively rare DSM-IV diagnosis of "Hallucinogen persisting perception disorder" (American Psychiatric Association, 1994a; Seymour & Smith, 1987; Wesson & Smith, 1978). "Flashbacks" are transient spontaneous occurrences of one or more of the perceptual aspects of the hallucinogenic drug intoxication following cessation of use. Resulting psychosis, depression, and persisting perceptual disturbances are generally treated pharmacologically.

Some beneficial effects of LSD have been documented. LSD has been shown to elicit robust antidepressant effects (Buckholtz, Zhou, Freedman, & Potter, 1990; Savage, 1952; Stolz, Marsden, & Middlemiss, 1983). In addition, it has been successful in the treatment of substance abuse, sociopathy, and prisoner recidivism, and in the supportive care of terminally ill patients (Strassman, 1995). Results of these studies contain methodological confounds, but they underscore the potential advantages of further research to clarify the benefits and dangers of hallucinogen use.

Strassman (1995) argues that there are several reasons why the continuing study of LSD and other hallucinogenic drugs is useful and important. First, hallucinogens affect characteristic brain functions, including affect, cognition, volition, interoception, and perception. If we can characterize the properties of hallucinogens, our understanding of mind–brain relationships will be enhanced. Second, because drug-induced psychoses share features with biologically based psychotic syndromes, examination of mechanisms and effects of hallucinogens can inform development of treatment interventions for those who suffer from endogenous psychoses. Third, early studies suggest that hallucinogens may be of significant use in treating refractory psychiatric patients; given the time-limited approach of managed care organizations, these interventions may hold value as an option for specific patient populations (Strassman, 1995). Eliminating the investigation of mechanisms, benefits, and risks of hallucinogen use closes the door on important learning opportunities. A harm reduction approach to drug policy advocates further research that is conducted safely and will benefit individuals suffering from mental illness or problematic hallucinogen use.

Additional harm reduction strategies regarding LSD and other hallucinogen use include widespread education on the effects of these drugs, including both benefits and dangers. To reach large audiences, publications, newsletters, and Internet resources are available on potential negative consequences resulting from mixing drugs, buying from unfamiliar sources, and overdosing. Information aimed at individuals who choose to experiment should highlight risk factors for unpleasant hallucinogen experiences, psychological and physiological effects (including set and setting), research findings, and treatment and support group referrals. The goal of the information exchange is to inform potential hallucinogen users of the dangers of use so that harm can be avoided. From a legal perspective, punitive consequences for hallucinogen possession should be commensurate with the wrongs committed, if any.

Peyote

Peyote is the most common name given to plant preparations obtained from the mescal cactus. It is the "buttons" that sit atop the unobtrusive and acrid-tasting cactus that contain the principal peyote hallucinogen. Peyote was used by native groups in the present-day southwestern United States and Mexico for religious ceremonies and practices until the arrival of the Spaniards and the introduction of Christianity, when the use of hallucinogens was prohibited. However, the native groups resisted, and the use of these hallucinogenic cacti in the Native American Church (NAC) and Native American spiritual ceremonies continues today in many states—as does the legal battle. Recently, the U.S. Supreme Court ruled that the use of peyote can be banned, despite the religious context of its use in the NAC (Bullis, 1990). It is used as a traditional method to achieve "visions" of the Great Spirit for religious ceremonies.

The principal active component of the peyote plant is mescaline. Its chemical resemblance to drugs such as amphetamine and DOM, and also to epinephrine and norepinephrine, has provoked much speculation. However, its mechanism of action is more similar to LSD, as are its effects. Evidence for this is supported by the fact that drugs that reverse the effects of LSD also reverse the effects of mescaline (Winger, Hofmann, & Woods, 1992).

The initial effects of peyote ingestion include nausea, vomiting, profuse perspiration, and static tremors resulting from an increase in pulse rate and blood pressure. The characteristic effects that follow this initial 1- to 2-hour phase include visual hallucinations, color and space perceptual disturbances, synesthesias, and occasional auditory and tactile hallucinations. Like LSD intoxication, peyote intoxication is characterized primarily by dose-related changes in perception, thinking, emotion, arousal, and self-image. The user typically retains insight, and the sensorium remains undisturbed during the experience. Over the next 4–6 hours, the "high" peaks and then descends. Lucid recognition of philosophical and personal realities is characteristic of the psychedelic experience. A typical response to this experience is the process of identifying aspects of oneself that need changing, and one that Native Americans claim has brought about a better life for many peyote users (Stafford, 1983).

Peyote can be ingested orally, by smoking, or by suppository. Doses vary from 1 to 40 buttons; each button contains approximately 25 µg of mescaline and has a reported half-life of 12–14 hours. There is no evidence for the development of physiological dependence to peyote or mescaline, although tolerance has been reported. There are no withdrawal symptoms with cessation of use.

Peyote has been used in the treatment of pneumonia, tuberculosis, diabetes, arthritis, influenza, intestinal problems, and venereal disease; it has also been applied topically for burns, wounds, persistent sores, bites, and stings (especially from poisonous creatures). For several years, editions of the U.S. Dispensatory contained information on its medical uses under the former botanical name of the mescal cactus, *Anhalonium lewinii*. In 1895, researchers suggested using peyote buttons as an antispasmodic for intestinal problems, irritable cough, nervous headache, restlessness, insomnia, hysteria, and convulsions (Peyote Foundation, 1996).

The NAC incorporates harm reduction strategies with its religious practices. The greatest harm reported with peyote use is the nausea and gagging that occur immediately after ingestion; therefore, a church official is designated as the "shovel man," prepared to assist anyone experiencing difficulties. Another strategy used is abstaining from food and alcohol before ingestion, which decreases the chances of vomiting (Stafford, 1983). Unlike other drugs, peyote is grown by a small number of farmers, and therefore the secondary effects of violence and crime (which are typically associated with the sale of cocaine and heroin, for example) do not exist for peyote buyers and sellers. Harm related to peyote use is also reduced by distribution of information regarding peyote's physiological and psychological effects on several World Wide Web sites. For instance, the Peyote Foundation's on-line journal provides information "concerning peyote and the peyote religion that is documented, scientifically accurate, and politically neutral" (Peyote Foundation, 1996).

PRESCRIPTION DRUGS

Millions of individuals in the United States are successfully treated each year for medical and mental health disorders with prescription drugs that have well-documented therapeutic benefits. However, a minority of individuals use these medications to experience pleasurable effects, and it is for this reason that we include a brief discussion of these "licit" drugs in a chapter on illicit substances. Many physicians refuse to prescribe painkillers to patients suffering unbearable pain, for fear that they will be prescribing to the aforementioned group. Addressing the issue of medication availability for those individuals requiring medical and mental health care, while limiting access for the purposes of misuse, is an important public health policy issue. The goals of such a policy require striking a delicate balance between minimizing abuse and maximizing the provision of relief (Wilford, Finch, Czechowicz, & Warren, 1994).

There are three components of prescription drug abuse: (1) a physician factor, pertaining to inappropriate prescribing or medication use instructions; (2) a patient factor (i.e., noncompliance); and (3) a physician–patient communication factor (Lurie & Lee, 1991). Misused psychoactive prescription drugs include analgesics, tranquilizers (including benzodiazepines), stimulants, and sedatives (including barbiturates). Analgesics, with the highest rate of abuse, are popular because of their pain relief properties and euphoric effects. Tranquilizers and sedatives are used for reducing anxiety and inducing sleep. Stimulants increase energy level and assist in focusing attention for some individuals, and are most commonly prescribed for attention-deficit/hyperactivity disorder and weight loss.

In 1996, it was estimated that almost 3% of the household population (over 6 million people) had used prescription psychotherapeutic drugs for nonmedical reasons. Only 13 of the 140 medications most prescribed in 1990 were psychoactive (Office of the Inspector General, 1990). Therefore, only a relatively small proportion of drugs is abused, and a larger percentage is used appropriately. According to Table 6.5, it appears that misuse rates declined slightly from 1988 to 1996. However, because of differences in sampling procedures (e.g., increase in sample size in 1996, and inclusion of individuals living in military installations, dormitories, or homeless shelters), changes should be considered with caution. Of note is the pattern of relative stability, which supports findings that programs aimed at reducing the abuse of prescription drugs have a minimal effect.

In 1974, Silverman and Lee proposed a series of policy approaches to reduce the abuse of prescription drugs (Lurie & Lee, 1991). In 1980, the White House Conference on Prescription Drug Abuse drew attention to the striking rates of death and illness associated with deliberate misuse of prescription drugs, and recommendations for combating the problem at the state and national levels were developed. Unfortunately, these efforts have yet to provide solutions. Some programs have attempted to regulate prescription writing through triplicate requirements. In Texas, one study demonstrated a reduction in prescribing Schedule II drugs and a corresponding increase in Schedule III analgesic use (Sigler et al., 1984). Overall, little empirical evidence supports the triplicate system or any other programs initiated as a result of the White House Conference. An unfortunate consequence of attempts to reduce misuse is that some physicians have

TABLE 6.5. Trends in Nonmedical Use of Psychotherapeutic Agents, 1988 to 1996

	1988		1996	
	Number	%	Number	%
Lifetime	22,258,000	11	20,409,000	10
Past year	9,151,000	5	6,652,000	3
Past month	4,076,000	2	3,082,000	1

Note. Data from SAMHSA (1989, 1997).

increased their prescribing of outdated, ineffective, or lethal drugs, such as meprobate and chloral hydrate, instead of benzodiazepines (Weintraub et al., 1991).

Generally, medications are used as prescribed and contribute to a better quality of life for those suffering from debilitating or life-threatening disorders. Nonintentional prescription drug abuse can be reduced by improved prescription practices, facilitated compliance, and better communication between physicians and patients. For many patients, the immediate focus needs to be on the negative consequences of medication misuse. Clear, fact-driven, nonpunitive communication between health care professionals and patients may itself help ameliorate prescription drug misuse.

RISK REDUCTION EFFORTS WITH OTHER SUBSTANCES: KEEP THE DOOR OPEN TO INJECTORS

Throughout this chapter, harm reduction methods have been described for a variety of substances. The majority of strategies described above were empirically developed for commonly abused substances. Other substances, such as amphetamines and methamphetamines, "designer drugs," and steroids, have been less well studied—particularly from a harm reduction perspective. Because their use is often associated with risky behavior, future research efforts should consider exploring treatment options with these substances. Indeed, there is evidence that efforts to reduce the risks associated with these "other" substances are needed.

Amphetamines and Related Drugs

Amphetamines and methamphetamines are central nervous system stimulant drugs with very similar psychoactive properties as cocaine, but with a longer duration of action. Methamphetamine ("crystal," "speed," or "crank") is chemically similar to amphetamine, but produces greater effects on the central nervous system. Methcathinone ("cat") is a cheap stimulant that is easily manufactured by amateur chemists from battery acid, drain cleaner, and over-the-counter asthma medication. These drugs tend to be cheaper than cocaine, are more accessible to youth, and have particularly affected the U.S. Midwest, California, truck drivers, and some gay subcultures. Amphetamines and methamphetamines can be snorted in powder form, injected, dissolved in beverages, or smoked (e.g., methamphetamine hydrochloride or "ice"). In 1996, 2.3% of the U.S. population over age 12 reported having tried methamphetamines. The highest rate of use was among those aged 26–34, with 4.2% reporting lifetime use (SAMHSA, 1997).

"Designer drugs" are substances that are chemically altered versions of existing drugs. Changing the makeup of a drug or combining existing substances results in a product with new effects, or, in some cases, with effects that overlap those of existing chemical compounds. 3,4-Methylene-dioxymethamphetamine (MDMA; called "Ecstasy" or "X" in the United States, and "E" in the United Kingdom), is a methoxylated amphetamine and is the best-known designer drug. It is fairly popular on college campuses and in "rave" subcultures. In 1996, 2.8% of college students reported using MDMA, and 0.7% reported its use during the past month (Johnston et al., 1997). Aside from the actual physiological risks of the substance, the most significant risks of designer drugs stem from the development of the drugs (these drugs are essentially the by-products of uncontrolled chemistry experiments). Because the user cannot know the specifications of such a concoction, dosing and side effects are virtually unpredictable. Hence, aside from any concerns about route of administration, stressing to users the inherent risks involved in taking a transmuted substance is of great importance.

Methamphetamine use is associated with high risk for HIV. Waldorf, Murphy, Lauderback, Reinarman, and Marotta (1990) surveyed 178 male prostitutes and discovered that 68% of the sample reported drug injection; of these, 92% had injected methamphetamines, 59% had injected cocaine, and 41% had injected heroin. Over 70% of injectors reported that they had shared needles with an average of 1.5 persons in the past week, 3.6 in the last month, 24.4 in the last year, and 148.1 persons over an entire career. Clearly, their HIV risk is high.

Waldorf et al.'s subjects were also asked about reasons for sharing needles. Seventy percent responded that "there was only one [needle] available" and 91% reported that "needles were not available." Convenience appeared to be a significant reason to share needles: 56% agreed that it was more convenient to use other people's needles, and 48% agreed that sometimes they "can't wait to use [their] own outfit." Legal concerns influenced needle sharing, with 37% endorsing "You don't want to be arrested by the police for paraphernalia laws." The authors conclude that some of the risks associated with needle sharing may be avoided "if needle-exchange programs are implemented and laws relating to drug paraphernalia . . . are repealed, relaxed or allowed to go unenforced" (Waldorf et al., 1990, p. 329).

If these individuals won't quit using methamphetamines, can they at least reduce their HIV risk? Darke, Cohen, Ross, Hando, and Hall (1994) interviewed 301 regular amphetamine users about changes in the route of administration. Although 66% had injected amphetamines during the past 6 months, 24% used both injection and noninjection methods. Of 62% who had injected in the past month, 27% had borrowed a used needle, 31% had lent their used needle to another user, and 41% had done both. Regarding transitions among route of administration, 58% of the amphetamine users reported that snorting was their first route of administration. However, 40% reported having made a transition from other routes of administration (i.e., snorting, swallowing, and smoking) to injecting. Males were twice as likely report a transition to injecting. Subjects' reasons for making the transition to injecting included liking the "rush" associated with injecting (88%), believing that injecting is more economical (23%), and believing that injecting is "healthier" or "cleaner" than snorting, since it avoids the development of nasal ulcers (22%). On the other hand, 9% reported a transition from injecting to other routes of amphetamine administration, due to concern about veins (39%), fear of HIV (23%), and feeling addicted to amphetamines (19%). After the transition from inject-ing, 39% reported using more amphetamines, while an equal 39% reported a decrease in their use.

Darke et al. (1994) conclude that this information has implications for harm reduction. First, injectors reported that they regarded injecting as a more economical means of administration. However, since tolerance devel-ops rapidly with injection administration, this is not true. The injectors also reported using amphetamines more often, being more dependent than noninjectors, and increasing their amphetamine use after the transition to injecting; the authors thus argue that this paradox needs to be explained to injectors. Furthermore, many users believed that injecting is a healthier means of amphetamine use. It may be necessary to emphasize the harmful effects associated with injecting. In fact, concern about vascular damage was more frequently endorsed than was concern about HIV. Since most prevention efforts focus on the risks of acquiring HIV, attention should also be given to the harmful effects of injecting on the veins (Darke et al., 1994). Finally, recall that 41% of subjects in this sample reported sharing equip-ment for injection. If use is going to continue, encouraging transitions to safer routes may be needed.

Anabolic Steroids

Although there are legitimate medical uses for anabolic steroids, they are also used in sports because of their potential to enhance muscle strength, alter physical appearance, and meet some psychological needs (Goldberg, Bosworth, Bents, & Trevisan, 1990). One often thinks of steroid users as bodybuilders or as individuals in athletic competition, but there is also use among members of typical gymnasiums (Goldstein, 1994, March). Steroid users often view many of the effects that physicians see as negative physical consequences as very positive. Goldstein asks, "If a particular consequence is not perceived as harmful, is there a harm to reduce?" Indeed, it is unlikely that users will see a harm to reduce if the immediate psychological and physical needs associated with improving their body images are met. If the most visible effects associated with steroid use are viewed as positive by users, they may become resistant if one tries to convince them otherwise. In fact, education alone about the effects of anabolic steroids may not be effective in changing behavior in steroid users.

Education programs may increase awareness of the adverse effects of steroids, but differences in attitudes do not tend to follow (Goldberg et al., 1990). Just as with other substances, the challenge remains to find a way to reduce the risks associated with use. The spotlight can be shifted to a consequence that is less debatable—risks associated with the route of administration. Because anabolic steroids are injected, needle sharing can take place. Research has suggested that a knowledge of risks can result in fewer needle-sharing behaviors. A questionnaire based on the 1989 Secondary School Health Risk Survey and the 1990 Youth Risk Behavior Survey of the Centers for Disease Control and Prevention assessed steroid use in students in compulsory health science classes (DuRant, Rickert, Ashworth, Newman, & Slavens, 1993). Although the students' average age was only 14.9 years, almost 7% of the boys and 2% of the girls reported using anabolic steroids. Among students who used anabolic steroids, 25% reported that they had shared needles for drug injection within the past month. Of note, only 19% of steroid users who had received school-based education about AIDS and HIV had shared needles, compared to 31% of steroid users who had not received such education.

In a survey of 130 syringe exchange programs within the United Kingdom, 88 programs had given syringes to steroid injectors (Lenehan, 1994). However, steroid users are often ignored because, given a dwindling supply of needles, equipment will be provided to individuals viewed as "high-priority." If needle exchanges welcome steroid users as worthy patrons, at least the risks associated with sharing needles can be diminished. The entire burden should not fall, however, on the needle exchange workers. The attitudes of steroid users must be changed; the typical steroid injector does not see himself or herself as a "drug user." For services to be utilized, the individual must realize that he or she is a candidate for the services.

CONCLUSION

The high prevalence of drug use in the U.S. adult population requires careful attention, because this substance use is likely to have associated problems. It is often accompanied by negative consequences that cause problems for the users themselves, their families and friends, and society. Thus, it is desirable to reduce the problems associated with substance use. Harm reduction is one vehicle for achieving this reduction.

In this chapter, we have reviewed methods to reduce the risk and harm associated with various drugs of abuse. Specific strategies, such as drug replacement for opiate addiction, are recommended on the basis of strong empirical support. Other general strategies, such as viewing drug addiction along a continuum and working with drug users in a nonjudgmental manner, are less well supported by empirical studies. In addition, drug-related harm may be reduced by increased public transportation, safe settings for drug experimentation, public education on drug effects, earlier detection of drug dependence, and efforts to decrease normative substance use in the general population. Open-minded examination of current drug policies may improve the current drug situation as well (See chapter 10). Part of this open-mindedness includes maintaining open dialogues with opponents of harm reduction.

NOTE

1. In this chapter (as in all other chapters of this book except Chapter 4), we use the terms "drug abuse" and "substance abuse" in their more general sense of "substance misuse," rather than the more restricted sense in which the fourth edition of the *Diagnostic and Statistical Manual of Mental Disorders* (DSM-IV; American Psychiatric Association, 1994) defines "substance abuse." However, we do use "drug dependence" and "substance dependence" in DSM-IV's sense of "substance dependence" unless indicated otherwise. See Chapter 4 for a discussion of DSM-IV's definitions of "abuse" and "dependence" in regard to alcohol use.

ACKNOWLEDGMENTS

We gratefully acknowledge the editorial comments of Ron Jackson and Don Calsyn on earlier versions of this chapter.

REFERENCES

Abraham, H. D., Aldridge, A., & Aldridge, A. M. (1993). Adverse consequences of lysergic acid diethylamide. *Addiction, 88,* 1327–1334.

Alterman, A. I., O'Brien, C., McLellan, A. T., August, D. S., Snider, E. C., Droba, M., Cornish, J. W., Hall, C. P., Raphaelson, A. H., & Schrade, F. X. (1994). Effectiveness and costs of inpatient versus day hospital cocaine rehabilitation. *Journal of Nervous and Mental Disease, 182,* 157–163.

American Psychiatric Association. (1994a). *Diagnostic and statistical manual of mental disorders* (4th ed.) Washington, DC: Author.

American Psychiatric Association. (1994b). Position statement on methadone maintenance treatment. *American Journal of Psychiatry, 151,* 792–794.

Anglin, M. D., & McGlothlin, W. H. (1984). Outcome of narcotic addict treatment in California. In F. M. Tims & J. P. Ludford (Eds.), *Drug abuse treatment evaluation: Strategies, progress, and prospects* (NIDA Research Monograph No. 51, pp. 196–128). Rockville, MD: U.S. Department of Health and Human Services.

Appel, P. W. (1982). Sustained attention in methadone patients. *International Journal of the Addictions, 17,* 1313–1327.

Appel, P. W., & Gordon, N. B. (1976). Digit–symbol performance in methadone-treated ex-heroin addicts. *American Journal of Psychiatry, 133,* 1337–1339.

Ball, J. C., & Ross, A. (1991). *The effectiveness of methadone maintenance treatment.* New York: Springer-Verlag.

Battjes, R. J., Sloboda, Z., & Grace, W. C. (Eds.). (1994). *The context of HIV risk among drug users and their sexual partners* (NIDA Research Monograph No. 143). Rockville, MD: U.S. Department of Health and Human Services.

Beck, A. T., Wright, F. D., Newman, C. F., & Liese, B. S. (1993). *Cognitive therapy of substance abuse.* New York: Guilford Press.

Bell, J., Caplehorn, J. R. M., & McNeil, D. R. (1994). The effect of intake procedures on performance in methadone maintenance. *Addiction, 89,* 463–471.

Bell, J., Chan, J., & Kuk, A. (1995). Investigating the influence of treatment philosophy on outcome of methadone maintenance. *Addiction, 90,* 823–830.

Besteman, K. J., & Brady, J. V. (1994). Implementing mobile drug abuse treatment: Problems, procedures, and perspectives. In B. W. Fletcher, J. A. Inciardi, & A. M. Horton (Eds.), *Drug abuse treatment: The implementation of innovative approaches* (pp. 33–42). Westport, CT: Greenwood Press.

Bickel, W. K., Johnson, R. E., Stitzer, M. L., & Bigelow, G. E. (1987). A clinical trial of buprenorphine: I. Comparison with methadone in the detoxification of heroin addicts. II. Examination of its opioid blocking properties. In *Problems of drug dependence, 1986: Proceedings of the 48th Annual Scientific Meeting, the Committee on Problems of Drug Dependence* (NIDA Research Monograph No. 76, pp. 182–188). Rockville, MD: U.S. Department of Health and Human Services.

Bickel, W. K., Stitzer, M. L., Bigelow, G. E., Liebson, I. A., Jasinski, D. R., & Johnson, R. E. (1988a). Buprenorphine: Dose-related blockage of opioid challenge effects in opioid dependent humans. *Journal of Pharmacology and Experimental Therapeutics, 247,* 47–53.

Bickel, W. K., Stitzer, M. L., Bigelow, G. E., Liebson, I. A., Jasinski, D. R., & Johnson, R. E. (1988b). A clinical trial of buprenorphine: Comparison with methadone in the detoxification of heroin addicts. *Clinical Pharmacology and Therapeutics, 43,* 72–78.

Blomberg, R. D., & Preusser, D. F. (1974). Narcotic use and driving behavior. *Accident Analysis and Prevention, 6,* 23–32.

Broderick, P. A., Phelan, F. T., & Berger, S. P. (1992). Ibogaine alters cocaine induced biogenic amine and psychostimulant dysfunction but not [3H]GBR-12935 binding to the dopamine transporter protein. In *Problems of drug dependence, 1991: Proceedings of the 53rd Annual Scientific Meeting, the Committee on Problems of Drug Dependence* (NIDA Research Monograph No. 119, p. 385). Rockville, MD: U.S. Department of Health and Human Services.

Broderick, P. S., Phelan, F. T., Eng, F., & Wechsler, T. (1994). Ibogaine modulates cocaine responses, which are altered due to environmental habituation: *In vivo* microvoltammetric and behavioral studies. *Pharmacology, Biochemistry and Behavior, 49,* 711–728.

Bryant, K. J., Rounsaville, B., Spitzer, R. L., & Williams, J. B. W. (1992). Reliability of dual diagnosis: Substance dependence and psychiatric disorders. *Journal of Nervous and Mental Disease, 180,* 251–257.

Buckholtz, N. S., Zhou, D., Freedman, D. X., & Potter, W. (1990). Lysergic acid diethylamide (LSD) administration selectively downregulates serotonin$_2$ receptors in rat brain. *Neuropsychopharmacology, 3,* 137–148.

Budd, R. D., Muto, J. J., & Wong, J. K. (1989). Drugs of abuse found in fatally injured drivers in Los Angeles County. *Drug and Alcohol Dependence, 23,* 153–158.

Bullis, R. (1990). Swallowing the scroll: Legal implications of the recent Supreme Court peyote cases. *Journal of Psychoactive Drugs, 22*(3), 325–332.

Bushnell, T. G., & Justins, D. M. (1993). Choosing the right analgesic: A guide to selection. *Drugs, 46,* 394–408.

Calsyn, D. A., Fleming, C., Wells, E. A., & Saxon, A. J. (1996). Personality disorder subtypes among opiate addicts in methadone maintenance. *Psychology of Addictive Behaviors, 10,* 3–8.

Calsyn, D. A., Meinecke, C., Saxon, A. J., & Stanton, V. (1992). Risk reduction in sexual behavior: A condom giveaway program in a drug abuse treatment clinic. *American Journal of Public Health, 82,* 1536–1658.

Calsyn, D. A., Wells, E. A., Saxon, A. J., Jackson, T. R., Wrede, A. F., Stanton, V., & Fleming, C. (1994). Contingency management of urinalysis results and intensity of counseling services have an interactive impact on methadone maintenance treatment outcome. *Journal of Addictive Diseases, 13,* 47–63.

Caplehorn, J. R. M. (1994). A comparison of abstinence-oriented and indefinite methadone maintenance treatment. *International Journal of the Addictions, 29,* 1361–1375.

Cappendijk, S. L. T., & Dzoljic, M. R. (1993). Inhibitory effects of ibogaine on cocaine self-administration in rats. *European Journal of Pharmacology, 241,* 261–265.

Carroll, K. M., Chang, G., Behr, H., & Clinton, B. (1995). Improving treatment outcome in pregnant, methadone-maintained women: Results from a randomized clinical trial. *American Journal on Addictions, 4,* 56–59.

Carroll, K. M., & Rounsaville, B. J. (1992). Contrast of treatment-seeking and untreated cocaine abusers. *Archives of General Psychiatry, 49,* 464–471.

Carroll, K. M., Rounsaville, B. J., & Keller, D. S. (1991). Relapse prevention strategies for the treatment of cocaine abuse. *American Journal of Drug and Alcohol Abuse, 17,* 249–265.

Carroll, K. M., Rounsaville, B. J., Nich, C., Gordon, L. T., Wirtz, P. W., & Gawin, F. (1994). One-year follow-up of psychotherapy and pharmacotherapy for cocaine dependence. *Archives of General Psychiatry, 51,* 989–997.

Chaisson, R. E., Bacchetti, P., Osmond, D., Brodie, B., Sande, M. A., & Moss, A. R. (1989). Cocaine use and HIV infection in intravenous drug users in San Francisco. *Journal of the American Medical Association, 261,* 561–565.

Chakko, S., & Myerburg, R. J. (1995). Cardiac complications of cocaine abuse. *Clinical Cardiology, 18,* 67–72.

Chang, G., Carroll, K. M., Behr, H. M, & Kosten, T. R. (1992). Improving treatment outcome in pregnant opiate-dependent women. *Journal of Substance Abuse Treatment, 9,* 327–330.

Chasnoff, I. J., Griffith, D. R., Freier, C., & Murray, J. (1992). Cocaine/polydrug use in pregnancy: Two-year follow up. *Pediatrics, 89,* 284–289.

Childress, A. R., Hole, A. V., Ehrman, R. N., Robbins, S. J., McLellan, A. T., & O'Brien, C. P. (1993). Cue reactivity and cue reactivity interventions in drug dependence. *In Behavioral treatments for drug abuse and dependence* (NIDA

Research Monograph No. 137, pp. 73–95). Rockville, MD: U.S. Department of Health and Human Services.

Cohen, E., Navaline, H., & Metzger, D. (1994). High-risk behaviors for HIV: A comparison between crack-abusing and opioid-abusing African-American women. *Journal of Psychoactive Drugs, 26,* 233–241.

Cohen, S. (1976). Marihuana: Does it have medical usefulness? *Drug Abuse and Alcoholism Newsletter, 5,* 1–4.

Cowan, A., Doxey, J. C., & Harry, E. J. R. (1977). The animal pharmacology of buprenorphine: An oripavine analgesic agent. *British Journal of Pharmacology, 60,* 547–554.

Cregler, L. L. (1991). The newest risk factor for cardiovascular disease. *Clinical Cardiology, 14,* 449–456.

Cregler, L. L., & Mark, H. (1986). Medical complications of cocaine abuse. *New England Journal of Medicine, 315,* 1495–1500.

Darke, S., Cohen, J., Ross, J., Hando, J., & Hall, W. (1994). Transitions between routes of administration of regular amphetamine users. *Addiction, 89,* 1077–1083.

D'Aunno, T., & Vaughn, T. E. (1992). Variations in methadone treatment practices. *Journal of the American Medical Association, 267,* 253–258.

Dawe, S., Gerada, C., & Strang, J. (1992). Establishment of a liaison service for pregnant opiate-dependent women. *British Journal of Addiction, 87,* 867–871.

Deschenes, E. P., Anglin, M. D., & Speckart, G. (1991). Narcotics addiction: Related criminal careers, social and economic costs. *Journal of Drug Issues, 21,* 383–411.

Diaz, J. (1997). *How drugs influence behavior: Neurobehavioral approach.* Upper Saddle River, NJ: Prentice-Hall.

Doberczak, T. M., Kandall, S. R., & Friedmann, P. (1993). Relationship between maternal methadone dosage, maternal–neonatal methadone levels, and neonatal withdrawal. *Obstetrics and Gynecology, 81,* 936–940.

Doblin, R. E., & Kleiman, M. A. R. (1991). Marijuana as antiemetic medicine: A survey of oncologists' experiences and attitudes. *Journal of Clinical Oncology, 9,* 1314–1319.

Dolan, M. P., Black, J. L., Penk, W. E., Robinowitz, R., & DeFord, H. A. (1985). Contracting for treatment termination to reduce illicit drug use among methadone maintenance treatment failures. *Journal of Consulting and Clinical Psychology, 53,* 549–551.

Dole, V. P., Nyswander, M., & Warner, A. (1968). Successful treatment of 750 criminal addicts. *Journal of the American Medical Association, 206,* 2708–2711.

Dole, V. P., Robinson, J. W., Orraca, J., Towns, E., Searcy, P., & Caine, E. (1969). Methadone treatment of randomly selected criminal addicts. *New England Journal of Medicine, 208*(25), 1372–1375.

Drake, R. E., Rosenberg, S. D., & Mueser, K. T. (1996). Assessing substance use disorders in persons with severe mental illness. *New Directions for Mental Health Services, 70,* 3–17.

Drug Abuse Warning Network. (1995). *Data from the Drug Abuse Warning Network (DAWN): Medical examiner data.* Rockville, MD: U.S. Department of Health and Human Services.

Drug Abuse Warning Network. (1996). *Data from the Drug Abuse Warning*

Network (DAWN), Medical examiner data. Rockville, MD: U.S. Department of Health and Human Services.

DuRant, R. H., Rickert, V. I., Ashworth, C. S., Newman, C., & Slavens, G. (1993). Use of multiple drugs among adolescents who use anabolic steroids. *New England Journal of Medicine, 328,* 922–926.

Dzoljic, E. D., Kaplan, C. D., & Dzoljic, M. R. (1988). Effects of ibogaine on naloxone-precipitated withdrawal syndrome in chronic morphine-dependent rats. *Archives of International Pharmacodynamics, 294,* 64–70.

Edlin, B. R., Irwin, K. L., Faruque, S., McCoy, C. B., Word, C., Serrano, Y., Inciardi, J. A., Bowser, B. P., Schilling, R. F., Holmberg, S. D., & the Multicenter Crack Cocaine and HIV Infection Study Team. (1994). Intersecting epidemics: Crack cocaine use and HIV infection among inner-city young adults. *New England Journal of Medicine, 331,* 1422–1427.

El-Bassel, N., Schilling, R. F., Turnbull, J. E., & Su, K. (1993). Correlates of alcohol use among methadone patients. *Alcoholism: Clinical and Experimental Research, 17,* 681–686.

Engelsman, E. L. (1989). Dutch policy on the management of drug-related problems. *British Journal of Addiction, 84,* 211–218.

Everingham, S., & Rydell, C. (1994). *Controlling cocaine.* Santa Monica, CA: Rand Corporation.

Fairbank, J. A., Dunteman, G. H., & Condelli, W. S. (1993). Do methadone patients substitute other drugs for heroin? Predicting substance use at 1-year follow-up. *American Journal of Drug and Alcohol Abuse, 19,* 465–474.

Fox, C. H. (1994). Cocaine use in pregnancy. *Journal of the American Board of Family Practice, 7,* 225–228.

Freedman, D. (1986). Hallucinogenic drug research—if so, so what?: Symposium summary and commentary. *Pharmacology, Biochemistry and Behavior, 24,* 407–415.

Frenken, G., & Nodelman, A. (1996, July). The necessity of addict self-help involvement in ibogaine treatment procedures. In *International Addict Self-Help (INTASH)* [On-line]. Available: http://www.ibogaine.org/intash.html [6/9/98].

Fudala, P. J., Jaffe, J. H., Dax, E. M., & Johnson, R. E. (1990). Use of buprenorphine in the treatment of opioid addiction: II. Physiologic and behavioral effects of daily and alternate-day administration and abrupt withdrawal. *Clinical Pharmacology and Therapeutics, 47*(4), 525–534.

Gaughwin, M., Kliewer, E., Ali, R., Faulkner, C., Wodak, A., & Anderson, G. (1993). The prescription of methadone for opiate-dependence in Australia, 1985–1991. *Medical Journal of Australia, 159,* 107–108.

Gawin, F. H., & Ellinwood, E. H. (1988). Cocaine and other stimulants: Actions, abuse and treatment. *New England Journal of Medicine, 318,* 173–182.

Gawin, F. H., & Kleber, H. D. (1986). Abstinence symptomatology and psychiatric diagnosis in cocaine abusers. *Archives of General Psychiatry, 43,* 107–113.

Gerstein, D. R., & Harwood, H. J. (Eds.). (1990). *Treating drug problems: A study of the evolution, effectiveness, and financing of public and private drug treatment systems* (Vol. 1). Washington, DC: National Academy Press.

Gilmore, T., & Bowers, C. (1995, October). Starting a patient run program. *National Alliance of Methadone Advocates Education Series* [On-line serial], 6. Available: http://www.methadone.org/es6.html [6/9/98].

Glick, S. D., Rossman, K., Rao, N. C., Maisonneuve, I. M., & Carlson, J. N. (1992). Effects of ibogaine on acute signs of morphine withdrawal in rats: Independence from tremor. *Neuropharmacology, 31*, 497–500.

Glick, S. D., Rossman, K., Steindorf, S., Maisonneuve, I. M., & Carlson, J. N. (1992). Effects and aftereffects of ibogaine on morphine self-administration in rats. *European Journal of Pharmacology, 195*, 341–345.

Gold, M. S. (1993). Opiate addiction and the locus coeruleus: The clinical utility of clonidine, naltrexone, methadone, and buprenorphine. *Psychiatric Clinics of North America, 16*, 61–73.

Gold, M. S. (1997). Cocaine (and crack): Clinical aspects. In J. H. Lowinsin, P. Ruiz, R. B. Millman, & J. G. Langrod (Eds.), *Substance abuse: A comprehensive textbook* (3rd ed., pp. 181–199). Baltimore: Williams & Wilkins.

Gold, M. S., & Kleber, H. D. (1979). A rationale for opiate withdrawal symptomatology. *Drug and Alcohol Dependence, 4*, 419–424.

Gold, M. S., & Miller, N. S. (1997). Cocaine (and crack): Neurobiology. In J. H. Lowinsin, P. Ruiz, R. B. Millman, & J. G. Langrod (Eds.), *Substance abuse: A comprehensive textbook* (3rd ed., pp. 166–181). Baltimore: Williams & Wilkins.

Gold, M. S., Sorensen, J. L., McCanlies, N., Trier, M., & Dlugosch, G. (1988). Tapering from methadone maintenance: Attitudes of clients and staff. *Journal of Substance Abuse Treatment, 5*, 37–44.

Goldberg, L., Bosworth, E. E., Bents, R. T., & Trevisan, L. (1990). Effect of an anabolic steroid education program on knowledge and attitudes of high school football players. *Journal of Adolescent Health Care, 11*, 210–214.

Goldstein, A. (1994). *Addiction: From biology to drug policy.* New York: W.H. Freeman.

Goldstein, P. (1994, March). *Performance enhancing drugs and sports.* Panel presentation at the 5th International Conference on the Reduction of Drug Related Harm, Toronto, Ontario.

Goldstein, P. (1989). Drugs and violent crime. In N. A. Weiner & M. E. Wolfgang (Eds.), *Pathways to criminal violence* (pp. 16–48). Beverly Hills, CA: Sage.

Gordon, N. B. (1970). Reaction times of methadone treated ex-heroin addicts. *Psychopharmacologia, 16*, 337–344.

Gorelick, D. A. (1992). Alcohol and cocaine: Clinical and pharmacological interactions. In M. Galanter (Ed.), *Recent developments in alcoholism: Vol. 10. Alcohol and cocaine: Similarities and differences* (pp. 37–56). New York: Plenum Press.

Gossop, M., Griffiths, P., & Strang, J. (1988). Chasing the dragon: Characteristics of heroin chasers. *British Journal of Addiction, 83*, 1159–1162.

Gossop, M., & Strang, J. (1991). A comparison of the withdrawal responses of heroin and methadone addicts during detoxification. *British Journal of Psychiatry, 158*, 697–699.

Goutarel, R., Gollnhofer, O., & Sillans, R. (1993). Pharmacodynamics and therapeutic applications of iboga and ibogaine. *Psychedelic Monographs and Essays, 6*, 71–111.

Gritz, E. R., Shiffman, S. M., Jarvik, M. E., Harber, J., Dymond, A. M., Coger, R., Charuvastra, V., & Schlesinger, J. (1975). Physiological and psychological effects of methadone in man. *Archives of General Psychiatry, 32*, 237–242.

Gunne, L., & Gronbladh, L. (1981). The Swedish methadone maintenance program: A controlled study. *Drug and Alcohol Dependence, 7*, 249–256.

Gutierrez-Cebollada, J., de la Torre, R., Ortuno, J., Garces, J. M., & Cami, J. (1994). Psychotropic drug consumption and other factors associated with heroin overdose. *Drug and Alcohol Dependence, 35,* 169–174.

Higgins, S. T., Budney, A. J., Bickel, W. K., Foerg, F. E., Donham, R., & Badger, G. J. (1994). Incentives improve outcome in outpatient behavioral treatment of cocaine dependence. *Archives of General Psychiatry, 51,* 568–576.

Higgins, S. T., Budney, A. J., Bickel, W. K., Hughes, J. R., Foerg, F., & Badger, G. (1993). Achieving cocaine abstinence with a behavioral approach. *American Journal of Psychiatry, 150,* 763–769.

Higgins, S. T., Budney, A. J., Bickel, W. K., Hughes, J. R., Foerg, F., & Badger, G. (1994). Alcohol dependence and simultaneous cocaine and alcohol use in cocaine-dependent patients. In S. Magura, A. Rosenblum, & B. Stimmel (Eds.), *Experimental therapeutics in addiction medicine* (pp. 177–189). New York: Haworth Press.

Higgins, S. T., Stitzer, M. L., Bigelow, G. E., & Liebson, I. A. (1986). Contingent methadone delivery: Effects on illicit-opiate use. *Drug and Alcohol Dependence, 17,* 311–322.

Hoffer, A. (1965). LSD: A review of its present status. *Clinical Pharmacology and Therapeutics, 6,* 183–255.

Hoffman, J. A., Caudill, B. D., Koman, J. J., Luckey, J. W., Flynn, P. M., & Hubbard, R. L. (1994). Comparative cocaine abuse treatment strategies: Enhancing client retention and treatment exposure. In S. Magura, A. Rosenblum, & B. Stimmel (Eds.), *Experimental therapeutics in addiction medicine* (pp. 115–128). New York: Haworth Press.

Hollister, L. E. (1986). Health aspects of cannabis. *Pharmacological Reviews, 38,* 1–20.

Hollister, L. E. (1992). Marijuana and immunity. *Journal of Psychoactive Drugs, 24,* 159–164.

Hubbard, R. L., Marsden, M. E., Rachal, J., Valley, H., & Henrick, J. (1989). *Drug abuse treatment: A national study of effectiveness.* Chapel Hill: University of North Carolina Press.

Hubbard, R. L., Rachal, J. V., Craddock, S. G., & Cavanaugh, E. R. (1984). Treatment Outcome Prospective Study (TOPS): Client characteristics and behaviors before, during, and after treatment. In F. M. Tims & J. P. Ludford (Eds.), *Drug abuse treatment evaluation: Strategies, progress, and prospects* (NIDA Research Monograph No. 51, pp. 42–68). Rockville, MD: U.S. Department of Health and Human Services.

Huber, G. L., First, M. W. & Gruber, O. (1991). Marijuana and tobacco smoke: Gas-phase cytotoxins. *Pharmacology, Biochemistry, and Behavior, 40,* 629–636.

Iguchi, M. Y., Stitzer, M. L., Bigelow, G. E., & Liebson, I. A. (1988). Contingency management in methadone maintenance: Effects of reinforcing and aversive consequences on illicit polydrug use. *Drug and Alcohol Dependence, 22,* 1–7.

Institute of Medicine. (1982). *Marijuana and health.* Washington DC: National Academy Press.

Institute of Medicine. (1995). *Federal regulation of methadone treatment.* Washington, DC: National Academy Press.

Isner, J. M., & Chokshi, S. K. (1991). Cardiovascular complications of cocaine. *Current Problems in Cardiology, 16,* 91–123.

Jaffe, J. H. (1995). Pharmacological treatment of opioid dependence: Current techniques and new findings. *Psychiatric Annals, 25,* 369–375.

Jaffe, J. H., & Martin, W. R. (1990). Opioid analgesics and antagonists. In A. G. Gilman, T. W. Rall, A. S. Nies, & P. Taylor (Eds.), *Goodman and Gilman's: The pharmacological basis of therapeutics* (8th ed., pp. 485–521). New York: Pergamon Press.

Jaffe, J. H., Schuster, C. R., Smith, B. B., & Blachly, P. H. (1970). Comparison of acetylmethadol and methadone in the treatment of long-term heroin users. *Journal of the American Medical Association, 211,* 1834–1836.

Jarvis, M. A. E., & Schnoll, S. H. (1994). Methadone maintenance during pregnancy. *Journal of Psychoactive Drugs, 26,* 155–161.

Jasinski, D. R., Pevnick, J. S., & Griffith, J. D. (1978). Human pharmacology and abuse potential of the analgesic buprenorphine. *Archives of General Psychiatry, 35,* 501–516.

Jenkins, A. J., Keenan, R. M., Henningfield, J. E., & Cone, E. J. (1994). Pharmacokinetics and pharmacodynamics of smoked heroin. *Journal of Analytical Toxicology, 18,* 317–330.

Joe, G. W., Simpson, D. D., & Hubbard, R. L. (1991). Treatment predictors of tenure in methadone maintenance for opioid dependence. *Journal of Nervous and Mental Disease, 181,* 358–364.

Johnson, R. E., Jaffe, J. H., & Fudala, P. J. (1992). A controlled trial of buprenorphine treatment for opioid dependence. *Journal of the American Medical Association, 267,* 2750–2755.

Johnston, L. D., O'Malley, P. M., & Bachman, J. G. (1997). *National survey results on drug use from the Monitoring the Future study, 1975–1996: Vol. I. Secondary school students* (NIH Publication No. 97-4139). Rockville, MD: U.S. Department of Health and Human Services.

Joseph, H. (1988). The criminal justice system and opiate addiction: A historical perspective. In *Compulsory treatment of drug abuse: Research and clinical practice* (NIDA Research Monograph No. 86, pp. 106–125). Rockville, MD: U.S. Department of Health and Human Services.

Kelley, D., Welch, R., & McKnelley, W. (1978). Methadone maintenance: As assessment of potential fluctuations in behavior between doses. *International Journal of the Addictions, 13,* 1061–1068.

Kidorf, M., Stitzer, M. L., Brooner, R. K., & Goldberg, J. (1994). Contingent methadone take-home doses reinforce adjunct therapy attendance of methadone maintenance patients. *Drug and Alcohol Dependence, 36,* 221–226.

Kleinman, P. H., Kang, S., Lipton, D. S., Woody, G. E., Kemp, J., & Millman, R. E. (1992). Retention of cocaine abusers in outpatient psychotherapy. *American Journal of Drug and Alcohol Abuse, 18,* 29–43.

Kosten, T. R., Kleber, H. D., & Morgan, C. (1989). Treatment of cocaine abuse with buprenorphine. *Biological Psychiatry, 26,* 637–639.

Kosten, T. R., Morgan, C., & Kleber, H. D. (1991). Treatment of heroin addicts using buprenorphine. *American Journal of Drug and Alcohol Abuse, 17,* 119–128.

Kosten, T. R., Rounsaville, R. J., & Kleber, H. D. (1987). A 2.5-year follow-up of cocaine use among treated opioid addicts. *Archives of General Psychiatry, 44,* 281–284.

Kosten, T. R., Schottenfeld, R., Ziedonis, D., & Falcioni, J. (1993). Buprenorphine versus methadone maintenance for opioid dependence. *Journal of Nervous and Mental Disease, 181,* 358–364.

Kotler, D. P. (1989). Malnutrition in HIV infection and AIDS. *AIDS, 3*(1), S175–S180.

Kreek, M. J. (1992). Rationale for maintenance pharmacotherapy of opiate-dependence. In C. P. O'Brien & J. H. Jaffe (Eds.), *Addictive states* (pp. 205–230). New York: Raven Press.

Kreek, M. J., Novick, D. M., Richman, B. L., Friedman, J. M., Friedman, J. E., Fried, C., Wilson, J. P., & Townley, A. (1993). The medical status of methadone maintenance patients in treatment for 11–18 years. *Drug and Alcohol Dependence, 33,* 235–245.

Landry, M. J. (1992). An overview of cocaethylene, an alcohol-derived, psychoactive, cocaine metabolite. *Journal of Psychoactive Drugs, 24,* 273–276.

Lane, M., Vogel, C. L., Ferguson, J., Krasnow, S., Saiers, J. L., Hamm, J., Salva, K., Wiernik, P. H., Holroyde, C. P., Hammill, S., Shepard, K., & Plasse, T. (1991). Dronabinol and prochlorperazine in combination for the treatment of cancer chemotherapy-induced nausea and vomiting. *Journal of Pain and Symptom Management, 6,* 352–359.

Lap, M. (1995). Pharmacology and substances: The opiates. In *Drug text* [On-line]. Available: http://www.calyx.com/mariolap/sub/opiat1.html.

Larrat, E. P., & Zierler, S. (1993). Entangled epidemics: Cocaine use and HIV disease. *Journal of Psychoactive Drugs, 25,* 207–221.

Lenehan, P. (1994, March). *Performance enhancing drugs and sports.* Panel presentation at the 5th International Conference on the Reduction of Drug Rekated Harm, Toronto, Ontario.

Lester, B. M., LaGasse, L., Freier, K., & Brunner, S. (1996). Studies of cocaine-exposed human infants. In *Behavioral studies of drug-exposed offspring: Methodological issues in human and animal* (NIDA Research Monograph No. 164, pp. 175–210). Rockville, MD: U.S. Department of Health and Human Services.

Levitt, M., Faiman, C., Hawks, R., & Wilson, A. (1984). Randomized double-blind comparison of delta-9-tetrahydrocannabinol (THC) and marijuana as chemotherapy antiemetics. *Proceedings of the American Society of Clinical Oncology, 3,* 91.

Liese, B. A., & Najavits, L. M. (1997). Cognitive and behavioral therapies. In J. H. Lowinsin, P. Ruiz, R. B. Millman, & J. G. Langrod (Eds.), *Substance abuse: A comprehensive textbook* (3rd ed., pp. 467–478). Baltimore: Williams & Wilkins.

Lillie-Blanton, M., Anthony, J. C., & Schuster, C. R. (1993). Probing the meaning of racial/ethnic group comparisons in crack cocaine smoking. *Journal of the American Medical Association, 269,* 993–997.

Ling, W., Rawson, R. A., & Compton, M. A. (1994). Substitution pharmacotherapies for opioid addiction: From methadone to LAAM and buprenorphine. *Journal of Psychoactive Drugs, 26,* 119–128.

Lombardo, W. K., Lombardo, B., & Goldstein, A. (1976). Cognitive functioning under moderate and low dosage methadone maintenance. *International Journal of the Addictions, 11,* 389–401.

Longshore, D., Hsieh, S., & Anglin, M. D. (1994). Reducing HIV risk behavior among injection drug users: Effect of methadone maintenance treatment on number of sex partners. *International Journal of the Addictions, 29,* 741–757.

Lotsof, H. S. (1995). Ibogaine in the treatment of chemical dependence disorders: Clinical perspectives. *Bulletin of the Multidisciplinary Association of Psychedelic Studies, 5,* 16–27.

Lotsof, H. S., Della Sera, E., & Kaplan, C. D. (1995, August). *Ibogaine in the treatment of narcotic withdrawal.* Paper presented at the 37th International Congress on Alcohol and Drug Dependence, La Jolla, CA.

Lurie, P., & Lee, P. R. (1991). Fifteen solutions to the problems of prescription drug abuse. *Journal of Psychoactive Drugs, 23*(4), 349–357.

Maddux, J. F., Desmond, D. P., & Vogtsberger, K. N. (1995). Patient-regulated methadone dose and optional counseling in methadone maintenance. *American Journal on Addictions, 4,* 18–32.

Maisonneuve, I. M., Keller, R. W., & Glick, S. D. (1991). Interactions between ibogaine, a potential anti-addictive agent and morphine: An in vivo microdialysis study. *European Journal of Pharmacology, 199,* 35–42.

Maisonneuve, I. M., Rossman, K. L., Keller, R. W., & Glick, S. D. (1992). Acute and prolonged effects of ibogaine on brain dopamine metabolism and morphine-induced locomotor activity in rats. *Brain Research, 574,* 69–73.

Majewska, M. D. (Ed.). (1996). *Neurotoxicity and neuropathology associated with cocaine abuse* (NIDA Research Monograph No. 163). Rockville, MD: U.S. Department of Health and Human Services.

Marek, P., Ben-Eliyahu, S., Gold, M., & Liebeskind, J. C. (1991). Excitatory amino acid antagonists (kynurenic acid and MK-801) attenuate the development of morphine tolerance in the rat. *Brain Research, 547,* 77–81.

Margolin, A., Kosten, T. R., Petrakis, I., Avants, S. K., & Kosten, T. (1991). Bupropion reduces cocaine abuse in methadone-maintained patients. *Archives of General Psychiatry, 48,* 87.

Marlatt, G. A., & Tapert, S. F. (1993). Harm reduction: Reducing the risks of addictive behaviors. In J. S. Baer, G. A. Marlatt, & R. J. McMahon (Eds.), *Addictive behaviors across the lifespan* (pp. 243–273). Newbury Park, CA: Sage.

Mash, D. C. (1995). *Ibogaine in drug detoxification: From preclinical studies to clinical trials.* Paper presented at the Symposium on Maturational Issues in Behavioral Disorders, Maastricht, the Netherlands.

Mash, D. C., Staley, J. K., Pablo, J. P., Holohean, A. M., Hackman, J. C., & Davidoff, R. A. (1995). Properties of ibogaine and its principal metabolite (12-hydroxyibogamine) at the MK-801 binding site of the NMDA receptor complex. *Neuroscience Letters, 192,* 53–56.

Mathias, R. (1997). Rate and duration of drug activity play major roles in drug abuse, addiction and treatment. *NIDA Notes, 12*(2), 8–11.

McCaul, M. E., Stitzer, M. L., Bigelow, G. E., & Liebson, I. A. (1984). Contingency management interventions: Effects on treatment outcome during methadone detoxification. *Journal of Applied Behavior Analysis, 17,* 35–43.

McLachlan, C., Crofts, N., Wodak, A., & Crowe, S. (1993). The effects of methadone on immune function among injecting drug users: A review. *Addiction, 88,* 257–263.

McLellan, A. T., Alterman, A. I., Metzger, D. S., Grissom, G. R., Woody, G. E., Luborsky, L., & O'Brien, C. P. (1994). Similarlity of outcome predictors across opiate, cocaine, and alcohol treatments: Role of treatment services. *Journal of Consulting and Clinical Psychology, 62,* 1141–1158.

McLellan, A. T., Woody, G. E., Luborsky, L., & Goehl, L. (1988). Is the counselor an "active ingredient" in substance abuse rehabilitation? *Journal of Nervous and Mental Disease, 176,* 423–430.

Metzger, D. S., Woody, G. E., McLellan, A. T., O'Brien, C. P., Druley, P., Navaline, H., DePhilippis, D., Stolley, P., & Abrutyn, E. (1993). Human immunodeficiency virus seroconversion among intravenous drug users in- and out-of-treatment: An 18-month prospective follow-up. *Journal of Acquired Immune Deficiency Syndromes, 6,* 1049–1056.

Milby, J. B. (1988). Methadone maintenance to abstinence: How many make it? *Journal of Nervous and Mental Disease, 176,* 409–422.

Miller, W. H., & Hyatt, M. C. (1992). Perinatal substabce abuse. *American Journal of Drug and Alcohol Aubse, 18,* 247–261.

Mitchell, S. W. (1896). The effects of *Anhalonium lewinii* (the mescal button). *British Medical Journal, ii,* 1625–1628.

Montoya, I. D., Hess, J. M., Preston, K. L., & Gorelick, D. A. (1994). A model for pharmacological research—treatment of cocaine dependence. *Journal of Substance Abuse Treatment, 12,* 415–421.

Morgan, J. P., & Zimmer, L. (1997). The social pharmacology of smokeable cocaine: Not all it's cracked up to be. In C. Reinarman & H. G. Levine (Eds.), *Crack in America: Demon drugs and social justice* (pp. 131–170). Berkeley: University of California Press.

Mueser, K. T., Bellack, A. S., & Blanchard, J. J. (1992). Comorbidity of schizophrenia and substance abuse: Implications for treatment. *Journal of Consulting and Clinical Psychology, 60,* 845–856.

Murphy, S., & Irwin, J. (1992). "Living with the dirty secret": Problems of disclosure for methadone maintenance clients. *Journal of Psychoactive Drugs, 24,* 257–264.

Nadelmann, E. A., & McNeely, J. (1996). Doing methadone right. *Public Interest, 123,* 83–93.

Nahas, G. (1977). Biomedical aspects of cannabis usage. *Bulletin on Narcotics, 29,* 13–27.

Naranjo, C. (1973). *The healing journey.* New York: Pantheon.

National Institute on Drug Abuse (NIDA). (1991). *NIDA capsules: Summary of findings from the 1990 National Household Survey on Drug Abuse.* Rockville, MD: U.S. Department of Health and Human Services.

National Institutes of Health. (1997). *Workshop on the medical utility of marijuana* [On-line]. Available: http://www.nih.gov/news/medmarijuana/MedicalMarijuana.htm.

Newman, R. G. (1995). Another wall that crumbled: Methadone maintenance treatment in Germany. *American Journal of Drug and Alcohol Abuse, 21,* 27–35.

Newman, R. G., & Peyser, N. (1991). Methadone treatment: Experiment and experience. *Journal of Psychoactive Drugs, 23,* 115–121.

Newman, R. G., & Whitehill, W. B. (1979). Double-blind comparison of methadone and placebo maintenance treatments of narcotic addicts in Hong Kong. *Lancet, ii,* 485–488.

Novick, D. M., Joseph, H., Salsitz, E. A., Kalin, M. F., Keefe, J. B., Miller, E. L., & Richman, B. L. (1994). Outcomes of treatment of socially rehabilitated methadone maintenance patients in physicians' offices (medical maintenance):

Follow-up at three and a half to nine and a fourth years. *Journal of General Internal Medicine, 9,* 127–130.

Novick, D. M., Richman, B. L., Friedman, J. M., Friedman, J. E., Fried, C., Wilson, J. P., Townley, A., & Kreek, M. J. (1993). The medical status of methadone maintenance patients in treatment for 11–18 years. *Drug and Alcohol Dependence, 33,* 235–245.

Noyes, R., Brunk, S., Baram, D. A., & Canter, A. (1975). Analgesic effects of delta-9-tetrahydrocannabinol. *Journal of Clinical Pharmacology, 15,* 139–143.

Nunes, E., Quitkin, F., Brady, R., & Post-Koenig, T. (1994). Antidepressant treatment in methadone maintenance patients. *Journal of Addictive Diseases, 13,* 13–24.

O'Brien, C. P. (1996). Recent developments in the pharmacotherapy of substance abuse. *Journal of Consulting and Clinical Psychology, 64,* 677–686.

Office of the Inspector General. (1990). *Initiative to improve states' internal controls over prescription drugs purchased under the medical program* (Publication No. A-30-90-000204). Washington, DC: U.S. Department of Health and Human Services.

O'Hare, P. A., Newcombe, R., Matthews, A., Buning, E. C., & Drucker, E. (Eds.). (1992). *The reduction of drug-related harm.* London: Routledge.

O'Hearn, E., & Molliver, M. E. (1993). Degeneration of Purkinje cells in parasagittal zones of the cerebellar vermis after treatment with ibogaine or harmaline. *Neuroscience, 55,* 303–310.

Onken, L. S., Blaine, J. D., & Boren, J. J. (1993). *Behavioral treatments for drug abuse and drug dependence* (NIDA Research Monograph No. 137). Rockville, MD: U.S. Department of Health and Human Services.

Pani, P. P., Pirastu, R., Ricci, A., & Geesa, G. L. (1996). Prohibition of take-home dosages: Negative consequences on methadone maintenance treatment. *Drug and Alcohol Dependence, 41,* 81–84.

Peyote Foundation. (1996, July–August). The medicine: Herbal uses. *Peyote Awareness Journal* [On-line serial], 1. Available: http://www.maps.org/paj/ [6/9/98].

Plasse, T. F., Gorter, R. W., Krasnow, S. H., Lane, M., Shepard, K. V., & Wadleigh, R. G. (1991). Recent clinical experience with dronabinol. *Pharmacology, Biochemistry and Behavior, 40,* 695–700.

Popik, P., Layer, R. T., & Skolnick, P. (1994). The putative anti-addictive drug ibogaine is a competitive inhibitor of [3H]MK-801 binding to the NMDA receptor complex. *Psychopharmacology, 114,* 672–674.

Pot smoking acceptable at S.F. club. (1995, March 26). *San José Mercury News,* p. 3B.

Powell, J., Gray, J., & Bradley, B. (1993). Subjective craving for opiates: Evaluation of a cue exposure protocol for use with detoxified opiate addicts. *British Journal of Clinical Psychology, 32,* 39–53.

Rainone, G. A., Deren, S., Kleinman, P. H., & Wish, E. D. (1987). Heavy marijuana users not in treatment: The continuing search for the "pure" marijuana user. *Journal of Psychoactive Drugs, 19*(4), 353–359.

Rand Corporation. (1995, Spring). Treatment: Effective (but unpopular) weapon against drugs. *Rand Research Review,* p. 4.

Ratner, M. S. (1993). *Crack pipe as pimp: An ethnographic investigation of sex-for-crack exchanges.* New York: Lexington.

Rawson, R. A., Shoptaw, S. J., Obert, J. L., McCann, M. J., Hasson, A. L.,

Marinelli-Casey, P. J., Brethen, P. R., & Ling, W. (1995). An intensive outpatient approach for cocaine abuse treatment: The Matrix model. *Journal of Substance Abuse Treatment, 12,* 117–127.

Ray, O., & Ksir, C. (1993). *Drugs, society, and human behavior* (6th ed.). St. Louis, MO: C.V. Mosby.

Ray, W. A., Fought, R. L., & Decker, M. D. (1992). Psychoactive drugs and the risk of injurious motor vehicle crashes in elderly drivers. *American Journal of Epidemiology, 136,* 873–883.

Regier, D. A., Farmer, M. E., Rae, D. S., Locke, B. Z., Keith, S. J., Judd, L. L., & Goodwin, F. K. (1990). Comorbidity of mental disorders with alcohol and other drug abuse: Results from the Epidemiologic Catchment Area (ECA) study. *Journal of the American Medical Association, 264,* 2511–2518.

Renner, J. A. (1984). Methadone maintenance: Past, present, and future. *Advances in Alcohol and Substance Abuse, 3,* 75–90.

Reynolds, I., & Magro, D. (1976). The use of methadone as a treatment tool for opiate addicts: A two-year follow-up study. *Medical Journal of Australia, 2,* 560–562.

Riley, E. P., & LaFiette, M. H. (1996). The effects of prenatal cocaine exposure on subsequent learning in the rat. *In Behavioral studies of drug-exposed offspring: Methodological issues in human and animal* (NIDA Research Monograph No. 164, pp. 53–77). Rockville, MD: U.S. Department of Health and Human Services.

Roffman, R. A., & Barnhart, R. (1987). Assessing need for marijuana dependence treatment through an anonymous telephone interview. *International Journal of the Addictions, 22,* 639–651.

Roffman, R. A., & George, W. H. (1988). Cannabis Abuse. In D. M. Donovan & G. A. Marlatt (Eds.), *Assessment of addictive behaviors* (pp. 325–363). New York: Guilford Press.

Roffman, R. A., & Stephens, R. S. (1993). Cannabis dependence. In D. L. Dunner (Ed.), *Current psychiatric therapy* (pp. 105–109). Philadelphia: W. B. Saunders.

Roffman, R. A., Stephens, R. S., Simpson, E. E., & Whitaker, D. L. (1988). Treatment of marijuana dependence: Preliminary results. *Journal of Psychoactive Drugs, 20,* 129–137.

Rosen, M. I., & Kosten, T. R. (1991). Buprenorphine: Beyond methadone? *Hospital and Community Psychiatry, 42,* 347–349.

Rosenblum, A., Magura, S., & Joseph, H. (1991). Ambivalence toward methadone treatment among intravenous drug users. *Journal of Psychoactive Drugs, 23,* 21–27.

Rothenberg, S., Schottenfeld, S., Gross, K., & Selkoe, D. (1980a). Specific oculomotor deficit after acute methadone: I. Saccadic eye movements. *Psychopharmacology, 67,* 221–227.

Rothenberg, S., Schottenfeld, S., Gross, K., & Selkoe, D. (1980b). Specific oculomotor deficit after acute methadone: II. Smooth pursuit eye movements. *Psychopharmacology, 67,* 229–234.

Rothenberg, S., Schottenfeld, S., Meyer, R. E., Krauss, B., & Gross, K. (1977). Performance differences between addicts and non-addicts. *Psychopharmacology, 52,* 299–306.

Rounsaville, B. J., Weissman, M. M., Kleber, H. D., & Wilber, C. (1982). Heterogeneity of psychiatric disorders in treated opiate addicts. *Archives of General Psychiatry, 39,* 161–166.

Savage, C. (1952). Lysergic acid diethylamide (LSD-25): A clinical-psychological study. *American Journal of Psychiatry, 108,* 896–900.

Saxon, A. J., Calsyn, D. A., Greenberg, D., Blaes, P., Haver, V. M., & Stanton, V. (1993). Urine screening for marijuana among methadone-maintained patients. *American Journal on Addictions, 2,* 207–211.

Saxon, A. J., Calsyn, D. A., Kivlahan, D. R., & Roszell, D. K. (1993). Outcome of contingency contracting for illicit drug use in a methadone maintenance program. *Drug and Alcohol Dependence, 31,* 205–214.

Schick, J. F., & Smith, D. (1970). Analysis of the LSD flashback. *Journal of Psychedelic Drugs, 3,* 13–19.

Schuckit, M. A. (1995). Chasing the dragon. In J. A. Inciardi & K. McElrath (Eds.), *The American drug scene* (pp. 144–146). Los Angeles: Roxbury.

Schwartz, R. H., & Beveridge, R. A. (1994). Marijuana as an antiemetic drug: How useful is it today? Opinions from clinical oncologists. *Journal of Addictive Diseases, 13,* 53–65.

Senay, E. C., Barthwell, A. G., Marks, T., Bokos, P., Gillman, D., & White, R. (1993). Medical maintenance: A pilot study. *Journal of Addictive Diseases, 12,* 59–76.

Serpelloni, G., Carrieri, M. P., Rezza, G., Morganti, S., Gomma, M., & Binkin, N. (1994). Methadone treatment as a determinant of HIV risk reduction among injecting drug users: A nested case–control study. *AIDS Care, 6,* 215–220.

Sershen, H., Hashim, A., Harsing, L., & Lajtha, A. (1992). Ibogaine antagonizes cocaine induced locomotor stimulation in mice. *Life Sciences, 50,* 1079–1086.

Sershen, H., Hashim, A., & Lajtha, A. (1993). Ibogaine reduces preference for cocaine consumption in C57BL/6By mice. *Pharmacology, Biochemistry and Behavior, 47,* 13–19.

Seymour, R. B., & Smith, D. E. (1987). *Drugfree: A unique, positive approach to staying off alcohol and other drugs.* New York: Facts on File.

Shaner, A., Eckman, T. A., Roberts, L. J., Wilkins, J. N., Tucker, D. E., Tsuang, J. W., & Mintz, J. (1995). Disability income, cocaine use, and repeated hospitalization among schizophrenic cocaine abusers. *New England Journal of Medicine, 333,* 777–783.

Shaner, A., Khalsa, M. E., Roberts, L., Wilkins, J., Anglin, D., & Hsieh, S. (1993). Unrecognized cocaine use among schizophrenic patients. *American Journal of Psychiatry, 150,* 758–762.

Sheppard, S. G. (1994). A preliminary investigation of ibogaine: Case reports and recommendations for further study. *Journal of Substance Abuse Treatment, 11,* 379–385.

Siddiqui, N. S., Brown, L. S., Jr., Meyer, T. J., & Gonzalez, V. (1993). Decline in HIV-1 seroprevalence and low seroconversion rate among injecting drug users at a methadone maintenance program in New York City. *Journal of Psychoactive Drugs, 25,* 245–250.

Sigler, K. A., Guernsey, B. G., Ingrim, N. B., Buessing, A. S., Jokanson, J. A., Galvan, E., & Doutre, W. H. (1984). Effect of a triplicate prescription law on prescribing of Schedule II drugs. *American Journal of Hospital Pharmacy, 41,* 108–111.

Smart, R. G. (1991). Crack cocaine use: A review of prevalence and adverse effects. *American Journal of Drug and Alcohol Abuse, 17,* 13–26.

Smith, D. E., Wesson, D. R., Sees, K. L., & Morgan, J. P. (1988). An epidemiological and clinical analysis of propylhexedrine abuse in the United States. *Journal of Psychoactive Drugs, 20,* 441–442.

Sorensen, J. L., Acampora, A., Trier, M., & Gold, M. (1987). From maintenance to abstinence in a therapeutic community: Follow-up outcomes. *Journal of Psychoactive Drugs, 19,* 345–351.

Sorensen, J. L., Batki, S. L., Good, P., & Wilkinson, K. (1989). Methadone maintenance program for AIDS-affected opiate addicts. *Journal of Substance Abuse Treatment, 6,* 87–94.

Spensley, J. (1974). The adjunctive use of tricyclics in a methadone program. *Journal of Psychedelic Drugs, 6,* 421–423.

Stafford, P. (1983). Peyote, mescaline, and San Pedro. In K. Stull, N. Sanford, & B. Eisner (Eds.), *Psychedelics encyclopedia* (pp. 103–155). Los Angeles: Tarcher.

Stapleton, J. M., Guthrie, S., & Linnoila, M. (1986). Effects of alcohol and other psychotropic drug on eye movements: Relevance to traffic safety. *Journal of Studies on Alcohol, 47,* 426–432.

Stephens, R. S., Roffman, R. A., & Simpson, E. E. (1993). Adult marijuana users seeking treatment. *Journal of Consulting and Clinical Psychology, 61,* 1000–1004.

Stephens, R. S., Roffman, R. A., & Simpson, E. E. (1994). Treating adult marijuana dependence: A test of the relapse prevention model. *Journal of Consulting and Clinical Psychology, 62,* 92–99.

Stitzer, M., Bigelow, G., Lawrence, C., Cohen, J., D'Lugoff, B., & Hawthorne, J. (1977). Medication take-home as a reinforcer in a methadone maintenance program. *Addictive Behaviors, 2,* 9–14.

Stitzer, M. L., Iguchi, M. Y., & Felch, L. J. (1992). Contingent take-home incentive: Effects on drug use of methadone maintenance patients. *Journal of Consulting and Clinical Psychology, 60,* 927–934.

Stolz, J., Marsden, C., & Middlemiss, D. (1983). Effect of chronic antidepressant treatment and subsequent withdrawal on [^{3}H]5-hydroxytryptamine and [3H]spiperone binding in rat frontal cortex and serotonin receptor mediated behavior. *Psychopharmacology, 80,* 150–155.

Strain, E. C., Stitzer, M. L., Liebson, I. A., & Bigelow, G. E. (1994). Comparison of buprenorphine and methadone in the treatment of opioid dependence. *American Journal of Psychiatry, 151,* 1025–1030.

Strassman, R. J. (1984). Adverse reactions to psychedelic drugs: A review of the literature. *Journal of Nervous and Mental Disease, 172,* 577–595.

Strassman, R. J. (1995). Hallucinogenic drugs in psychiatric research treatment: Perspectives and prospects. *Journal of Nervous and Mental Disease, 183,* 127–138.

Substance Abuse and Mental Health Services Administration (SAMHSA). (1989). *National Household Survey on Drug Abuse: Population estimates, 1988.* Rockville, MD: U.S. Department of Health and Human Services.

Substance Abuse and Mental Health Services Administration (SAMHSA). (1997). *National Household Survey on Drug Abuse: Population estimates, 1996.* Rockville, MD: U.S. Department of Health and Human Services.

Swan, N. (1994). Research demonstrates long-term benefits of methadone treatment. *NIDA Notes, 9*(4), 1, 4–5.

Sweetnam, P. M., Lancaster, J., Snowman, A., Collins, J. L., Perschke, S., Bauer, C., & Perkany, J. (1995). Receptor binding profile suggests multiple mechanisms of actions are responsible for ibogaine's putative anti-addictive activity. *Psychopharmacology, 118,* 369–376.

Tashkin, D. P., Gorelick, D., Khalsa, M. E., Simmons, M., & Chang, P. (1992). Respiratory effects of cocaine freebasing among habitual cocaine smokers. *Journal of Addictive Behaviors, 11*(4), 59–70.

Titievsky, J., Seco, G., Barranco, M., & Kyle, E. M. (1982). Doxepin as adjunctive therapy for depressed methadone maintenance patients: A double-blind study. *Journal of Clinical Psychiatry, 43,* 454–456.

Trujillo, K. A., & Akil, H. (1991). Inhibition of morphine tolerance and dependence by NMDA receptor antagonist MK-801. *Science, 251,* 85–87.

Umbricht-Schneiter, A., Ginn, D. H., Pabst, K. M., & Bigelow, G. E. (1994). Providing medical care to methadone clinic patients: Referral vs. on-site care. *American Journal of Public Health, 84,* 207–210.

Ungerleider, J. T., & Andrysiak, T. (1985). Therapeutic issues of marijuana and THC (tetrahydrocannabinol). *International Journal of the Addictions, 20,* 691–699,

U.S. Department of Health and Human Services. (1993). *State methadone treatment guidelines* (DHHS Publication No. SMA 93-1991). Rockville, MD: Author.

U.S. General Accounting Office (GAO). (1996). *Cocaine treatment: Early results from various approaches* (GAO Publication No. GAO/HEHS-96-80). Gaithersburg, MD: Author.

Vanichseni, S., Wongsuwan, B., The Staff of BMA Narcotics Clinic No. 6, Choopanya, K., & Wongpanich, K. (1991). A controlled trial of methadone maintenance in a population of intravenous drug users in Bangkok: Implications for prevention of HIV. *International Journal of the Addictions, 26,* 1313–1320.

Vincent, B. J., McQuiston, D. J., Eihorn, L. H., Nagy, C. M., & Brames, M. J. (1983). Review of cannabinoids and their antiemetic effectiveness. *Drugs, 25*(Suppl. 1), 52–62.

Vinciguerra, V., Moore, T., & Brennan, E. (1988). Inhalation marijuana as an antiemetic for cancer chemotherapy. *New York State Medical Journal, 88,* 525–527.

Waldorf, D., Murphy, S., Lauderback, D., Reinarman, C., & Marotta, J. (1990). Needle sharing among male prostitutes: Preliminary findings of the Prospero Project. *Journal of Drug Issues, 20,* 309–334.

Wallace, B. C. (1991). *Crack cocaine: A practical treatment approach for the chemically dependent.* New York: Brunner/Mazel.

Walsh, S. L., Preston, K. L., Stitzer, M. L., Cone, E. J., & Bigelow, G. E. (1994). Clinical pharmacology of buprenorphine: Ceiling effects at high doses. *Clinical Pharmacology and Therapeutics, 55,* 569–580.

Ward, C. F., Ward, G. C., & Saidman, L. J. (1983). Drug abuse in anesthesia training programs: A survey, 1970 through 1980. *Journal of the American Medical Association, 250,* 922–925.

Ward, J., Mattick, R., & Hall, W. (1992). *Key issues in methadone maintenance treatment.* Sydney, New South Wales, Australia: New South Wales University Press.

Washton, A. M. (1989). *Cocaine addiction: Treatment, recovery, and relapse prevention.* New York: Norton.

Weddington, W. W. (1992). Use of pharmacologic agents in the treatment of addiction. *Psychiatric Annals, 22,* 425–429.

Weil, A., & Rosen, W. (1993). *From morphine to chocolate: Everything you need to know about mind-altering drugs.* Boston: Houghton Mifflin.

Weintraub, M., Singh, S., Bryne, L., Maharaj, K., & Guttmacher, L. (1991). Consequences of the 1989 New York State triplicate benzodiazepine prescription regulations. *Journal of American Medical Assocation, 266,* 2392–2397.

Weiss, R. D., Mirin, S. M., Griffin, M. L., & Michael, J. L. (1988). Psychopathology in cocaine abusers: Changing trends. *Journal of Nervous and Mental Disease, 176,* 719–725.

Weller, R. A., & Halikas, J. A. (1980). Objective criteria for the diagnosis of marijuana abuse. *Journal of Nervous and Mental Disease, 168,* 98–103.

Wesson, D. R., & Smith, D. E. (1978). Psychedelics. In A. Schecter (Ed.), *Treatment aspects of drug dependence* (pp. 201–231). West Palm Beach, FL: CRC Press.

Wilford, B. B., Finch, J., Czechowicz, D. J., & Warren, D. (1994). An overview of prescription drug misuse and abuse: Defining the problem and seeking solutions. *Journal of Law, Medicine, and Ethics, 22*(3), 197–203.

Wilson, B. K., Spannagel, V., Thomson, C. P. (1976). The use of L-acetylmethadol in treatment of heroin addiction: An open study. *International Journal of the Addictions, 11,* 1091–1100.

Winger, G., Hofmann, F. G., & Woods, J. H. (1992). *A handbook on drug and alcohol abuse: The biomedical aspects* (3rd ed.). New York: Oxford University Press.

Woody, G. E., Luborsky, L., McLellan, A. T., O'Brien, C. P., Beck, A. T., Blaine, J., Herman, I., & Hole, A. (1983). Psychotherapy for opiate addicts: Does it help? *Archives of General Psychiatry, 40,* 639–645.

World Health Organization. (1995, March 14). *Publication of the largest global study on cocaine use ever undertaken.* Geneva: Author.

Yancovitz, S. R., Des Jarlais, D. C., Peyser, N. P., Drew, E., Friedmann, P., Trigg, H. L., & Robinson, J. W. (1991). A randomized trial of an interim methadone maintenance clinic. *American Journal of Public Health, 81,* 1185–1191.

Young, G. A., Moreton, J. E., Meltzer, L. T., & Khazan, N. (1977). L-alpha-acetylmethadol (LAAM), methadone and morphine abstinence in dependent rats: EEG and behavioral correlates. *Drug and Alcohol Dependence, 2,* 141–148.

Zacny, J. P. (1995). A review of the effects of opioids on psychomotor and cognitive functioning in humans. *Experimental and Clinical Psychopharmacology, 3,* 432–466.

Zias, J., Stark, H., Seligman, J., Levy, R., Werker, E., Breuer, A., & Mechoulam, R. (1993). Early medical use of cannabis. *Nature, 363,* 215.

Zimmer, L., & Morgan, J. P. (1997). *Marijuana myths, marijuana facts: A review of the scientific evidence.* New York: Lindesmith Center.

Zimmerman, S., & Zimmerman, A. M. (1990). Genetic effects of marijuana. *International Journal of the Addictions, 25,* 19–33.

Zinberg, N. E. (1979). Nonaddictive opiate use. In R. I. DuPont, A. Goldstein, & J. O'Donnel (Eds.), *Handbook on drug abuse* (pp. 303–313). Rockville, MD: U.S. Department of Health and Human Services.

Zuckerman, B., Frank, D. A., Hingson, R., Amaro, H., Levenson, S. M., Kayne,

H., Parker, S., Vinci, R., Aboagye, K., Fried, L. E., Cabral, H., Timperi, R., & Bauchner, H. (1989). Effects of maternal marijuana and cocaine use on fetal growth. *New England Journal of Medicine, 320,* 762–768.

Zweben, J. E., & O'Connell, K. (1988). Strategies for breaking marijuana dependence. *Journal of Psychoactive Drugs, 20*(1), 121–127.

Zweben, J. E., & Sorensen, J. L. (1988). Misunderstandings about methadone. *Journal of Psychoactive Drugs, 20,* 275–281.

CHAPTER SEVEN

Harm Reduction and HIV/AIDS Prevention

PEGGY L. PETERSON
LINDA A. DIMEFF
SUSAN F. TAPERT
MARTIN STERN
MIKE GORMAN

OVERVIEW

Harm reduction approaches for HIV/AIDS prevention grew out of grassroots community efforts to stem the frightening rate of HIV infection among members of certain at-risk populations. Community groups representing and working with these populations made use of harm reduction strategies naturally, although the strategies may not have been specifically labeled as such. Translating what was known about HIV transmission into pragmatic approaches, the groups began risk reduction efforts such as distributing condoms or promoting needle exchanges.

Initially identified as a problem of socially marginalized groups, including men who have sex with men (MSM), injection drug users (IDUs), and sex workers, AIDS was viewed by many mainstream observers as a moral issue rather than as a public health problem. Public animosity intensified the gaps between affected and unaffected groups, as the former were seen as "vectors of disease" that threatened society. Impassioned to prevent the spread of HIV infection, community activists intervened with courageous and pragmatic innovation. These individuals and groups mobilized to provide an effective and compassionate response to HIV/AIDS— one that was not forthcoming from mainstream society. Because of their position as "insiders," these activists were able both to access their communities directly and to tailor programs to the specific needs and culture of their communities.

Many of the innovative risk reduction methods that evolved out of community efforts have been adopted and disseminated by public health programs, which use members of the target groups as street outreach workers. Since the people most at risk for exposure to HIV infection tend to be members of the most mobile and/or socially marginalized groups, they are the most difficult to reach by traditional or mainstream strategies, communication channels, or professionals. Outreach programs conducted by members of a target group reduce the barriers commonly encountered by traditional public health programs (e.g., establishing trust and credibility, locating and reaching individuals in the target group). These programs also carry the potential for increasing both specific and global access to public health services by putting people in contact with public health providers in a safe forum.

The harm reduction model and principles applied to alcohol use, smoking, and drug use, as described in earlier chapters, also apply to HIV/AIDS risk reduction. The goal remains reducing risk for harm; in the case of HIV/AIDS, this translates into reducing the risk for HIV infection. Shared principles include meeting people where they are in the risk reduction process and helping them move along the risk continuum from higher-risk to lower-risk behaviors. Harm reduction principles that are unique to HIV/AIDS intervention include recognition of the following: (1) the ability and competence of marginalized people to make choices and changes in their lives; (2) the need for individuals and communities affected by AIDS risk behavior to be involved in the organization and creation of strategies for harm reduction interventions; and (3) the diversity of people affected by HIV/AIDS, and the necessity for outreach and services that reflect this diversity. Not all injection drug use behaviors or sexual behaviors carry the same degree of risk. Harm reduction programs advocate that individuals engage in behaviors that afford the highest level of protection and the lowest level of risk possible. Particularly when abstinence is not a realistic goal, it is important to use a hierarchy of risks and to encourage individuals to move incrementally along this continuum.

One of the ways in which HIV exposure differs from alcohol use or noninjection drug use is that one occurrence of unprotected sex or use of a "dirty" needle can cause seroconversion and can ultimately be life-threatening. One "slip" in HIV/AIDS risk behavior can thus have more severe consequences than one "slip" in alcohol or drug use behavior. Harm reduction programs do not eliminate risk; rather, they provide realistic options for people for whom total abstention from HIV/AIDS risk behaviors is often not possible. In this way, harm reduction programs constitute a pragmatic public health response to a complex health issue.

In the beginning of the AIDS epidemic, HIV risk was thought of in terms of distinct risk groups (e.g., MSM and IDUs as noted above). Within these groups, interventions typically focused on one category of risk behavior, such as sexual risk for MSM and needle risk for IDUs. But the reality of HIV risk is much more complex. MSM may also inject drugs, and IDUs may also transmit HIV through unprotected sex. Furthermore, these risk behaviors may well occur within a political, economic, cultural, and social context that limits options for risk reduction. Harm reduction programs, in meeting people where they are, need to be cognizant of these contextual variables and to address multiple risk factors.

This chapter begins by discussing harm reduction programs for IDUs; we focus on the pros and cons of needle exchange programs (NEPs) and bleach distribution programs, and the contextual factors that have affected the implementation of these programs. The second section discusses harm reduction programs for MSM; both sexual and injection risk reduction programs are discussed. Most of the harm reduction strategies, broadly defined (e.g., NEPs, bleach distribution, outreach, condom distribution), are covered in the first two sections. The remaining three sections focus on harm reduction for women, adolescents, and prison populations. The specific contextual factors that are important for understanding each group's HIV risk, and that may influence the development, implementation, or effectiveness of harm reduction programs for each group, are discussed. We also describe existing harm reduction programs and strategies, and, in cases where they have been evaluated, provide evidence of their effectiveness.

This chapter is thus an attempt to convey the complexity of HIV/AIDS risk behaviors and to provide an overview of harm reduction strategies and programs. Although this chapter is organized around different groups, we wish to emphasize that behaviors are what place people at risk, not group membership per se.

HIV RISK REDUCTION FOR INJECTION DRUG USERS

Nearly 3 million people in the United States alone are estimated to have injected illicit drugs at some point in their lifetimes (SAMHSA, 1997), and over 1.1 million Americans are estimated to be current IDUs (Turner, Miller, & Moses, 1989). The particular drug injected varies by geographic region and other individual factors. For example, cocaine is reported as the most frequently injected drug in such cities as Toronto, Honolulu, and Boulder, Colorado; amphetamines are most common in Lund, Sweden; and heroin is most common in San Francisco and the United Kingdom. In most cities, mixtures of different drugs (e.g., heroin and cocaine, or "speedballs") are common among IDUs (Lurie et al., 1993). Thirty-six percent of all documented adult/adolescent U.S. AIDS cases through 1997 have been attributed to injection drug use. This includes 31% of all male cases (8% of whom are both MSM and IDUs) and 61% of all female cases (Centers for

Disease Control and Prevention [CDC], 1997a). Not only is sharing needles with a seropositive person the quickest and most efficient route for HIV transmission; it also increases risk of hepatitis and transmission of other bacteria and viruses, which can result in such life-threatening conditions as abscesses, endocarditis, and cellulitis.

Injection drug use also plays an indirect role in HIV seroconversion, particularly for women sexual partners of IDUs (see the section on women below). For example, 41% of all pediatric HIV cases are related to maternal injection drug use via prenatal exposure; 19% of these pediatric cases have been reported to result from primary maternal exposure through sexual contact with an IDU (CDC, 1995).

Clearly, injection drug use poses a major public health risk in the transmission of HIV. IDUs, as well as their sexual partners and offspring, are at risk for HIV and other health problems. Because of the prevalence of injection drug use and the life difficulties often facing this population (e.g., homelessness, mental illness, financial and legal problems), simple, affordable, and accessible prevention approaches are necessary. We explore two such approaches in this section: bleach distribution programs and NEPs. As described in Chapter 6, drug replacement treatments, such as methadone maintenance, buprenorphine, and L-alpha-acetylmethadol (LAAM) programs, have also proven efficacious in reducing HIV infection rates (Baker, Kochon, Dixon, Wodak, & Heather, 1995).

Bleach Distribution Programs

Commonly a part of street outreach programs, bleach distribution was the first harm reduction approach applied to the prevention of HIV infection among IDUs in the United States. In 1986, San Francisco's Mid-City Consortium to Combat AIDS distributed the first instructions to IDUs on how to deactivate HIV in syringes by flushing with bleach (Gleghorn, 1994). These instructions were based on a study (Resnick, Veren, & Salahuddin, 1986) demonstrating viral inactivity after bleach exposure in laboratory settings. Users were taught to clean their drug injection equipment to kill HIV as follows: first rinsing the syringe with water; then filling it with bleach and allowing the bleach to remain in the syringe barrel at least 60 seconds; rinsing the syringe again with clean water; and repeating the process (CDC, 1994). Bleach distribution programs were chosen initially over needle exchange because bleach is legal and easily obtained.

In spite of the documented practical value of this accessible approach (Flynn et al., 1994; McCusker et al., 1992; Siegel, Weinstein, & Fineberg, 1991), bleach distribution has been downplayed by public health and national campaigns (Broadhead, 1991). Some public officials have viewed distributing bleach to IDUs as a form of "catering to drug users." Others have attacked these programs as a "social policy copout" or an insufficient response to the real problems of drug addiction. For example, NEP advocates have expressed skepticism about the effectiveness of bleach distribution to reduce the spread of HIV, noting that lower-functioning IDUs may have difficulty in fully sanitizing their equipment and may thereby be better served by replacing each dirty syringe with a clean unit. Furthermore, the use of bleach in cleaning injection equipment presents additional health risks when the bleach is not sufficiently flushed from the injection unit (Gleghorn, Doherty, Vlahov, Celentano, & Jones, 1994; Haverkos & Jones, 1994; U.S. Preventive Services Task Force, 1996). In the midst of this controversy, explicit reference to bleach distribution has been prohibited by many state and local funding agencies for fear of public disapproval.

Despite public perceptions, studies of bleach distribution programs nonetheless support the efficacy of this harm reduction approach. In fact, some have used the effectiveness of bleach distribution programs as an argument against the need for NEPs (see Broadhead, 1991). Studies have demonstrated that street outreach efforts to distribute bleach do increase the incidence of IDUs' cleaning injection equipment (McCusker et al., 1992; Moss et al., 1994). In one longitudinal study of IDUs receiving bleach distribution services, seroprevalence rates of HIV remained relatively stable throughout the late 1980s, suggesting that outreach services such as bleach distribution may have helped to prevent an increase in the rate of HIV (Moss et al., 1994).

Bleach distribution programs may be most effective in areas with low HIV prevalence. Using survey data and medical information on HIV disease progression, Siegel et al. (1991) created a statistical model of HIV transmission and mortality rates; they estimated that bleach distribution programs save 2.3 years per HIV-negative user in a low-HIV-prevalence area, compared to 1.7 and 1.3 life-years in medium- and high-prevalence areas, respectively.

Use of bleach by IDUs as a means of preventing HIV infection is not without its disadvantages. The bleach and water required to clean needles are difficult to transport, particularly for homeless IDUs; moreover, bleaching entails effort and inconvenience, and it may damage the injection equipment. In addition, detection of possession of bleach can result in a police search, even though many city police departments have agreed not to define bleach as drug paraphernalia (Broadhead, 1991). Because HIV can also be transmitted through sharing of other components involved in the injection process (e.g., the water used to dilute drugs, the cooker used to prepare the drugs, the cotton used to filter the dissolved intoxicant, and the rinse water), IDUs may believe that they have taken sufficient precautions to minimize risk, when in fact exposure through less direct sharing may still pose significant risk for infection. Proper cleaning of the syringe can be particularly difficult for some users, who rely on public facilities that are themselves unclean. Finally, bleach can cause a variety of health problems, including chest pain, vomiting, and blood coagulation, if the syringe is not adequately flushed with water prior to injection (Morgan, 1992).

Several factors have been found to influence the overall effectiveness of this harm reduction approach. Obviously, bleaching is only effective if consistently and properly used. In one study, 450 IDUs were instructed on the proper procedure for disinfecting injection equipment. Only 36% successfully performed the necessary steps (McCoy et al., 1994). In a study of 117 African American IDUs, dramatic variations in cleaning practices were observed as a function of the IDUs' attitudes toward cleaning needles with bleach. Forty-three percent of the variance in frequency and duration of bleach use was predicted by IDUs' ratings of how "pleasant," "wise," "safe," and "good" bleach cleaning is. Furthermore, 12% of the variance in bleach use was predicted by IDUs' perception of normative peer bleach use, and 10% by perceived self-efficacy in cleaning needles with bleach (Krepcho, Fernandez-Esquer, Freeman, Magee, & McAlister, 1993).

In summary, the effectiveness of bleach distribution programs in reducing HIV seroconversion among IDUs is seriously compromised by the number of required conditions, including time, knowledge, feasibility of transporting bleach and water, and proper implementation of the required steps for cleaning. Overall, such programs must be regarded as minimal interventions, particularly in communities and in circumstances where other resources are lacking or are prohibited. Bleach distribution programs alone are not likely to bring a halt to the AIDS epidemic in this population.

Needle Exchange Programs

Description

NEPs are HIV prevention services that provide IDUs with new, sterile syringes in exchange for their used syringes. It is important to note that NEPs exchange needles for those clients who already possess syringes; most NEPs do not give out needles. NEPs use a variety of outreach strategies to ensure accessibility of services. Distribution locations include folding tables on streets, storefronts, cafés, clinics, drive-through windows, and mobile vans. Some NEPs offer "starter kits" for IDUs new to the programs; these kits commonly contain information, bleach, condoms, alcohol prep pads, and sometimes syringes. Although some programs require registration of participants, either in fulfillment of legal requirements or for purposes of data collection, other programs allow users to remain anonymous. Used syringes are dropped into "sharps containers," which are disposed of through medical disposal services. This method helps keep used syringes off streets and out of parks and dumpsters, where they might otherwise be discarded. Overall, NEPs operate differently according to the local needs and available resources, and are most effective when they take into account the unique circumstances and features of the community they aim to serve.

As noted in Chapter 2, the first NEP was started in Amsterdam in 1984 by the local *Junkiebond* (Junkie League), an organization formed by and for illicit drug users (Buning, 1991). Two years later, NEPs were operating in other parts of Europe, including England and Sweden (Christensson & Ljungberg, 1991; Lart & Stimson, 1990), but they did not reach the United States for several more years. The first NEP in the United States was founded in 1988 by David Purchase, a former drug treatment counselor in Tacoma, Washington. In January 1989, the program began receiving its funding through the county health department, as public health officials saw an opportunity to reduce a variety of health problems associated with injection drug use (Hagan, Des Jarlais, Purchase, Reid, & Friedman, 1991; Sorge, 1990).

Serving as a model for other communities, the Tacoma NEP led to similar programs in other cities. By 1990, a range of cities from Connecticut to Alaska had initiated NEPs. Whereas some of these programs were openly operated through health departments or clinics, others were run by underground networks of AIDS activists who risked arrest. The number of NEPs operating in the United States is growing rapidly. Major cities in Canada, New Zealand, Australia, Thailand, Nepal, Brazil, and Europe also have NEPs. Despite these advances, syringes are still available only through medical prescriptions in many areas throughout the United States and the world.

New York City has an estimated 168,300 IDUs and the nation's highest HIV seroprevalence for street IDUs at 41% (Holmberg, 1995); thus, it has been the scene of much controversy over needle exchange. Temporarily legalized in 1988, an NEP was first operated out of the Manhattan office of the city health department. Predictably, many IDUs were put off by the location of the service, resulting in its underuse. By 1990, the program was discontinued. Despite its short life and limited utility, this project served as an important bridge to drug abuse treatment (Firlik & Schreiber, 1992), and activists continued to operate underground needle exchanges in neighborhoods with high drug use levels. In July 1992, the New York State Health Commissioner granted waivers from state law, which required prescriptions for possession of syringes. Former New York City Mayor David Dinkins announced formal support for privately funded pilot NEPs after reviewing encouraging results from other NEPs, such as the New Haven exchange. In 1992, the city overstepped state paraphernalia laws and made needle exchange legal because of the AIDS crisis and the effectiveness demonstrated in the New Haven study. Since then, NEPs have expanded rapidly in New York City (Kochems et al., 1996).

The NEP in Seattle, Washington provides a good example of how urban NEPs operate. The program was launched in March 1989 by the Seattle AIDS Coalition To Unleash Power (ACT/UP), and was taken over by the Seattle/King County Department of Public Health 2 months later. The program is situated in a heavy-drug-use area of downtown Seattle and is operated by a knowledgeable health department staff member and two volunteers, who set up a folding table on an accessible street corner. Staff and volunteers are encouraged to treat clients with respect and without judgment. The table contains a medical waste disposal container for used syringes, a variety of new syringes, a bin of condoms, boxes of sterile alcohol pads and cotton, a bin of small bleach bottles and empty bottles to be used for water, and a display rack filled with brochures and information. The table is set up during regular hours every day of the week except Sunday, rain or shine, regardless of holidays.

A line quickly forms once the table is set up in the early afternoon. The user at the head of the line counts his or her used syringes for the NEP volunteer, drops them into the sharps container, and is handed an equal number of clean syringes. The syringes distributed by the Seattle NEP bear a small red identification band, indicating that they originated from the NEP. Another volunteer records the client's gender and race, the number of syringes exchanged, and the number of exchanged syringes bearing the Seattle NEP band. The health department staff member answers clients' questions, and provides general health-related advice and treatment referrals for interested clients. Although most clients appear comfortable with using the exchange, the presence of police near the exchange table virtually halts its operation. Clients without used syringes who request syringes are offered bleach and information, but are not given a syringe.

In addition to the folding table located in downtown Seattle, health department staff members also operate needle exchanges out of a van in three other locations in the county on a weekly basis. This facilitates access to a greater range of IDUs. Clients at these locations tend to be employed females with stable housing; they also tend to exchange larger numbers of syringes, usually for friends or neighbors. A fourth needle exchange van site, run under the auspices of the health department's Project NEON (Needle and Sex Education Outreach Network), targets gay and bisexual men who are drug (primarily methamphetamine) users. Project NEON site is the first gay/bisexual needle exchange in the United States. In all, the Seattle/King County Department of Public Health exchanged approximately 780,000 syringes in 1994, averaging 65,000 syringes per month (M. Hanrahan, personal communication, 1995). Health department staff members report that it takes years for exchange sites to build the trust of users and accumulate large numbers of clients, primarily via outreach efforts and word of mouth.

Evidence of Effectiveness

Do NEPs reduce HIV in the communities they serve? Lurie et al. (1993) conducted an extensive literature review of NEP evaluations. They noted that the design of the studies severely limited the conclusions that could be drawn. In order to have enough statistical power to detect differences in seroconversion rates, evaluation of the effectiveness of community-based NEPs would require large longitudinal cohorts, estimated by Lurie et al. at 2,500 IDUs randomly assigned to conditions (i.e., needle exchange or no needle exchange) and followed for a number of years. This type of study is extremely expensive and clearly raises political and ethical dilemmas.

Evidence for the effectiveness of needle exchange is also derived by comparing the rates of HIV seroconversion among IDUs in cities with and without NEPs. Although the incidence of HIV infection among IDUs has increased worldwide, incidence of seroconversions among IDUs in areas with NEPs has remained at a stable level, suggesting that NEPs are associated with the prevention of HIV infection in the following cities: Amsterdam (Coutinho, 1990); Lund, Sweden (Ljungberg & Christensson, 1991); Liverpool, England (Home Office, 1992; Newcombe, 1990); San Francisco (Watters et al., 1990); Sydney, Australia (Tsai, Goh, Webeck, & Mullins, 1988); Toronto (Millson et al., 1993); Montreal (Hankins, Gendron, Rouah, & Lepine, 1993); Portland, Oregon (Des Jarlais & Maynard, 1992); and Tacoma, Washington (Hagan, Des Jarlais, Friedman, Purchase, & Reid, 1992). In the following areas, HIV has shown decreasing incidence rates: Glasgow, Scotland (Goldberg et al., 1988); Honolulu (Department of Health, State of Hawaii, 1992); England in general (Dolan, Donoghoe, Jones, & Stimson, 1991) and London in particular (Hart et al., 1991); and Zurich, Switzerland (Hornung, Alvo, Fuchs, & Grob, 1994). Evaluation of HIV rates based on availability of NEPs worldwide revealed that cities with NEPs enjoy decreased rates of seroconversion by 6% annually, while cities without NEPs experience 6% increases per year (Hurley, Jolley, & Kaldor, 1997).

Another means of gauging the effectiveness of NEPs is to evaluate the influence of syringe availability. This is done by comparing rates of HIV infection in cities with comparable IDU populations that have different policies regarding the availability of clean syringes. In Scotland, two cities with similar injection drug use epidemics handled syringe availability differently in the 1980s and had quite different outcomes (Brettle, 1991). Edinburgh's city government made it illegal to buy syringes from pharmacies without a prescription in 1981, in an attempt to reduce drug use. This led to considerable needle sharing. Over 50% of all IDUs in Edinburgh were HIV-positive by 1984, and an epidemic of hepatitis B occurred simultaneously. Glasgow had a larger number of IDUs, but did not restrict syringe availability and did not suffer HIV or hepatitis B epidemics, with fewer than 2% of its IDUs testing HIV-positive.

Cities that allowed syringe purchase without a prescription prior to the AIDS epidemic, such as St. Louis (Compton, Cottler, Decker, Mager, & Stringfellow, 1992) and Seattle (Calsyn, Saxon, Freeman, & Whittaker, 1991), have suffered lower rates of HIV among IDUs than have metropolitan areas where syringe purchase remains illegal (Des Jarlais & Friedman, 1990). In San Juan, Puerto Rico, more than 40% of IDUs are estimated to be HIV-positive (Holmberg. 1996; Tellado et al., 1997) compared to approximately 20% in Seattle (Holmberg, 1996), where harm reduction approaches were instigated early in the epidemic. As Lurie et al. (1993) noted, seroprevalence among IDUs entering treatment is higher in U.S. states that require prescriptions for syringes (median = 15%) than in states that do not have such requirements (median = 2.7%).

Although other factors could account for these differences in HIV incidence rates, the consistency of the patterns across studies and communities supports the effectiveness of needle exchange programs. Other evidence also supports the link between seroconversion and syringe availability (DePhilippis & Metzger, 1993; Espinoza, Bouchard, & Ballian, 1988; Ingold & Ingold, 1989; Jones et al., 1990; Lurie et al., 1993; Magura et al., 1989; Valleroy, Weinstein, Groseclose, Kassler, & Jones, 1993). In one study, Nelson et al. (1991) found that nondiabetic IDUs were almost three times more likely than diabetic IDUs to be HIV-positive, despite similar patterns of drug use. They attributed this difference to diabetics' legal access to clean needles.

A rigorous examination of the effectiveness of the New Haven NEP was conducted by the Yale School of Medicine (Heimer, Kaplan, Khoshnood, Jariwala, & Cadman, 1993; Kaplan, Khoshnood, & Heimer, 1994; Kaplan & O'Keefe, 1993; Kaplan, O'Keefe, & Heimer, 1991). Estimates of HIV prevalence were made from tests on returned syringes. Using a mathematical model of HIV transmission, Des Jarlais and Friedman (1992) estimated the New Haven NEP to have reduced new HIV infections among clients by 33%.

Data collected in Tacoma and New York also support the effectiveness of NEPs. The Point Defiance AIDS Project evaluated 154 Tacoma NEP clients and found substantial reductions in HIV-risky injection behaviors. Clients reported the following changes in risky behaviors: (1) a decrease in the number of occasions used syringes were obtained, from an average of 57 times in the month before starting the exchange to 36 times in the most recent month (Hagan, Des Jarlais, Purchase, Reid, & Friedman, 1991); (2) a decrease in passing used syringes to others, from an average of 100 times to an average of 65 times; (3) a marked increase in bleach use; and (4) a significant overall reduction in unsafe injection behavior. Incidence of hepatitis B virus, another blood-borne virus, is a good indicator that needle-sharing practices decreased significantly shortly after introduction of the NEP (Hagan, Des Jarlais, Purchase, Friedman, & Bell, 1991). The same group also reported a sixfold reduction in risk of contracting hepatitis B or hepatitis C for IDUs using the NEP, compared to IDUs who did not use the NEP (Hagan, Des Jarlais, Friedman, Purchase, & Alter, 1995).

Results from studies of the effectiveness of NEPs in the Bronx–Harlem and Lower East Side areas of New York City are also encouraging. Steady declines of injections with used syringes were observed (from 28% to 11%), along with significant declines in other high-risk injection behaviors (e.g., attending shooting galleries and passing used syringes to other IDUs) and no cases of increased drug use (Paone, Des Jarlais, Caloir, & Friedman, 1993). Lower HIV incidence was observed among NEP participants, compared to IDUs that do not use an NEP (1.38 vs. 5.26 per 100 person-years; Des Jarlais et al., 1996). Taking both the consistency in reported reductions in high-risk injection behavior and the low HIV seroconversion rate among NEP clients, Des Jarlais et al. (1994) estimated that regular participation in NEPs reduces the risk of new HIV infection by 50%.

Some authors have suggested that changes in injection behaviors may serve to promote safer sex behaviors and enhanced concern about general health (Lloyd et al., 1994; Reinfield, 1994). In addition, the nonjudgmental social exchange between outreach workers and clients may enhance IDUs' motivation to reduce HIV risk behaviors (Wenger & Murphy, 1994).

Evaluating the Pros and Cons

NEPs have the capacity to reach populations whose members may not be ready to seek treatment for drug problems, or may not have the resources to obtain such treatment once they are ready to do so. Particularly for hard-to-reach populations, NEPs provide more than sterile injection equipment. Many help network users into other needed services, including HIV testing, legal advocacy, referral to primary medical care, and housing. The Tacoma NEP administers tuberculosis testing (Hagan, Des Jarlais, Purchase, Friedman, & Bell, 1991), and tuberculosis treatment by medical staff members, in a health department vehicle parked near the needle exchange van (D. Purchase, personal communication, 1994). As previously described, most programs also offer educational materials and other supplies to reduce the risk of HIV infection. In addition, NEPs are generally more popular among users than bleach-only programs because a new needle is sharper and penetrates the skin more easily, and because the prevention strategy is more convenient than toting around bleach bottles.

As a result of the lack of drug treatment slots, and the difficulty many users face in abstaining from injecting drugs for lengthy periods, needle exchange is a simple and practical behavioral change to reduce the spread of HIV. Through contact with an NEP volunteer, some individuals may eventually be willing to initiate other health behaviors to avoid the risks from injection or use of harmful drugs. Some may "step up" to methadone maintenance or other drug treatment programs. Furthermore, NEPs are cost-effective in preventing HIV infection. Multiple mathematical models demonstrate that NEPs can prevent significant numbers of HIV seroconversions among NEP clients, their injection and sex partners, and their offspring (Kaplan, 1993; Kaplan & O'Keefe, 1993; O'Keefe, Kaplan, & Khoshnood, 1991; U.S. General Accounting Office, 1993). The cost of operating an NEP for each HIV conversion averted is estimated at approximately $9,000 (Lurie et al., 1993)—much less than the estimated $119,000 average lifetime cost of treating an HIV-infected individual (Hellinger, 1993) and the estimated $40,000 average annual cost for treating one child born with AIDS (Hsia, Fleishman, East, & Hellinger, 1995). Needless to say, harm reduction approaches such as NEPs have major economic implications and the number of programs has continued to expand (CDC, 1997b).

The most common argument against NEPs—one voiced by many federal and state politicians, is that needle exchange will encourage or increase illicit drug use (Office of National Drug Control Policy, 1990). This argument, however, has never been supported empirically. In 1986, a Sydney methadone clinic added an NEP to its services and reported no increase in illicit drugs in the urine specimens of clinic clients, compared to clients of a methadone clinic without an NEP (Wolk, Wodak, Guinan, Macaskill, & Simpson, 1990). A San Francisco study found a decrease in frequency of injecting by IDUs, corresponding temporally to the initiation of San Francisco's NEP (Watters, Cheng, Clark, & Lorvick, 1991). The San Francisco group also found a slowly aging population of IDUs, indicating that new, younger users were not starting drug injection as a result of the NEP. A New York study produced similar results (Des Jarlais et al., 1994); an evaluation of a London NEP likewise failed to show an increase in drug use (Hart et al., 1989). In a 1991 survey of 154 Tacoma NEP clients, the mean number of injections per month remained the same following the initiation of the NEP, indicating no evidence that the NEP increased the clients' frequency of injection (Hagan, Des Jarlais, Purchase, Friedman, & Bell, 1991). There also was no evidence that NEPs recruited non-IDUs into shooting drugs.

Evaluations of Amsterdam's NEP indicate that the HIV seroprevalence rate of IDUs has remained stable since 1989, and that the incidence of new hepatitis B cases has declined. Concomitantly, no increase in consumption of injectable drugs has been observed. The average age of IDUs increased between 1983 and 1988, with a concurrent decrease in the number of young IDUs. For example, 14.4% of Amsterdam's IDUs in 1983 were under 22, but by 1988, only 3.4% were under 22 (Buning, 1991).

An examination of all the data available, including emergency room mentions of illicit drugs, drug possession arrests, frequency of positive toxicology screens among arrestees, and responses of IDUs participating in focus groups, has provided no support for the fear that NEPs are associated with an increase in illicit drug use (DeWitt, 1992; Drug Abuse Warning Network, 1989; Federal Bureau of Investigation, 1988; Lurie et al., 1993). It appears that the potential benefits NEPs provide in terms of reaching IDUs and reducing the spread of AIDS greatly outweigh the potential cost, which seems to be the unsubstantiated fear of increased drug use.

Tailoring Programs to Target Populations

NEPs are most successful when they address the special needs of the population they target. The modal NEP client is male, with a mean age of 35–40 years, and has a long history of injection drug use. The future success of NEPs will require further tailoring them to meet the needs of women, ethnic minorities (including speakers of languages other than English), adolescents and young adults, and MSM. Some NEPs have used creative strategies in accessing different populations. An NEP in Portland, Oregon, was located in a trendy café to reach younger users. A Boulder NEP set up its outreach site near a gymnasium to target steroid injectors. A San Diego outreach worker targeted transgender individuals who inject hormones. NEPs could also be placed in women's health clinics to provide discreet needle exchange for female clients who inject drugs.

Certain populations have multiple risk factors. MSM often inject amphetamines, thus placing themselves at additional risk for HIV. In addition, amphetamine and cocaine injectors are at higher risk for contracting HIV than heroin injectors, because these drugs tend to be injected more frequently and are often associated with higher-risk sexual activity (Hando & Hall, 1994). These men are often reluctant to visit NEPs geared toward opiate users and may be better served through gay/bisexual men's organizations, or at places where they meet socially, such as bars. Information relevant to their specific needs could then be provided more effectively.

AIDS has disproportionately affected minorities in the United States, especially cases related to injection drug use. African-Americans comprise 12% of the U.S. population but account for 49% of injection drug-related AIDS cases, and Hispanics account for 24% (CDC, 1997a). These populations must be targeted with prevention strategies more effectively. The Seattle NEP evaluated Latino clients' service utilization and found a marked increase in use while a Latino staff member was present (C. Price, personal communication, 1993). Individuals may feel more comfortable utilizing a service when someone of their own cultural and language group is available. These factors should be taken into consideration when programs are designed. In addition, issues beyond drug use may need addressing. For example, successful HIV prevention programming may also require self-esteem enhancement and assertion training. Ethnic minority women who inject drugs may have greater difficulty in negotiating safer sex and requiring condom use (Schilling, El-Bassel, Gilbert, & Schinke, 1991), and are therefore at greater risk for HIV through unsafe sexual contacts. (See the section on women, below.)

Summary

Injection drug use is the fastest-growing risk factor for HIV infection. Every IDU who contracts HIV puts others at risk, and many IDUs are highly sexually active to support their drug habits; thus, dramatic measures are necessary to reduce HIV/AIDS risk in this group. Yet, to be effective, HIV/AIDS prevention programs must be tailored to their target populations. More creative methods are required to reach IDUs and to keep them in contact with public health programs. Education alone is clearly insufficient. The often troubled and disorganized nature of the injection drug use lifestyle requires repeated education, easy access to the tools necessary for safety, and low-threshold programs so that everyone can participate in risk reduction. If IDUs are ready to reduce risks further and are willing either to administer drugs through safer routes or to quit drugs altogether, services to aid in these changes must be made available. Ample data are available to support the conclusion that NEPs reduce the harm of injection drug use to individuals and communities. Research efforts must now focus on maximizing utilization and effectiveness of NEPs for all IDUs.

The National Research Council and the Institute of Medicine of the National Academy of Sciences organized a panel in September 1993 to examine the benefits and risks of NEPs and bleach distribution programs. Summarizing the effectiveness of NEPs, Dr. Peter Selwyn of the AIDS Program Section of Infectious Diseases, Yale University School of Medicine, concluded:

> They do not cause people to use drugs, they seem in many instances to promote positive behavioral change, they definitely help provide access to vulnerable and sometimes otherwise inaccessible populations, and they may reduce the risk of transmission of HIV. But . . . needle exchange programs should not be looked at as a single or simple solution. . . . It is not simply a matter of handing out clean needles. The behavioral and social factors underlying drug use must also be addressed. (Institute of Medicine, 1994, p. 110)

We agree that the empirical evidence for bleach distribution as an HIV prevention strategy does not support its widespread use when other, more effective approaches are available. NEPs have strong empirical support for lowering HIV transmission rates; moreover, not a single study has supported the notion that NEPs increase drug use or cause other harm to the community. Many local governments have heeded the data. Other cities need to implement NEPs as soon as possible, in order to reduce the harm injection drug use causes to both users and the community at large, in terms of financial cost and quality of life.

REDUCING HIV RISK AMONG MEN WHO HAVE SEX WITH MEN

AIDS was first identified in the United States among MSM. Initial case reports from Los Angeles and New York described several men who had developed rare opportunistic infections because of unusually compromised immune systems. The association of gay men with the symptoms that would soon be called "AIDS" was so apparent in the beginning that the syndrome was originally called "gay-related immune deficiency" or "GRID." And though the incidence of HIV infection has risen more rapidly in recent years among other risk groups, gay and bisexual men continue to have the highest prevalence of HIV in the United States (CDC, 1997a).

As of 1997, MSM represented 55% of the cumulative U.S. AIDS cases, as well as 39% of the adults newly diagnosed with AIDS in 1997 (CDC, 1997a). Unprotected sex is the largest category of risk exposure for MSM. Though controversy continues over the relative risk of transmission through other routes (e.g., oral sex), among sexual behaviors HIV infection is known to be most highly associated with unprotected anal intercourse (Coates et al., 1988; Detels et al., 1989). For example, Kingsley et al. (1987) found that unprotected receptive anal intercourse with only one partner increases the risk of seroconversion by 300%.

The other area of concern with respect to gay and bisexual men (including those who do not identify with these labels) has to do with substance abuse, including injection drug use. As of December 1997, 20% of those individuals diagnosed with AIDS and having a history of injection drug use were also homosexually active men. Despite attention to general issues of injection drug use and HIV, the epidemiological nexus between injection drug use and homosexual activity has received considerably little attention. According to Battjes (1994), "with regard to [gay and bisexual IDUs] little research has been conducted except for that focused on male prostitutes: It appears that very few of this dual risk group are reached through primary prevention initiatives that target drug abusers" (p. 84). Injection drug use in particular and substance abuse in general warrant more attention in this population, especially with respect to HIV.

Gay and bisexual men dramatically decreased their frequency of unprotected anal intercourse during the 1980s (Joseph et al., 1987; Martin, 1987; Winkelstein et al., 1987). However, research in the 1990s has indicated an increased prevalence of unprotected sexual behavior. In the San Francisco Young Men's Health Study, about 25% of the 18- to 29-year-old gay and bisexual men had engaged in unprotected anal intercourse in the previous month (Osmond et al., 1994). In another study of gay and bisexual men in Portland, Oregon, 50% of the men reported unprotected intercourse during the previous year (M. Stark, personal communication, 1995). There has been a corresponding resurgence of seroconversion, particularly among young MSM. Two San Francisco studies found high HIV rates among young gay and bisexual men (Lemp et al., 1993; Osmond et al., 1994), and these findings are being replicated in a number of other studies in different geographical locations: midsized university towns, a small Southern city, and three medium-sized West Coast cities (Hays, Kegeles, & Coates, 1990; Kelly, St. Lawrence, et al., 1992;

Stall et al., 1992; Catania, Coates, Stall, et al., 1992). Moreover, several studies suggest that gay men of African American and Latino descent may be at elevated risk (Peterson et al., 1992; Lemp et al., 1993). Thus, risk reduction efforts among MSM will continue to be critically important in the 1990s and beyond.

Risk reduction and other important behavioral changes have been attributed to a variety of efforts within the gay community. Using differing strategies—from grassroots outreach to formal behavior change interventions—programs have sought to educate men about the probable risks of HIV exposure from sexual acts, to alter community norms surrounding sexual behavior, and to teach strategies for achieving and maintaining safer sexual practices (Becker & Joseph, 1988; Coates, 1990; Stall, Coates, & Hoff, 1988). In the sections below, we review several types of programs aimed at reducing the incidence of HIV among gay/bisexual men.

As is true of the risk behaviors of alcohol and other drug use, not all forms of sexual activity lead to harm (in this case, HIV infection). Although most sexual behaviors carry some risk of infection, some, such as receptive anal intercourse, are more risky than others. Recognizing this continuum of risk, most programs for MSM seek the reduction of the highest-risk behaviors while encouraging the adoption of lower-risk behaviors. Moreover, rigid abstinence goals are generally avoided; individuals are largely "met where they are" and encouraged to set their own goals for risk reduction. Thus, for some, simply increasing condom use during intercourse may represent a desirable (though clearly not risk-free) outcome. Others may seek a monogamous relationship with a seronegative-concordant partner, avoid anal intercourse altogether, or limit their sexual activity to mutual masturbation and other forms of touching. In short, harm reduction serves as the working goal in all of these efforts.

A Historical Perspective: The Gay Community's Early Response to HIV/AIDS

Mainstream community and governmental agencies were initially slow to respond to the AIDS epidemic. The multiple reasons for these tardy responses have been explored in depth by several authors, most notably Randy Shilts (1987). A likely contributing factor is that in many countries, including the United States, the general public remains quite ambivalent about sexual issues and is particularly uncomfortable with the topic of homosexuality. Fortunately, when the first signs of the emerging epidemic became clear, established gay communities in major U.S. cities (e.g., New York City, San Francisco, Los Angeles) quickly mobilized their organizational resources to provide information on known AIDS risk behaviors, as well as to provide services to those men initially diagnosed with AIDS. A number of health education campaigns were started in these cities, including those operated by the Gay Men's Health Crisis (GMHC) in New York, the

STOP AIDS program in San Francisco and other cities, and the SafetyNet program in Boston. We describe the GMHC and STOP AIDS below.

Gay Men's Health Crisis

The GMHC was founded in 1981 as a grassroots organization by six men in New York City (Katoff & Dunne, 1988). Originally organized by these volunteers to provide information as well as to raise funds for research, it grew over the years to include over 5,000 volunteers providing education, outreach, financial, legal, domestic, and medical referral services to more than 6,000 of those infected with HIV in New York.

Not surprisingly, GMHC programs have not proceeded without encountering obstacles. Operating within the larger social and governmental spheres of mainstream culture, the GMHC was forced to tailor its activities with an eye toward potentially hostile public reaction. For example, in 1985 the GMHC began to advertise its "800 Men Study" (described below), a large project designed to engage men in one of four safer sex educational programs. Many of the project's educational media were appropriately sexually explicit. In a 1988 article, former 800 Men Study director James D'Eramo documented the difficulties experienced by the GMHC as its members prepared to disseminate promotional and educational materials to the public. For example, D'Eramo described how the original promotional campaign had included an explicit drawing of two men engaged in masturbation. However, prior to distribution this drawing was edited so that the penises would not be seen.

The removal of this erotic content was explained by D'Eramo as partly a response to the Helms amendment, a then-recent U.S. federal appropriations bill rider stating that federal funds should not be used to "promote homosexuality." Senator Jesse Helms of North Carolina had displayed existing GMHC educational materials (which had been partly funded from federal sources) as examples of such "promotion" during his arguments for the adoption of his amendment. D'Eramo suggested that the sanitation of these materials served both to undermine the recruitment of participants and to send messages to the at-risk gay community associating the GMHC with "sex phobia and internalized homophobia" (1988). From a harm reduction perspective, moral judgments regarding a stigmatized group, as well as aspects of risk behavior, began to interfere with the promotion of effective, realistic risk reduction.

This behind-the-scenes story was published soon after the Fourth International Conference on AIDS was held in Stockholm in 1988. At that meeting, D'Eramo, Quadland, Shatts, Schuman, and Jacobs (1988) presented a paper describing their evaluation of the effectiveness of the four educational strategies in GMHC's 800 Men Study. Over 600 men participated in the evaluation, completing questionnaires prior to and three months following the intervention. The four conditions were as follows: (1)

informational sessions describing AIDS and the transmission of HIV; (2) a "visual menu" of sexually explicit videos and slides, which presented safer sex behavior in an "affirmative, erotically appealing manner"; (3) a didactic presentation (without the audiovisual materials), consistent with the theme in condition 2 of eroticizing safer sex; and (4) distribution of printed safer sex guidelines. The authors concluded that the erotic program (the one that included the sexually explicit visuals) was most effective in helping to shift men to low-risk or no-risk sexual behavior. Unfortunately, because of the intolerance of homosexually explicit materials fostered by the Helms amendment, the safer sex video that the authors found so effective was not made available to other investigators or clinicians.

It would appear that the goal of governmental policies such as the Helms amendment is to encourage abstinence from homosexual behavior altogether. By taking a moral rather than a public health approach, the U.S. government has hampered the harm reduction effort. Clearly, abstinence from sexual activity was not a goal of the 800 Men Study. Instead, abstinence from high-risk activity (particularly unprotected anal intercourse) and the adoption of lower-risk behavior were the project's primary aims. Consistent with the principles of harm reduction, clients were "met where they were" and encouraged to proceed downward on a risk behavior continuum.

Changes in public policy may be needed to enable programs like the 800 Men Study to expand to serve other groups of gay and bisexual men. A persistent discomfort with explicit erotic images of gay men hampers HIV prevention campaigns aimed at the gay community. In light of the recent ascendance of conservative political power in the United States, this discomfort is likely to intensify and lead to further prohibitions. Yet, with evidence that erotic elements are effective aspects of safer sex education, their use in future prevention efforts should nevertheless be strongly encouraged.

STOP AIDS

The STOP AIDS project was started in San Francisco in 1984, following comprehensive survey research designed to assess the HIV prevention needs of gay and bisexual men. An explicit goal of this grassroots effort was the changing of community norms consistent with a harm reduction approach—in particular, helping gay and bisexual men reduce high-risk sex and increase lower-risk activities. Operating for about 2½ years, STOP AIDS–San Francisco (STOP AIDS-SF) enrolled approximately 7,000 men in a one-evening-long, peer-led discussion group intervention. Discussions in these nonprofessional groups focused on AIDS prevention, safer sex guidelines, attitudes about AIDS, and strategies for adopting and enhancing safer sex. Bye (1990) reported the results of a telephone survey, which estimated that by that time about 20% of the gay men in San Francisco had attended a STOP AIDS group and 51% were aware of the program. Thus, a significant portion of San Francisco's gay community had been affected at some level by STOP AIDS-SF. Over the same period of time, HIV seroconversion rates among gay and bisexual men dropped from 18% to almost zero. Buoyed by these figures and community word of mouth that safer sex had indeed become the norm, the leaders of STOP AIDS-SF discontinued the project.

Although STOP AIDS-SF was a possible contributor to the changes in community norms and the coincident drop in seroconversion, given the climate of emergency in which it developed, no formal plans were made for an evaluation of the efficacy of this approach. However, a STOP AIDS group in Orange County, California did conduct an assessment of pre- to postintervention change in AIDS knowledge, attitudes, and behavioral intentions among its participants. Miller, Booraem, Flowers, and Iversen (1990), using the AIDS Prevention Test (APT), reported significant pre–post positive shifts in knowledge, attitudes, and sexual behavioral intentions among 148 gay and bisexual men who attended the group discussions. The authors failed, however, to find significant associations between posttest knowledge or attitudes and posttest behavioral intentions. Unfortunately, since there was no measure of actual behavior following group participation, the impact of behavioral intentions on actual future behavior could not be determined.

A much larger evaluation of the STOP AIDS approach was conducted by Flowers et al. (1991). These investigators studied 327 gay and bisexual men equally divided among STOP AIDS projects in Orange County, Chicago, and Phoenix. As in the Miller et al. (1990) study, the APT was used to assess pre- to posttest changes in AIDS-related knowledge, attitudes, and intentions regarding future sexual behavior. Participants in all three areas demonstrated the same level of HIV risk behavior prior to the group, and committed to the same amount of change in risk behavior at the group's conclusion. As in Miller et al. (1990), no correlations were found between posttest AIDS knowledge or attitudes and posttest intentions regarding sexual behavior; these findings were consistent with the outcomes of many health promotion evaluations (see Becker & Joseph, 1988, and Kelly & St. Lawrence, 1988, for reviews). The authors stressed that AIDS prevention should concentrate on demonstrable changes in behavior, rather than on alterations in knowledge or attitudes. Again, however, a follow-up measure of actual behavior change was not administered, so that conclusions regarding the overall behavioral efficacy of STOP AIDS must await further study.

Despite the general lack of evaluation data and the limitations of the few evaluations performed thus far, grassroots programs targeted to gay and bisexual men do have significant advantages. They maximize the ownership of interventions by the community at risk, as well as the overall level of trust and acceptance. Furthermore, they are relatively low-cost and are easily adapted to fit the various social, cultural, and economic circumstances experienced by gay and bisexual men.

Community-Level Coordinated Campaigns: The Case of San Francisco

Because San Francisco was hit early and hard by AIDS, a sense of urgency propelled responses in all sectors of the community. In addition to the grassroots efforts aimed at groups of individuals, academic and public health experts in San Francisco joined forces to outline a coordinated community-wide HIV prevention campaign. As described by Coates (1990), the San Francisco model attempted to address the emerging crisis of AIDS by applying principles and strategies that had been used successfully in programs designed to reduce cardiovascular disease risk.

Coates (1990) describes seven major domains that were identified as equally important components of a larger effort to meet the pressing need for rapid and effective risk reduction. These domains included (1) promulgation of HIV transmission and risk behavior information via print, radio, and television media; (2) provision of information, guidance, and advice by health care professionals to their at-risk patients; (3) provision of printed material, guest speakers, and condoms in schools; (4) provision of printed material, videos, and condoms at work sites; (5) provision of HIV risk assessments, instruction in safer sex and safer injection drug use, and counseling at sexually transmitted disease (STD), family planning, and drug abuse clinics; (6) use of guest speakers, examples of community members infected with HIV, and classes for churches, clubs, and similar groups; and (7) provision of comprehensive HIV risk assessments and risk reduction classes at HIV antibody testing centers. An attempt was also made within each domain to educate staff members and clients about the importance of personally relevant public policy and legislative issues, such as sex education in schools, safeguards for persons with HIV in the workplace, lobbying for drug abuse treatment, and maintaining confidentiality and nondiscrimination for persons testing for HIV.

The approach developed in the early years of the HIV/AIDS epidemic in San Francisco exemplifies the principles of harm reduction through its emphasis on risk reduction (instead of abstinence), community involvement, tailoring interventions to differing groups), establishing trust through the use of credible role models, and lobbying for governmental policies consistent with a public health model of HIV disease.

Group Clinical Interventions

Although community-level prevention and brief educational programs have been helpful in reducing HIV risk among many gay and bisexual men, some individuals have continued to engage in high-risk sexual behavior across several years of follow-up (Becker & Joseph, 1988; Stall et al., 1988). This should not be surprising, given the highly reinforcing nature of sex and the difficulties typically encountered in efforts to maintain lower risk in virtually all potentially health-damaging behaviors (Brownell, Marlatt, Lichtenstein, & Wilson, 1986). For these individuals, a more intensive skills training model of behavior change may be most helpful in bringing about and maintaining reduced HIV risk. By the middle to late 1980s, several groups were attempting to address the problems encountered by those men who were aware of HIV transmission risks and protective strategies, yet had difficulty limiting themselves to safer sex. These more intensive behavioral interventions also provided services for at-risk men that were consistent with a harm reduction approach.

Starting in early 1986, Valdiserri et al. (1989) designed a mostly peer-led AIDS risk reduction intervention for gay and bisexual men. A randomized, controlled evaluation of 584 initially enrolled men was included in their program, allowing them to test the efficacy of two approaches. The first condition consisted of a 60- to 90-minute small-group lecture focused on a number of topics, including HIV transmission, risk behavior, proper condom use, and HIV testing. This was compared to a second intervention that began with the small-group lecture and was then followed by a skills training session (geared toward practice in negotiating safer sex encounters) and a therapist-led group process session.

The authors found that both groups significantly reduced their number of sexual partners for nearly all sexual behaviors (insertive and receptive anal intercourse, insertive and receptive oral intercourse, and mutual masturbation). A concomitant increase in condom use across both conditions was not seen, which implies that participants may have regarded unprotected sex as risky, rather than protected sex as desirable. Moreover, condom use during insertive anal intercourse increased significantly in the skills training/group process condition relative to the small-group-lecture-only condition. This effect was maintained at both 6- and 12-month follow-up assessments. Overall, participants in the skills training/group process condition increased their frequency of condom use during insertive anal intercourse 33% more than those in the small-group-lecture-only condition.

Valdiserri et al.'s failure to find significant increases in condom use during the riskiest behavior (receptive anal intercourse) is cause for concern. It suggests that future interventions should be clearly targeted toward very specific behaviors. In addition, in keeping with harm reduction principles, the importance of both reducing higher-risk behaviors and increasing lower-risk behaviors in HIV prevention efforts should be emphasized.

Rigorous intervention and evaluation programs for gay men have been conducted by Kelly, St. Lawrence, and colleagues (Kelly, St. Lawrence, Hood, & Brasfield, 1989; Kelly, St. Lawrence, Brasfield, & Hood, 1990). These researchers developed a 12-session treatment protocol that focused on education, behavioral management, group support for condom use assertion skills, and reinforcement of alternatives to high-risk behavior. In an evaluation of their program, Kelly et al. (1989) studied 104 gay men who were randomly assigned to either the immediate 12-session treatment or a waiting-list control group. Those participating in the immediate intervention, compared to control subjects, significantly decreased their frequency of unprotected anal intercourse and significantly increased the proportion of anal intercourse occasions where they used condoms. These changes were maintained during an 8-month follow-up assessment and were confirmed by both retrospective assessments and biweekly behavioral monitoring.

Although the effectiveness of this intervention is impressive, 12 weeks may be too lengthy and expensive for easy implementation in other communities. However, this same research group reported that a shorter intervention, focused on similar strategies for risk reduction, was also successful in producing meaningful changes in behavior. Kelly et al. (1990) reported an evaluation of 15 gay men who attended a 7-session treatment group. Significant changes were seen in the frequency of unprotected anal intercourse (which decreased to nearly zero) and in condom use (which increased to almost 90% of all anal intercourse occasions).

Another intervention for MSM was designed by Roger Roffman and colleagues at the University of Washington. Roffman et al. (1989) offered gay and bisexual men a 4-month treatment program focused on reducing high-risk sexual behavior. This program included components of the relapse prevention model developed by Marlatt and Gordon (1985); treatment content emphasized education, identification of "triggers" for risky sex, role playing of condom use assertion skills, and the anticipation and management of relapse. A waiting-list control condition was employed. Preliminary data (Roffman et al., 1997) indicated that the intervention subjects, relative to the waiting-list control subjects, significantly reduced their frequency of unprotected oral intercourse. However, the intervention subjects in this early sample did not report greater reductions in unprotected anal intercourse or increases in condom use over control subjects.

Overall, the Valdiserri et al., Kelly et al., and Roffman et al. treatment programs show promise as effective approaches to HIV risk reduction among gay and bisexual men. Such programs could be enhanced by employing peer group instruction and by attempting to make key program components (e.g., skills training) more "portable." These alterations could increase trust, acceptance, and program use among marginally accessible at-risk men.

Reducing Barriers to Access

The majority of programs described above were conducted with men who were predominantly European American, urban, and primarily self-identified as gay. This population may continue to represent the majority of MSM who are affected by HIV/AIDS, as well as those who continue to be at risk for HIV infection. However, few early programs addressed the needs of gay and bisexual men of color and or those of lower socioeconomic status (including gay/bisexual homeless individuals)—a gap pointed out by Peterson and others (Peterson et al., 1992; Peterson & Marin, 1988). In recent years, this situation has begun to change; several studies and interventions have focused on ethnic minority gay/bisexual populations (Becker & Joseph, 1988; Kelly, Murphy, & Roffman, 1992). Yet there remain continuing research needs in this area. In the past, few programs had the resources to target populations outside the major HIV epicenters. This has slowly begun to change with the availability of additional resources for men in smaller suburban and rural communities. In the final analysis, another population that remains to be targeted adequately consists of those who are bisexual or do not identify themselves as gay.

The harm reduction components that have been useful as part of mainstream efforts are likely to be even more important for MSM groups that are further marginalized by factors of ethnicity, economics, geography, or a more "closeted" life. These groups must truly be "met where they are" in an atmosphere of trust, safety, confidentiality, and empowerment. Programs should ideally emanate from within each community; if this is not possible, they need at least to be carefully tailored to culturally specific norms, customs, and forms of communication. Creative strategies will be needed in order to maximize accessibility. Described below are two programs that have attempted to meet some of these important challenges.

One approach to the problem of accessibility is outreach by telephone. In conjunction with their in-person safer sex counseling program, Roffman et al. (1989) also offered men an option of participating in anonymous telephone groups. The telephone format featured therapist-led group counseling, which also incorporated the relapse prevention components of Marlatt and Gordon (1985). During recruitment, those MSM who chose the telephone rather than in-person groups were more likely to identify themselves as bisexual, to be more "closeted," and to indicate that it was important for them to conceal their sexual preference from others (Roffman et al., 1989). Moreover, the telephone group members were more likely than the in-person subjects to reside in smaller, outlying communities without local gay organizations. Thus, this project appears to have reduced some barriers of sexual identity, fear of exposure, and geographical isolation.

Roffman, Beadnell, Gordon, Stern, and Siever used a pre–post design (1991) to evaluate the effectiveness of this telephone program. Of the 92 participants, 63% had engaged in at least one instance of unprotected anal intercourse in the 3 months prior to counseling. Following the intervention, significant reductions were observed in both unprotected anal and oral intercourse. Although increases were not seen in condom use, participants reported significantly more encounters consisting only of mutual masturbation, as well as significantly fewer anonymous partners.

Because a control group was not used in the Roffman et al. (1991) study, the efficacy of the telephone format cannot be determined. However, this research group is currently conducting a randomized trial of similar therapist-led telephone groups and using a waiting-list control condition. This project features a nationwide recruitment effort with local coordination in several U.S. cities. We hope that the potential of telephone outreach and intervention can be more thoroughly assessed in this and other studies.

A more direct approach to the problems faced by men who live outside HIV epicenters has been employed by Kelly and colleagues. Noting the importance of peer support for behavior change (Fisher, 1988), these investigators implemented a unique peer-mediated intervention designed to reduce high-risk sexual behavior in three small Southern U.S. cities (populations between 50,000 and 75,000). Applying the theory of "diffusion of innovation" (Rogers, 1973), Kelly, St. Lawrence, Diaz, et al. (1991) identified popular peers among gay bar patrons in the three smaller cities to serve as behavior change agents for their communities. These "trend setters" then received training in HIV education, social influence, and the initiation and conduct of safer sex conversations with peers.

Kelly, St. Lawrence, Diaz, et al. (1991) designed their intervention as an experimental evaluation, in which one of the cities served as the target community and the other two as control cities. The three cities were geographically isolated from one another (i.e., separated by at least 60 miles), which minimized crossover effects. Population surveys of baseline measures (knowledge, attitudes, and behavior) were conducted in all cities prior to and following the intervention in the target city. The authors reported significant reductions in the proportion of men who engaged in unprotected anal intercourse (from 36.9% to 27.5%) in the target city. In addition, they noted a 16% increase in condom use during anal intercourse. Over the same period of time, little or no change was seen among surveyed men in the control communities.

Kelly, St. Lawrence, et al. (1992) conducted a subsequent study that replicated and extended the design described above. Using a multiple-baseline design, the authors assessed sexual behavior in all three of the Southern communities and then introduced the same intervention sequentially over time in all cities. Results were similar to the earlier investigation, with significant reductions observed in unprotected anal intercourse (15–29% decreases from baseline levels) following intervention in each city.

Taken together, the Kelly et al. studies suggest that trained peer leaders can be effective in helping to reduce risky sexual behavior among gay and bisexual men. This innovative technique has distinct advantages over more traditional educational efforts. It can be easily tailored to the needs of other groups (e.g., MSM of color and adolescents) through the use of community members as key mediators of change. Moreover, it is an approach that combines several components necessary to reach marginalized groups, such as trust, credibility, sensitivity to cultural norms, and compatible styles of communication.

Returning to High-Risk Sex: The Need for Relapse Prevention

Although significant reductions in high-risk sexual behavior have taken place among MSM since the beginning of the HIV epidemic, research in the 1990s has indicated an increased prevalence of unprotected sexual behavior. Studies also indicate that a significant proportion of men who had initially reduced their frequency of unprotected anal intercourse have begun to report increases in this behavior (Ekstrand & Coates, 1990; Joseph, Montgomery, Kessler, Ostrow, & Wortman, 1988; Kelly, St. Lawrence, & Brasfield, 1991; Stall, Ekstrand, Pollack, McKusick, & Coates, 1990). Factors associated with vulnerability to relapses into high-risk sex include younger age, an earlier history of frequent unprotected anal intercourse with multiple partners, unprotected anal intercourse as a favorite sexual activity, a greater belief that HIV infection is due to external factors (e.g., chance), and positive feelings about a sexual partner (Ekstrand & Coates, 1990; Kelly, St. Lawrence, & Brasfield, 1991; Kelly, Kalichman, et al., 1991; McKusick, Coates, Morin, Pollack, & Hoff, 1990; Stall et al., 1990).

Although relapse is common following other health-related behavior changes (Brownell et al., 1986; Jeffrey, 1989), occasional slips into high-risk sexual behavior carry the potential for tragic consequences. For this reason, future education and intervention programs need to anticipate that some men will experience problems with safer sex maintenance, and thus to include relapse prevention components. In this sense, HIV prevention campaigns among MSM need to be ongoing efforts of engagement, reinforcement, and support for essential behavior changes.

Dual Risks: Unprotected Sex and Drug Use

In the United States as a whole, one in five AIDS cases among individuals with a history of injection drug use were among MSM; very little has been written about this issue (Battjes, 1994). Even among adolescent and young male adult AIDS cases, a surprising 11% had these same dual risk factors. Among those adolescent and adult cases with an injection drug use history, about 32% were homosexually active males.

In a review of the published scientific literature on the relationship between illicit drug use and sexual HIV risk behaviors, Ostrow (1996) noted that studies demonstrated significantly higher baseline prevalence rates of HIV infection among users of illicit drugs than among nonusers (Gorman, 1996; Gorman, Morgan, & Lambert, 1995; Sadownick, 1994). An analysis of sexual risks for HIV transmission in gay men attending a substance abuse treatment program (Paul, Stall, & Davis, 1993) found that amphetamine users in particular had difficulty recognizing the HIV risks resulting from using drugs (especially "speed") and having unprotected sex. Another HIV study by the CDC found that methamphetamine use was highest among IDUs who were MSM, especially in the Western part of the United States (Diaz et al., 1994).

Only a few harm reduction programs to date have targeted MSM who use drugs. Substance Use Counseling and Education (SUCE) is a program conducted by the GMHC that describes itself as a peer-based model of harm reduction and recovery readiness (Feldman & Elovich, 1989). The goals of the program are twofold: to help HIV-negative gay men who use alcohol and/or drugs remain uninfected, and to assist HIV-positive gay men who use alcohol and drugs in staying healthy and accessing appropriate health and support services. This program provides a range of educational interventions, including an explicit relapse prevention approach based on the work of Marlatt and Gordon (1985), for men who do not have resources to obtain gay-positive counseling or gay-sensitive alcohol or drug counseling. Specific subgroups targeted by the program include African American and Latino gay and bisexual men. SUCE also has a lesbian outreach component targeted to lesbian drug and alcohol users.

Two other notable programs influenced by harm reduction and targeted to gay and bisexual men include Seattle's Project NEON, mentioned earlier in this chapter, and Operation Recovery, a relapse-prevention-based substance abuse treatment program in San Francisco. Project NEON is targeted especially to gay and bisexual men who inject methamphetamines. The program entails community outreach on the streets and in the bars and clubs of Seattle's lower Capitol Hill neighborhood; an ongoing harm reduction group facilitated by a health educator and a substance abuse counselor; and the provision of the first gay needle exchange located in a gay neighborhood, so as to facilitate use of clean needles in this hidden population. Operation Recovery, located in the oldest gay and lesbian mental health agency in San Francisco, utilizes a relapse prevention model for treating substance abuse among gay and bisexual men and lesbians. Although the ultimate goal of the program is clearly abstinence from harmful behavior, this unique program allows clients to begin treatment before they have stopped using.

Summary

The gay community has risen to the challenge and developed innovative and effective programs to reduce risk for HIV infection among MSM. The activism of the community has made a tremendous difference in reducing risk behavior among gay/bisexual men and slowing the rate of HIV seroconversion. However, gay and bisexual men still constitute the majority of the cumulative AIDS cases in the United States, and a significant proportion of men who had initially reduced their frequency of unprotected anal intercourse have shown increases in this behavior (Ekstrand & Coates, 1990; Joseph et al., 1988; Kelly, St. Lawrence, & Brasfield, 1991; Stall et al., 1990). As shown by recent epidemiological data, there are also subgroups of MSM who are at high HIV/AIDS risk and have not yet been adequately reached, particularly younger gay/bisexual men and methamphetamine users. Harm reduction approaches that combine street outreach with pragmatic behavioral alternatives, that meet people where they are, and that work with multiple and interrelated risks provide a feasible and promising direction for the future.

REDUCING HIV RISK FOR WOMEN

As of 1994, HIV infection was the third leading cause of death among women aged 25–44 in the United States, and it was the leading cause of death among African American women in this age group (CDC, 1996). Although more men than women have AIDS, the rate of new AIDS cases is growing faster among women (CDC, 1995). In 1997, women made up 15.5% of the cumulative U.S. AIDS cases and 21.8% of the new AIDS cases for that year (CDC, 1997a).

Before 1993, injection drug use was the predominant route of HIV infection for women. The rates of infection due to heterosexual contact have rapidly increased, with the largest proportionate increase in AIDS occurring among people infected through heterosexual contact (CDC, 1997c). Of new AIDS cases among women reported in 1997, 32% were attributed to injection drug use and 38% to heterosexual contact with a partner at risk for or known to have HIV infection or AIDS; for 28%, the transmission category was unidentified and for 1% the transmission category was blood transfusions, blood components, or tissue (CDC, 1997a).

AIDS disproportionately affects inner-city women of color, many of whom live in poverty. In 1997, nearly 80% of the new AIDS cases were among African American and Latina women. The annual rate per 100,000 people of AIDS was 58.8 for African American women and 21.5 for Latina women compared to 3.0 for European American women (CDC, 1997a).

In order to be effective, harm reduction programs need to be placed within the larger context of women's lives. They need to recognize the ways in which poverty impinges upon the abilities of many women at high HIV risk to protect themselves. O'Leary (1994) cogently argues that several factors associated with poverty decrease women's ability to protect themselves from harm. These factors include (1) higher risk for drug use and drug addiction, (2) high prevalence of STDs (see Aral & Holmes, 1991), (3) life concerns that compete with HIV protection for priority, and (4) the economic dependence of some women on their partners.

The ways in which the dynamics of power and issues of trust are expressed within sexual relationships critically affect the opportunities for women to reduce their individual risk (Amaro, 1995). Cultural factors regarding gender roles and beliefs; beliefs about and attitudes toward condom use; adherence to folk beliefs about disease etiology; and distrust in the medical profession also influence the success of reducing women's risk for harm from HIV transmission. If harm reduction efforts are to be able to meet women where they are, the ways in which contextual factors influence women's lives and behavior change opportunities must be understood.

Heterosexual Transmission of HIV

Women are at greater risk for HIV infection through heterosexual transmission than men are, as HIV appears to be more efficiently transmitted from men to women than from women to men. One study reported that HIV was transmitted 12 times more efficiently from men to women (Padian, Shiboski, & Jewell, 1990). This trend, however, appears most prominent in developed countries and in areas with particularly high seroprevalence rates. Recent research has questioned whether the difference in transmission efficiency is real or an artifact of the progression of the HIV epidemic in the United States (Inciardi, 1994). In addition, because the prevalence of HIV infection is higher among men, women are more likely to have sexual partners who are HIV-positive than men are (Ickovics & Rodin, 1992).

Other factors that increase women's risk for contracting HIV through unprotected heterosexual sex include having multiple sexual partners or having STDs (CDC, 1995). In fact, a woman who has multiple sexual partners in an area of high HIV seroprevalence is more likely to contract HIV than is a woman who has the same number of sexual contacts but with the same HIV-positive partner. This is because HIV is most readily transmitted during two points in the disease progression: when a person is initially infected, and when the person is in the final stages of AIDS. As Des Jarlais (quoted in Kolata, 1995, p. B6) has explained,

> If a woman, for example, has sex 100 times with a man who is infected with HIV, but is in the long latent stage when the virus is more difficult to transmit, she is much less likely to get infected than if she has sex just once with one man who may be in the infectious stage. So a woman is at much greater risk having sex once with 100 partners, most of whom are infected, than having sex 100 times with a man who is infected but in the latent stage.

Unprotected sexual behavior also increases the risk of acquiring STDs, the lesions of which have been found to facilitate acquisition of HIV. Although syphilis and gonorrhea have been steadily declining in most developed countries, they have been increasing in recent years among inner-city ethnic minority populations in the United States (Aral & Holmes, 1991). Because of the higher prevalence of STDs and HIV, the risk of acquiring HIV through unsafe sex is higher in these inner-city areas.

Harm Reduction Strategies

A primary method for sexually active women to reduce their risk of HIV infection through heterosexual sex is for their partners to use condoms. Achieving consistent condom use is a formidable challenge, however. As noted by DeCarlo (1994),

> Women do not wear the condom. For women to protect themselves from HIV infection, they must not only rely on their own skills, attitudes, and behaviors regarding condom use, but also on their ability to convince their partner to use a condom. (p. 1)

Men do not like using condoms for a variety of reasons, including that they interfere with the pleasure and spontaneity of sex; the most frequent reason women give for not using condoms is that their partners do not like them (Allen, 1994; Catania et al., 1989; Morrison, Gilmore, & Baker, 1995; Weissman & the National AIDS Research Consortium [NARC], 1991). The use of condoms also carries important symbolic meaning, particularly in regard to trust. Based on results from an in-depth interview study of young women in England, Holland, Ramazanoglu, Scott, Sharpe, and Rhomson (1992) noted:

> Although women can and do make demands for safer sex, asking young men to use condoms is not easy in unequal relationships, and where desire is constructed by eroticizing inequality and relationship. Where these relationships are defined in terms of love and trust, sexual safety can become a contradictory practice. (p. 278)

A woman's asking her partner to use a condom can be construed as either lack of trust in his faithfulness or an indication that she has not been faithful or is infected with HIV. The power structure of heterosexual relationships may also make it very difficult for women to insist on condom use. This power dynamic is perhaps most salient for women in abusive relationships, who may be unable to negotiate or enforce condom use safely.

The methods to enhance condom use discussed in the previous section on MSM, such as eroticizing condom use, have been used with women as well. Condom use has also been increased through teaching women negotiation and other skills (Schilling et al., 1991). Some street outreach programs teach sex workers skills to put condoms on men during sex without their being aware of it. This strategy however, could, backfire if discovered and could put women at risk for physical harm; it should therefore be used cautiously. Another approach is for programs to work to change male attitudes toward condom use and increase their willingness to use condoms, or to work with both partners. After all, it still is the man who needs to use the condom.

Another set of harm reduction strategies provide women with more control over protection than that afforded by the male condom. The recently developed female condom has been long awaited by many women's advocates. Its major advantage is that the woman is the one using the condom and thus has more control. However, the female condom faces some of the same attitudinal barriers to its use as does the male condom. In addition, the female condom may be obvious to the partner, and thus women may run into similar obstacles with partners who do not want the use of any barrier. Nevertheless, more needs to be done to improve the female condom and make it more accessible for those women who are able to use it. Other methods of self-protection over which women have control also need to be developed.

A controversial HIV risk reduction method advocated by some groups is the use of spermicides with nonoxynol-9 when women are unable to use condoms. Although nonoxynol-9 has been shown to kill HIV and STDs, there is some concern that it disrupts the outer lining of the cervix and vagina in some women and may thus facilitate transmission of infection (Ickovics & Robin, 1992; O'Leary, 1994). In light of these risks, more research on this method of protection is needed to determine its merits.

In outreach efforts to increase use of condoms or spermicides, it is important to make it clear to women that contraception per se does not equal protection from HIV. In particular, there is concern that women may believe that the birth control pill may offer protection (Ickovics & Rodin, 1992). It is important that this and other misconceptions be dispelled, in order for women to be able to make informed decisions about their lives.

An Example of a Program to Reduce Heterosexual HIV Transmission

To date, few empirically validated studies of HIV/AIDS prevention efforts among adult heterosexual women have been conducted. Similarly, the effectiveness of strategies described in prevention materials disseminated by public health departments and other organizations remains largely unevaluated (Beadnell, Baker, Gordon, Collier, & Ryan, 1997). One program, the Women's Health Project, is an innovative treatment outcome study of women at high risk for HIV infection, currently in progress at the University of Washington's School of Social Work.

The Women's Health Project (Beadnell et al., 1997) is a 5-year study that aims to test the efficacy of an intervention to decrease high-risk sexual behaviors in women. This intervention is based on Marlatt and Gordon's (1985) cognitive-behavioral relapse prevention model, and has been adapted from an effective HIV prevention intervention developed by Roffman and colleagues for MSM (described earlier in this chapter). The adaptation has been based on extensive interviews, focus groups, and a needs assessment of high-risk women, along with input from an advisory board of community members who work with high-risk men.

Participants for the study are being recruited through local STD clinics in surrounding urban centers. The clinical intervention is provided by trained professionals and is held in a group format. The group meets for 16 sessions and focuses on helping women to identify their own risk behaviors, to develop goals and motivation for change, and to learn specific strategies for change. Maintenance of behavioral change is included to assist women in learning how to manage "slips," improve their lifestyle, and enhance their social support network. Consistent with the relapse prevention model, coping skills and assertiveness training are taught and practiced within the group context, where new behaviors can be practiced, modeled, and reinforced by the group members, and where participants can receive feedback and "coaching" from peers and the group's therapists. This program is consistent with harm reduction principles, in that it explicitly seeks to meet women where they are in the change process; provides them with information about their risk, so that they can make informed choices about how to reduce this risk; and provides them with opportunities to develop and practice risk reduction skills.

HIV Transmission in Women through Injection Drug Use

Understanding the social context of women's injection drug use is critical to developing effective harm reduction programs for women. The few studies that focus explicitly on women IDUs highlight the structural and personal difficulties women face in reducing their risk for HIV (Amaro, 1995). Women are often introduced to drugs and maintain access to them through men (Amaro, Zuckerman, & Cabral, 1989; Anglin, Hser, & McGlothlin, 1987). The illicit drug distribution system is dominated by men and may restrict women's ability to obtain their own drugs. In addition, women who obtain their own drugs may have to pay with both money and sex, often with no reduction in the price (Braine, 1994). As a result, drug-dependent women become reliant on men to get their drugs and are often more difficult to access at the usual outreach locations, such as "drug-copping" sites (Hartel, 1994; Weissman & NARC, 1991).

Women are more likely to report sharing drugs only with their partners, whereas men are more likely to report sharing with others in addition to sharing with their sexual partners (Barnard, 1993). The nature of the relationship between women IDUs and their partners, including issues of trust, may limit women's ability to exert control over using "clean works." Some women IDUs are dependent on their partners for shelter and money, in addition to drug procurement, and may not have their own works. Furthermore, it appears that there are high rates of domestic violence in these relationships, also affecting women's ability to exert influence over protective behaviors (Weissman & NARC, 1991).

In addition to the risk of contracting HIV through the use of infected needles, women IDUs are also placed at risk for HIV from unprotected sex. They are more likely to be involved in street prostitution and may face economic incentives to perform higher-risk sex (e.g., no condom use, anal intercourse, etc.) in exchange for higher wages (Jackson, Highcrest, & Coates, 1992). Finally, they are more likely to have sexual partners who inject drugs than are women who do not inject drugs.

Partners of Injection Drug Users

Women partners of IDUs constitute another high-HIV-risk group about which relatively little is known. These women can be a relatively hidden and difficult group to reach. If they do not themselves inject drugs, they may or may not know that their partners inject drugs.

Partners of male IDUs who are not themselves IDUs may use other drugs that increase their risk behavior (Allen, 1994; Corby, Wolitski, Thornton-Johnson, & Tanner, 1991; Tortu, Beardsley, Deren, & Davis, 1994). In a national demonstration project of partners of IDUs in 63 sites, Weissman and NARC (1991) found that partners of IDUs, whether or not they themselves injected drugs, reported frequent use of alcohol, cocaine, and marijuana. A particular cause for concern was that half of the women partners of IDUs who did not inject drugs reported using crack in the 6 months prior to the interview, and 35% of these women reported trading sex for drugs.

In another study of partners of IDUs, Tortu et al. (1994) compared three groups of partners who were not themselves IDUs in terms of their risk behavior: those with a single partner, those with multiple partners, and those with multiple partners who exchanged sex for drugs or money. They found that the women who exchanged sex were significantly more likely than either of the other two groups to use crack, to be homeless, to have been incarcerated, and to have had more frequent unsafe sex. Tortu et al. commented:

> On nearly all of the characteristics examined, even when major demographic variables were controlled, . . . women who traded sex for drugs and/or money lead lives that are the most chaotic, the least healthy, and the most risky . . . of a magnitude that is very dramatic in terms of what they mean in "real" life. (p. 1249)

Harm Reduction Strategies

Bleach distribution and NEPs as harm reduction strategies for IDUs have been discussed earlier in this chapter (methadone treatment is discussed in Chapter 6). Three key issues need to be addressed in implementing these programs for women IDUs and partners of IDUs.

1. *Improving outreach to women.* As others have suggested, outreach to women IDUs or to partners of male IDUs needs to extend to other sites, such as welfare offices, health clinics, and food banks. Because many women do not buy their own drugs or have their own injection equipment, some women may not be reached through sites located at drug-copping areas. The consequences of drug use for a woman are also different from those for a man. For one, female drug users are more likely to have primary care responsibilities for children, and are therefore more at risk for having their children removed by children's protective services. Second, addiction among women is often taken as an indication of sexual availability. Thus, some needle exchange and outreach sites need to be located in areas that are more private than a street corner.

2. *Tailoring drug treatment programs to women.* In addition to the lack of affordable substance abuse treatment programs, those that do exist seldom address the unique needs of women seeking treatment, such as child care or domestic violence. Male partners who are drug users may block women's access to treatment or eventually undermine their partners' successful participation in treatment. Women seeking substance abuse treatment may also require special attention to addressing sexual abuse, given its prevalence within this population. For example, in a review of the literature, Wilsnack, Wilsnack, and Klassen (1984) found that between 41% and 74% of women in alcohol or drug treatment had been sexually abused as children. Treatment programs are needed that work with these issues in women's treatment process.

3. *Recognizing the power dynamics and inequities in women's relationships.* Power disparities between women and their male partners in particular may interfere with their ability to adopt and maintain risk reduction efforts. Where it is possible and appropriate, harm reduction may best be achieved by directing outreach and risk reduction efforts toward both partners.

Intersection of Unsafe Sex and Drug Use

Sex Workers

Contrary to commonly held views, men's risk of contracting HIV through sex with a female prostitute in the United States is relatively low (Wallace,

Mann, & Beatrice, 1988; Chiasson, Stoneburner, Lifson, Hildebrandt, & Jaffe, 1988). Female sex workers, however, are at heightened risk of contracting HIV through high-risk sexual behaviors with customers and sexual intimates, as well as through injection drug use. The risk of these behaviors is heightened even further through a number of co-occurring factors: (1) living and working in high-seroprevalence areas, where partners are more likely to be HIV-positive; (2) the efficiency of transmission from males to females; and (3) living and working conditions among sex workers, which often limit their control over self-protection.

At the beginning of the AIDS epidemic, many feared that prostitutes would become vectors for the transmission of HIV from the gay male and drug-addicted communities to the "straight" communities. Prostitutes, particularly poor women and women of color, were viewed as "reservoirs" of infection—a social and public health liability. Public concern resulted in an increased stigmatization of sex workers and, in some places, adoption of restrictive legislation intended to deter sex workers—including mandatory HIV testing if arrested, increased police surveillance of common "strolls" (areas frequented by street workers), and increased arrests (Estebanez, Fitch, & Najera, 1993). Possession of a large number of condoms became sufficient evidence for arrest on prostitution charges.

Several studies have found a general increase in condom use among sex workers within the context of their trade (CDC, 1987; Estebenez et al., 1993). This trend appears to be particularly robust in countries or regions where commercial sex is legal or tolerated (Smith & Smith, 1986; Hooykaas, van der Pligt, van Doornum, van der Linden, & Coutinho, 1989). However, rates of reported use of condoms with nonpaying sexual intimates remain considerably lower (Day, Ward, & Harris, 1988; CDC, 1987; McKeganey & Barnard, 1992). Of 500 sex workers living in the San Francisco area, 38% reported always using a condom with paying customers, compared to 14% who sometimes used them with their personal intimates (Cohen et al., 1989). Similarly, in studies in London and Glasgow, virtually all sex workers surveyed (98%) reported condom use for commercial clients, but low rates were reported for nonpaying partners (12–17%) (Green et al., 1993; Ward et al., 1993).

A number of factors may account for the differential use of condoms. The issue of the symbolic meaning of condoms, mentioned earlier in this section, is particularly salient for female sex workers. Use of condoms with paying customers may serve as a psychological barrier, thereby creating a clear distinction between professional and private acts (Jackson et al., 1992). Providing narratives from interviews with sex workers in Glasgow, McKeganey and Barnard (1992) include the following comments from one participant:

> I think they think to themselves, "Well I don't want to do it if it feels like I'm still working." I felt like that wi' ma [sic] boyfriend. I didnae [sic] want to use

a condom. Mostly girls that don't use condoms it's because they've got that at the back of their mind about working the town. (p. 403)

Green et al. (1993) reported that one woman's romantic partner refused to wear condoms "because it made him feel like a client" (p. 330). Finally, some observe that because condom use negotiation goes to the core of societal sexism, sociocultural pressures may make it especially difficult for women to insist on safer sex practices with their sexual intimates.

Although there has been an increase in condom use by sex workers with customers, many sex workers face barriers to using condoms, ranging from economic incentives to have unprotected sex to the real threat of physical harm by male customers (Goldsmith, 1993). Estebanez et al. (1993) reported that one of the main reasons for not using condoms is client refusal; another is fear of arrest in areas where possession of condoms may be used as evidence of intent to commit prostitution. Drug-dependent women who sell sex to support their drug addiction may be particularly vulnerable to client requests for unsafe sex (McKeganey & Barnard, 1992; see below).

A number of commonly held assumptions about female sex workers have significantly shaped the course of research and service delivery to this population. Perhaps the most salient is the belief that all sex workers are alike. Female sex workers are in reality a diverse group with varied lifestyles, reasons for involvement in the sex industry, places of work, and conditions associated with their work setting (Miller, Turner, & Moses, 1990). Although street prostitution is clearly the most visible form of sex work, it accounts for about only 20% of all sex work in the United States (Campbell, 1991). Female sex workers are often viewed as psychologically deviant rather than socially underprivileged.

Rates of drug use among sex workers vary greatly from country to country, and depend on the type of sex work. Generally, rates of injection drug use are highest among women who work the streets, ranging from 50% to 80% (Estebanez et al., 1993; Green et al., 1993; McKeganey & Barnard, 1992). A multisite study of female sex workers in the United States found that 693 of the 1,396 women surveyed reported that either they or their sex partners were IDUs. Of the 693, 138 (20%) were seropositive, compared to 35 (5%) of women who reported that neither they nor their partners were IDUs (CDC, 1987). Studies have found, however, that prostitution by itself does not significantly increase the risk of contracting HIV for female IDUs (Miller et al., 1990; Padian, 1988; Rhodes, Donoghoe, Hunter, & Stimson, 1994; Tirelli et al., 1989).

In a review of the use of prostitution and drug use, Donoghoe (1992) concludes that use of drugs and alcohol does increase the probability of engagement in high-risk sexual activity and other risky behaviors. Reasons for this include the disinhibiting effects of the drugs, the drugs' direct pharmacological effects on cognitive and motor functioning (both of which are involved in proper use of a condom), and the milieu in which sexual opportunities are interwoven with drugs and alcohol (e.g., bars, clubs, etc.). Donoghoe also notes differences in drugs used, depending on the kind of sex work performed.

Trading Sex for Crack

As previously mentioned, the rapid increase in heterosexual transmission of HIV among women in the United States is tightly linked to drug use, particularly the use of crack cocaine. The CDC recently estimated that about half of the new infections among heterosexuals are occurring among crack cocaine users (Holmberg, cited in Kolata, 1995). Crack users tend to have a greater number of sexual partners, to have more STDs, and to be less likely to use condoms than people from comparable sociodemographic backgrounds who are not crack users (Cohen, Navaline, & Metzger, 1994; Dwyer et al., 1994; Edlin et al., 1992, 1994; Weatherby et al., 1992).

Crack is most widely used by young, poor, inner-city members of ethnic minorities, and in many of the same areas where HIV prevalence is highest. There is strong evidence that crack use is linked to HIV transmission through users' exchanging sex for crack, often with IDUs (Edlin et al., 1994). Both ethnographic and quantitative studies have found that the majority of women who use crack exchange sex for crack or for money to buy crack. In one study, crack users were four times more likely to exchange sex for drugs than were heroin users (Cohen et al., 1994). Edlin et al. (1992) found that women who used crack were 16 times more likely to have exchanged sex for crack, and nearly three times as likely to be HIV-positive, as other street-involved people who were not crack users. When exchanging sex for drugs was controlled for, the HIV prevalence was the same for crack users as for other street-involved people who were not crack users (Edlin et al., 1994). Thus, for crack users who are not themselves IDUs, exchanging unsafe sex for crack poses the greatest HIV risk

An Example of a Harm Reduction Program for Sex Workers

Sex workers have effectively organized in various parts of the world to share information to prevent the spread of HIV/AIDS within their communities (e.g., California AIDS Prevention and Education Project in San Francisco, the Red Thread Organization in Amsterdam, and the Australian Prostitutes Collective). CAL-PEP began as a joint enterprise between the San Francisco-based Association for Women's AIDS Research and Education (AWARE) and an existing prostitutes' rights organization, Call Off Your Old Tired Ethics (COYOTE). The primary aim of CAL-PEP is to form nonjudgmental partnerships with women sex workers, in order to help them understand their individual risks and particular risk behaviors, to facilitate the development of new behaviors that reduce these risks, and to make referrals to drug treatment programs available when appropriate. The program was founded on three basic beliefs; (1) that sex workers are unlikely to respond to public health authorities; (2) that sex workers will be more receptive to education and services if these are provided by their peers; and (3) that to encourage ongoing participation in the study, the project should provide a number of health services in exchange for provision of data. The outreach staff is composed primarily of former sex workers (Dorfman, Derish, & Cohen, 1992).

The CAL-PEP program consists of two primary components. First, street outreach workers walk along the strolls, distributing safety kits that contain condoms, bottles of bleach for cleansing needles, and instructions for reducing risk of HIV infection. Second, monthly "outings" are held to allow women receiving street outreach to participate in more intensive risk reduction training. Outings are typically held in local hotel rooms near the strolls and involve participation of all members of the CAL-PEP staff, including researchers. The primary goal of the outings is to provide women sex workers with more extensive information about HIV and specific techniques tailored to their needs to prevent its transmission. In addition to this informational component, skills-based training demonstrations and role plays provide an opportunity for women to put the information into practice. Demonstrations include techniques to clean injection drug equipment, effective strategies for using condoms for different sexual acts in ways that minimize breakage, and approaches to negotiate use of condoms and other safer sex practices with clients and intimate partners.

Summary

Women at risk for contracting HIV and AIDS face multiple and overlapping risk factors. As Weissman and NARC (1991) have noted,

> While prevention programs for women may be organized around or funded for a single specific issue . . . the women with whom the programs are trying to work cannot be categorized so neatly. . . . women are afflicted by multiple problems. Among these are drug abuse, homelessness, lack of financial support, dysfunctional or destructive interpersonal relationships, lack of effective social support systems, legal problems, and poor health. In designing programs for these women, it appears crucial to remember that neither they nor AIDS exist in a vacuum. . . . programs need to be mindful of the many contexts that shape the lives of these women, including psychological, familial, social economic, cultural, political, medical, and spiritual. (pp. 60–61)

Generally speaking, the women most at risk for HIV infection are poor members of ethnic minorities who live within urban centers. These women are less likely to have control over the means to reduce their risks of harm, largely as a result of economic hardship and diminished power in relation to their male counterparts. Concomitantly, risks for women are frequently multidetermined and seldom fall into one neat category.

If HIV harm reduction programs are to be effective for women, these programs must also meet women where they are and within a context that is safe, nonthreatening, and easily accessible. Most importantly, it is essential to recognize the contexts and factors where women have sufficient power and control to change behaviors, and those where they have less control over effecting change.

REDUCING HIV RISK AMONG ADOLESCENTS

The number of U.S. adolescents with AIDS is relatively low; 3,130 youth aged 13–19 were diagnosed with AIDS as of December 1997 (CDC, 1997a). However, there are substantially more young adults aged 20–24 with AIDS—people who were almost certainly infected with HIV as adolescents. Moreover, recent estimates are that one in four new HIV infections in the United States occurs among people under the age of 20 (Fleming, 1996).

Youth are obviously not all at equal risk for contracting HIV infection. For many, adolescence is a time of experimentation with alcohol, drugs, and/or sex, and this experimentation is often combined with perceptions of invulnerability (Cates, 1991; Irwin & Millstein, 1986; Dryfoos, 1990). Rates of STDs are high among adolescents—evidence that safer sex practices are not being consistently used (Cates, 1991; Bell & Hein, 1984). Whereas the rates of STDs (e.g., gonorrhea) decreased during the 1980s for most age groups, these statistics increased for sexually active adolescents (Cates, 1991; Bell & Hein, 1984). Overall, 75% of STDs occur among people between the ages of 15 and 24 (Bell & Hein, 1984). In 1996, the highest age-specific gonorrhea rates among women, and the second highest rates among men, were in the 15- to 19-year-old group (Division of STD Prevention, 1997). These statistics are a cause for alarm, because once HIV enters the social networks of adolescents more generally, the conditions are ripe for a rapid increase in rates of infection unless safer sex practices are adopted.

As with adults, by 1997, a larger proportion of adolescents and young adults (aged 13–24) with AIDS were male (72%) than female (28%) (CDC, 1997a). Of the young males, most (59.6%) were exposed through sex with other men, followed by exposure through injection drug use (11.8%). Another 10% of male adolescents were exposed through the dual risk avenues of sex with men and injection drug use. For young females with AIDS, unprotected heterosexual sex accounted for over half of the cumulative AIDS cases through 1997 (53.7%) and about a quarter were exposed through injection drug use (26%). Risk factors were either unknown or not reported for 17% of the female adolescent AIDS cases and 7% of the male cases (CDC, 1997a).

One group of adolescents at particularly high risk for HIV infection is that of street-involved youth, many of whom are gay or bisexual. "Street-involved youth" is a term used here to refer to adolescents who spend a substantial amount of time on the streets and who are not under the consistent care and supervision of a parental figure. It includes runaway, "throwaway," and homeless youth. Many of these youth have been forced to leave their homes, sometimes because of conflict involving a young person's gay or bisexual identity, or because home life is intolerable and/or abusive. Many have been in and out of foster homes and have dropped out of school. Often alienated from the system, these young people frequently do not receive HIV prevention education in school, from family members, or through traditional media. For many street-involved youth, the needs for food, shelter, clothing, protection, and a sense of belonging outweigh the need for reducing HIV risk. Motivation to prevent HIV is often less pressing than the more immediate needs of survival (Luna, 1991; Overby & Kegeles, 1994).

Street youth typically congregate in areas of drug use and prostitution, and are thus more likely to have sexual partners who are HIV-positive. In addition, many street youth engage in "survival sex," exchanging sex for food, shelter, or drugs. Studies have found that between 25% and 50% of street youth using health clinics have engaged in survival sex (Cohen, MacKenzie, & Yates, 1991; Farrow, Deisher, Brown, Kulig, & Kipke, 1992; Kennedy, 1991; Stricof, Kennedy, Nattell, Weisfuse, & Novick, 1991; Yates, MacKenzie, Pennbridge, & Swofford, 1991). Thus, inconsistent or no condom use increases their risk for HIV relative to that of other adolescents, whose partners are less likely to be HIV-positive.

The estimated prevalence of use for *all* types of drugs is higher among street youth than among other youth, and multiple-drug use is common (Koopman, Rosario, & Rotheram-Borus, 1994; Green, Ennett, & Ringwalt, 1997; Yates, MacKenzie, Pennbridge, & Cohen, 1988). Although in national samples of adolescents, about 1% of youth report a history of injection drug use, reports among street youth are substantially higher (CDC, 1994). In Los Angeles, 35% of street youth in one study reported a history of injection drug use, as did approximately 22% of street youth in the Seattle area (Carlin & Wagner, 1995; Yates et al., 1988). Approximately 28–38% of street youth in New York use crack cocaine (Rotheram-Borus, Koopman, Haignere, & Davies, 1991; Yates et al., 1988). As noted in a previous section, crack cocaine is indirectly associated with higher HIV risk through the link of exchanging sex for drugs or money.

A CDC seroprevalence study found that about 5% of males and 1.3% of females between the ages of 15 and 24 were HIV-positive (Allen et al., 1994), which is consistent with estimates found in other studies (New York State Department of Health, 1989, cited in Miller et al., 1990, p. 165; Stricof et al., 1991). Allen et al. (1994) also reported a disturbingly high percentage of gay/bisexual youth who were HIV-positive (26%); even higher proportions were found at one site among homeless male youth with the dual risks of having sex with men and injection drug use (45%). Even though these figures come from a nonprobability sample, seroprevalence studies do provide warning and indications of where risk reduction efforts need to be focused.

The current epidemiology of AIDS and STDs among adolescents in the United States thus points to an unfortunate reality: The youth at highest risk of contracting AIDS are those who are likely to be most disenfranchised and difficult to reach. They include street-involved youth, urban low-income youth of color, and gay/bisexual youth (obviously, these categories are not mutually exclusive).

Harm Reduction Strategies Targeting Adolescents

Harm reduction strategies to prevent HIV among adolescents are similar to those for adults discussed elsewhere in this chapter. Strategies include increasing access to condoms (including female condoms) and clean needles; teaching appropriate skills to reduce risk, including sexual and condom use negotiation, needle cleaning, and condom use skills; and fostering social norms that support adoption of risk reduction behaviors.

The Abstinence versus Risk Reduction Debate

Harm reduction programs for adolescents face moralistic hurdles similar to those faced by programs for adults. In addition, programs for adolescents must overcome societal denial that adolescents are engaging in sexual and drug use behaviors. Moral arguments against harm reduction programs in general are often based on the belief that they condone or promote immoral behavior that contributes to societal deterioration. These same arguments are directed against adolescent harm reduction programs with even greater fervor, because of the fear that harm reduction programs will in fact lure youth to *initiate* such behavior.

One need look no further than the uproar of opposition to the direct and realistic remarks of former U.S. Surgeon General Joycelyn Elders— remarks that ultimately resulted in her dismissal. Elders's comments on the importance of pragmatic approaches to sex education rekindled a national debate about the role of government in promoting safer sex behaviors among the nation's youth.

In an op-ed article in *The New York Times*, Elders (1994) wrote,

> Our country is engaged in a wrenching debate about . . . the role of government in keeping our nation healthy. Our streets and jails are teeming with children and young people nobody wants. The rates of sexually transmitted diseases continue growing. As parents, teachers and leaders, we cannot stand by and let our children slip away because of ignorance or a failure of courage.

This means telling the truth to our young people about the risks of their behavior and giving them ways to reduce these risks.

I regret that some of the words I have uttered about these and other matters have caused discomfort. But I regret even more the realities they describe. Sexual practices are, of course, best left to consenting adults, behind closed doors. But sex becomes a proper subject for government when sexual behavior endangers public health, as is clearly the case with AIDS and other diseases, or when it leads to increased poverty, ignorance and enslavement, as is the case with unplanned, unwanted children. (p. A19)

Those opposing her views argued that such an approach would promote sexual promiscuity among youth.

As is illustrated by the politics of Elders's removal from public office, harm reduction strategies applied to adolescent programs have faced vociferous and visible opposition, particularly in the area of government enforcement of abstinence-only messages in sex education. The official policy of the federal government has largely functioned in support of abstinence-only sex education programs (Miller et al., 1990). It is unfortunate that the controversy is portrayed as an abstinence versus nonabstinence debate, because most adolescent sexual risk reduction programs do support sexual abstinence as an important and appropriate goal for youth. It is the abstinence-*only* approach, wherein education on methods to protect oneself from STDs and pregnancy is not provided to adolescents, that those in favor of risk reduction consider problematic. As Carole Chervin, an attorney for the Planned Parenthood Federation (quoted in Gibbs, 1993, p. 64) stated, "All parents I know are absolutely in favor of abstinence. It's the abstinence *only* approach that's bothersome. We believe sex education should be comprehensive."

To be most effective, programs to delay age of sexual initiation and maintenance of abstinence need to begin in childhood or early adolescence. Once adolescents become sexually active, very few become abstinent, although they may not have sex on a regular basis (Hayes, 1987; Leigh, Morrison, Trocki, & Temple, 1994; Maticka-Tyndale, 1991). It is irresponsible for programs to ignore the reality that the majority of adolescents, particularly those in their middle to late teens, are sexually active (CDC, 1995). National surveys conducted in 1988 reported that over 82% of African American men, 71% of European American men, and 52% of Latino men had initiated sex by age 18 (National Survey of Adolescent Males, cited in Miller et al., 1990), and that approximately 66% of African American women and 49% of European American women had initiated sex by age 18 (National Survey of Family Growth, cited in Miller et al., 1990).

As already noted, one of the objections to adolescent programs that provide risk reduction information (e.g., information or skills training about how to use condoms, explicit discussion of sexual behaviors that pose HIV or STD risk) is that they will encourage youth to initiate sexual involvement. Empirical evidence suggests otherwise. A recent review of school-based programs to reduce sexual risk behavior found that programs providing information on contraceptives or safer sex, including condoms, were successful at delaying sexual initiation (Kirby et al., 1994). Furthermore, there was no evidence that the risk reduction programs increased the frequency of sexual behavior among those who had initiated such behavior before the programs. These education programs did not, however, result in an increase in contraceptive use, indicating once again that education alone is not enough to change behavior.

Programs whose only message is abstinence may even have unintended negative consequences for youth who have already initiated sex. For example, "Success Express" was an abstinence-only pregnancy prevention program that targeted low-income and minority middle school youth (Christopher & Roosa, 1990). The five-session program had education components on self-esteem and family values, growth and reproductive development, media and peer pressures, assertiveness skills, and setting life goals. Participants in the intervention group showed a *greater* increase in sexual behavior than the comparison group did, and there was no evidence that the program was effective in delaying initiation. An equally important finding was that youth who dropped out of the program were more likely to be sexually active than those who remained. Thus, it appears that the program may have missed youth most at risk for adverse outcomes from sexual behavior. Similar unintended consequences have been found in drug prevention programs, where drug use was found to increase in the intervention condition relative to the control condition among youth who had already initiated use (Ellickson & Bell, 1990).

One way to understand the "boomerang" effect of the abstinence-only education programs is that this abstinence message may alienate young people who have already initiated risk behavior. Such a message further defines these youth as deviant, and lessens the ability of a program to influence them. It may also lessen adults' credibility in general. The harm reduction approach may emphasize abstinence as an important option, but it also provides youth for whom abstinence is not a realistic goal with strategies to reduce their risk of AIDS, STDs, and pregnancy. In this way, it empowers youth to make decisions about their lives based on complete information.

Condom Distribution

Condom distribution for adolescents is a controversial harm reduction strategy, particularly when it is linked to school programs or school-based clinics (Sellers, McGraw, & McKinlay, 1994). It is, however, only one component of an HIV/AIDS harm reduction approach. The condom distribution programs increase the visibility of safer sex methods and make condoms more readily accessible, thus potentially reducing some barriers to safer sex (Wight, 1992). When coupled with peer education or street outreach programs, these programs have the potential to reach youth at high risk. Condom distribution programs do not, as feared by some, appear to increase the rate of sexual initiation or to increase the frequency of sexual behavior among youth (Sellers et al., 1994). Currently, an untested but desirable outcome of condom distribution would be that it results in attitudes and social norms that are more favorable toward safer sex among those who are sexually active.

How effective condom distribution has been in actually increasing condom use is as yet unknown. It is likely to take more than distribution per se to get the maximal payoff from this approach. In fact, most school-based condom distribution programs are embedded within more comprehensive programs (Sellers et al., 1994). For adolescents and adults alike, achieving consistent use of condoms is a difficult task (Catania, Coates, & Kegeles, 1992). Condom use appears to have increased during the later 1980s and into the early 1990s (CDC, 1995b; Sonenstein, Pleck, & Ku, 1989; Hingson, Strunin, & Berlin, 1990), with the percentage of adolescents who reported using condoms at time of first sexual intercourse and most recent sexual intercourse nearly doubling (Sonenstein et al., 1991). Unfortunately, more recent surveys of adolescents have found that slightly more youth have never used condoms than always use condoms (Brown, DiClemente, & Park, 1992; Strunin & Hingson, 1992; Leigh et al., 1994; Sonenstein et al., 1991).

Several studies have sought to uncover the main factors determining whether or not adolescents use condoms. It is clear that knowledge of AIDS risk factors and of preventive measures alone is not associated with condom use (Brown, DiClemente, & Park, 1992; DiClemente et al., 1992; Walter et al., 1992). Most of these studies have tested theoretical variables from the health belief model (Janz & Becker, 1984) or the theory of reasoned action (Ajzen & Fishbein, 1980), although few studies have been directly comparable in terms of which constructs were actually assessed and how they were assessed. In general, adolescents are less likely to use condom consistently if they (1) believe that condoms decrease sexual pleasure (Catania et al., 1989; Hingson et al., 1990; Sonenstein et al., 1991); (2) believe that condoms are not very effective in preventing HIV/AIDS (Brown, DiClemente, & Beausoleil, 1992; Catania et al., 1989; DiClemente et al., 1992; Hingson et al., 1990; Sonenstein et al., 1991); (3) do not feel personally susceptible to HIV infection (Hingson et al., 1990; Sonenstein et al., 1991); (4) do not perceive the norms of their peers as favorable toward safer sex or condom use (Walter et al., 1992); or (5) use drugs or drink alcohol during sex (Brown, DiClemente, & Beausoleil, 1992; Hingson et al., 1990). Younger adolescents and youth who are early initiators of sexual behavior are also less likely to use condoms (Sonenstein et al., 1991; Hingson et al., 1990). Youth also may not use condoms because they are in a monogamous relationship and they believe they are not at risk (Overby & Kegeles, 1994). Many youth, however, go through a series of monogamous relationships of varying duration, and the cumulative risk may not be recognized.

In summary, although condom distribution may reduce one important barrier to condom use, having a condom in hand does not necessarily mean that it will be used. Many of the relationship issues that interfere with condom use have been discussed in the section on women, and these are also relevant for adolescents; they include issues of trust, discomfort with asking one's partner to use condoms, and power disparities in a relationship. Condom distribution is but one important step in promoting HIV/AIDS protective behaviors. It needs to be part of a comprehensive program that addresses the factors inhibiting the use of condoms, and that provides skills training in negotiating condom use and using condoms effectively.

Skills Training

Few rigorous evaluations of HIV/AIDS prevention programs for adolescents exist. Some have not used comparison groups, and most have examined only AIDS knowledge gains or attitude changes without assessing behavior change (Brown, Fritz, & Barone, 1989; DiClemente et al., 1989). Studies from across a range of health-related behaviors indicate that knowledge is necessary but not sufficient for effecting behavioral change. At least one study that did evaluate behavior found that the knowledge adolescents demonstrated about HIV and AIDS did not coincide with the adoption of safer sex practices (Strunin & Hingson, 1992). Clearly, assessing only knowledge or attitudes and not behavior brings the value of any conclusions into question.

The most promising HIV/AIDS prevention programs among those studied combine information and education about safer sex behaviors (e.g., condom use) with skills training, social norm changes, and motivational efforts encouraging youth to implement new, safer behaviors (see Fisher & Fisher, 1992, for a review). Jemmott, Jemmott, and Fong (1992) conducted an AIDS prevention program among adolescent inner-city African American males recruited from a number of community settings. Participants were stratified by age, then randomly assigned to either an experimental or a control condition. Participants in the experimental condition practiced safer sex-related skills in role plays, in addition to watching educational videos and playing interactive informational games. In the control condition, participants discussed career opportunities. Intervention participants showed greater AIDS knowledge, less favorable attitudes toward risky sexual behavior, and less intention to engage in those behaviors than the control group. These differences remained at a 3-month follow-up. Some differences in sexual behavior were also observed between the two groups.

Although no difference in rates of abstinence was found between the two groups, subjects receiving the intervention reported having fewer partners, less anal sex, and fewer occasions of unprotected sex, compared to subjects in the control condition.

Many HIV prevention programs for adolescents are school-based. Given that the majority of adolescents are enrolled in schools, outreach in schools can provide an effective avenue to reach a large and heterogeneous group of adolescents and young adults. Unfortunately, those at highest risk for contracting HIV have often dropped out of school. Street youth and young MSM—two groups at particularly high risk—may be either unreachable through, or alienated or threatened by, school-based programs. Street outreach programs and clinic-based programs (e.g., STD clinics, MSM-oriented agencies, public health clinics, and HIV testing and counseling centers) are especially important for reaching these otherwise hard-to-reach at-risk youth.

Rotheram-Borus et al. (1991) conducted a comprehensive HIV risk reduction intervention among street youth housed in two shelters in New York City. The intervention consisted of 20 sessions over the course of 3 weeks and had four components: (1) AIDS education, wherein youth developed AIDS-related videos or reviewed commercial HIV/AIDS videos; (2) training in coping skills targeted at high-risk situations; (3) access to health care and resources, including visits from public health nurses; and (4) an individual counseling session to modify attitudinal barriers to reducing behavioral risks. Rates of consistent condom use were compared between the youth receiving the intervention and youth staying in another (control) shelter in the city. Consistent condom use and reduction of other high-risk sexual behavior were positively associated with the number of intervention sessions attended, at both the 3- and 6-month follow-ups. No differences emerged between the groups in the percentage of youth who abstain from sex—a finding suggesting that encouraging abstinence is perhaps not effective as an HIV/AIDS prevention strategy among youth who are already sexually active.

Peer Education Programs

Peer education programs are a promising method of reaching adolescents. Adolescents spend an increased amount of time with their peers, and peers have an increased influence on their attitudes and behaviors. From studies of attitude change and persuasion, we know that the credibility and similarity of the communicator to the person receiving the information can result in greater attitude change (Petty & Cacioppo, 1981). Using peers of similar background (e.g., ethnicity, age, gender, sexual orientation, class) to deliver risk reduction messages may be important for increasing youth's receptivity to harm reduction messages and for helping youth to feel that they and their life situations can be understood. Using youth who are

HIV-positive as educators can be particularly effective in breaking through the myth of invincibility that is so common during adolescence.

Peer education and outreach may be a particularly pragmatic mode of intervention for marginalized youth, such as street youth. Peer outreach is "a faster, easier way to reach subpopulations who did not trust workers or agencies. Peers have instant credibility, know the culture, speak the correct language, know where the target population 'hangs out' and . . . know the streets" (Springer, 1992, p. 2).

The New York Peer AIDS Education Coalition (NYPAEC) is a peer education and outreach program for street youth. Begun in 1990, it is one of the first programs for youth that has identified itself as a harm reduction program. It started out in New York City's Times Square—an area with a high concentration of prostitution and drug use, and an area where street youth tended to congregate. Many of the target youth have since moved out of the area because the authorities boarded up the hangout and prostitution areas; NYPAEC has followed the youth to new hangouts.

Street youth are recruited and trained to provide HIV/AIDS education and to teach other youth how to use condoms, dental dams, and bleach kits to reduce their HIV risk. The peer educators receive 12 hours of training over 3 weeks that includes HIV/AIDS education, outreach strategies, harm reduction, and role playing. A weekly meeting of peer educators and staff is used to provide clinical supervision, discuss outreach efforts, solve problems, and provide support; the youth also eat a hot meal with the staff as a family. Some of the peer educators have developed a brochure to use during outreach, called "Stop! In the Name of Love." In addition to pictures of the Supremes, the brochure includes illustrations of how to clean needles and clear instructions on how to use a condom.

One of the defining characteristics of the program is the involvement of youth at all levels of decision making. Peer educators are allowed to choose the areas where and the people with whom they work. Each year, each peer educator works together with a staff member to develop a personal contract, which describes the number of outreach contacts and other tasks (such as documentation of outreach and attendance at meetings) that will be completed each week in order for the young person to receive a stipend. A third of the board of directors and two executive officers are peer educators.

Social influence theories assert that members of social groups who hold attitudes or values in conflict with those of the majority of the social group (e.g., youth who promote condom use) are most likely to influence the behavior of other members in the social group when they are similar to the majority (except in the particular position they are advocating), are consistent in their views over time, and are not rigid or dogmatic in upholding their views (Fisher & Mosovich, 1990). NYPAEC's harm reduction program is consistent with these social influence principles. Peer educators are similar to the youth with whom they do outreach work. Far from being rigid or dogmatic, they are trained to meet youth where they are in the behavioral risk reduction process—to help youth who are already sexually active to have safer sex, and to help those who are already using drugs to use them more safely.

In contrast to many traditional outreach programs, abstinence, or being in recovery, is also not required of the peer educators. In the view of the clinical director, Edith Springer, this is another way that the harm reduction philosophy is expressed in organizational policy. Drug use is not viewed as inherently harmful. The goal of the organization is HIV prevention; as long as drug use is not getting in the way of conducting outreach, the drug use of peer educators is not the concern of NYPAEC staff (E. Springer, personal communication, 1995).

In the first 2 years of NYPAEC's operations, between 2,500 and 5,000 street youth were reached; many of these were among the most marginalized youth. NYPAEC thus appears successful at being able to reach youth, although the population it is reaching is dependent to a large extent on the networks and hangouts of the peer educators. There is also evidence that the program is having a positive effect on the peer educators themselves. When the program began, nearly all of the peer outreach workers were homeless, using drugs, selling sex, and using safer sex methods inconsistently (if at all). After 2 years, none were homeless (although some were living in single-room occupancy hotels), two were working, and two were in school. Educators also reported that they were consistently practicing safer sex; about half had given up drugs, and half had stopped selling sex.

NYPAEC has recently received funding to expand the outreach program and add an evaluation component; the latter will provide a more systematic assessment of the outreach program, assess the effects of the program on peer educators, and examine the impact of the program on behavioral outcomes. Although an impact evaluation has not been conducted for NYPAEC, another study conducted among IDUs provides evidence that peer educators (who may still be using drugs) can effectively teach and disseminate AIDS risk reduction information to peers (Broadhead et al., 1995). Peer education and outreach thus appear to constitute a promising approach for harm reduction interventions and a particularly good method for reaching disenfranchised youth.

Summary

Although adolescents currently make up only a small proportion of AIDS cases, the estimated prevalence of adolescents infected with the HIV virus highlights the urgency of HIV among this population. Childhood and early adolescence are important windows of opportunity for interventions to delay the onset of sexual and drug use behavior, and to educate youth on safer behaviors before they have developed risky patterns. For the sake of the health and safety of our youth, it is time to move beyond the abstinence versus nonabstinence debate and to develop pragmatic interventions—ones that empower youth to make informed decisions about their lives, and that facilitate the development of skills and access to resources to enact those decisions. Comprehensive programs are needed that are tailored to youth at highest risk, such as street youth, urban minority youth, and gay/bisexual youth. These programs need to meet youth where they are developmentally and behaviorally, as well as to fit with their cultural and social reality. Programs that include peer outreach, education, and skill training are promising approaches for reaching youth and helping them reduce harm in their lives.

HIV HARM REDUCTION APPROACHES IN PRISON POPULATIONS

Since the outbreak of AIDS, prison inmates, like sex workers, have been viewed throughout the world as vectors for the spread of disease (both within and outside the prison setting). A number of factors account for this belief, including a high proportion of IDUs among prisoners, the prevalence of homosexual activity among male inmates, and prisoners' lack of access to preventive measures (e.g., bleach, clean needles, and condoms) while incarcerated. Despite widespread concern about the potential for a spread of HIV infection within prisons, several barriers to the implementation of effective prevention practices exist; not the least of these is the collision of public health pragmatism with the criminal justice system's goal of eliminating illegal behavior. More specifically, how can the very institution that serves to deter illegal actions and punish offenders openly acknowledge the occurrence of illegal acts, or "tolerate" such abuses of the law by accepting their inevitability and resorting to harm reduction approaches? Similarly, how can a society that maintains the sanctity of heterosexuality justify the distribution of condoms to male inmates without somehow sending a message that condones homosexual acts?

History of HIV/AIDS and Related Policy in U.S. Correctional Facilities

The problem of HIV infection and AIDS in U.S. prisons was first recorded by Wormser et al. (1983) when seven cases of AIDS were diagnosed in previously healthy males serving sentences in New York State correctional facilities between September 1981 and June 1982. All subjects denied engaging in homosexual behaviors, and all acknowledged being IDUs prior to incarceration. By November 1990, 4,519 cases of AIDS had been reported within the U.S. federal and state systems. Between 1991 and 1995, the number of confirmed AIDS cases among prison inmates more than tripled to 5,099 (4,965 cases within state prisons and 134 within federal prisons)(Bureau of Justice Statistics, 1997). While some of this rise was likely due to the Centers for Disease Control and Prevention expansion of the surveillance case definition for AIDS in January, 1993, the bulk of the increase was not. The majority of AIDS and HIV-positive cases are concentrated in several AIDS epicenters, most notably New York, Florida, Texas, California, and New Jersey (Bureau of Justice Statistics, 1997). The overall rate of confirmed AIDS cases among inmates in state and federal prisons (0.51%) was more than six times the U.S. population rate (0.08%). Table 7.1 summarizes the number of confirmed AIDS and HIV-positive cases among state and federal prisons within the five major epicenters at the year's end in 1995 (Bureau of Justice Statistics, 1997).

By the end of 1995, 23,404 state prison inmates were HIV-positive (2.4% of the total state prison population), and 822 (0.9%) in the federal prisons. A greater proportion of female state inmates were HIV-positive (4.0%) compared to male inmates (2.3%; Bureau of Justice Statistics, 1997). The total number of male seropositive inmates increased by 28% between 1991 and 1995 while the number for HIV-infected females increased by 88%. HIV seroprevalence was higher among Latinos/Latinas (3.2%) and African Americans (2.6%) than among inmates of European descent (1.4%), and higher among inmates 35 years or older (6.8%) than 34 and younger (2.8%).

The rate of AIDS-related death is approximately three times higher among state and federal inmates than in the total population of individuals between the ages of 15 and 54, and comprises about a third of all deaths of state inmates (Bureau of Justice Statistics, 1997). In 1995, death resulting from *Pneumocystis carinii* pneumonia, Kaposi's sarcoma, or other AIDS-related illnesses was the second leading cause of death among state inmates, after death resulting from non-AIDS illnesses and natural causes (1,010 deaths vs. 1,569 deaths, respectively). AIDS-related illness accounted for over half of all inmate deaths in certain states during 1995, including New

TABLE 7.1. Prevalence of HIV and AIDS Cases in State and Federal Prisons within AIDS Epicenters at Year's End, 1995

State	No. confirmed AIDS cases (% custody population)	No. HIV-positive inmates (% custody population)
New York	1,182 (1.7%)	9,500 (13.9%)
Florida	692 (1.1%)	2,193 (3.4%)
Texas	495 (0.4%)	1,890 (1.5%)
California	385 (0.3%)	1,042 (0.8%)
New Jersey	343 (1.5%)	847 (3.7%)

York (65%), Florida (59%), Connecticut (57%), and South Carolina (54%).

High seroprevalance in U.S. corrections facilities is largely associated with an increase in arrests for drug offenses. This trend began during 1986, when legislators responded to public concern over the spread of crack cocaine by instituting tougher sentences against drug dealers and users. As a result, the nation's prisons began to fill quickly with drug-abusing and drug-addicted offenders (Wexler, 1994). From 1986 to 1991, inmates sentenced for a drug offense rose from 9% to 21% and accounted for a 44% increase in the prison population. Within this 5-year period, rates for women imprisoned on drug offenses increased by 432%, from 2,400 in 1986 to 12,600 in 1991; 22% of first-time offenders were arrested on drug charges, including 7% for possession and 15% for drug trafficking. Sixty percent of those arrested had used drugs in the month prior to committing their offenses; 37% were under the influence of drugs when committing their crimes; and 22% reported committing their offenses to secure money for drugs (compared to 50%, 31%, and 17%, respectively, for all inmates) (U.S. Department of Justice, 1993). Of the 116,376 federal inmates imprisoned at the start of 1998, the majority (59.1%) had been sentenced for drug offenses. Robbery was the second most common offense (9.3%) among federal inmates (Federal Bureau of Prisons, 1998).

In response to the high risk for HIV infection in correctional facilities, the National Commission on AIDS (1991) conducted a visit to several federal, state, and local correctional facilities during August 1990, in order to assess the impact of HIV and AIDS in these facilities and to make recommendations for ensuring adequate prevention of infection and treatment of affected persons. The commission's findings included the following:

- Prisoners with HIV were rapidly acquiring tuberculosis; many more were at increased risk from the resurgent tuberculosis epidemic in the nation's prisons.
- Prisoners with HIV were often subject to automatic segregation from the rest of the prison community, despite the fact that there is no public health basis for this practice.
- Lack of education of inmates and staff created fear and discrimination against individuals with HIV; unjust policies directed toward inmates living with HIV were often the result of this ignorance.
- Despite high rates of HIV infection and an ideal opportunity for prevention and education efforts, former prisoners typically reentered their communities with little or no added knowledge about HIV or how to prevent it.

Recommendations by the commission largely advocated the creation of prevention programs and the active involvement of inmates in developing and implementing these prevention efforts. To ensure the maximal impact of a prevention approach, the commission further recommended that such programs reach all persons in the system, from detainees to persons on parole, in probation programs, or in halfway houses. Additionally, recommendations included mandatory participation in HIV/AIDS education and information programs by all inmates and prison staff, the opportunity for confidential HIV counseling and testing, the opportunity to participate in ongoing informational groups, and the development of programs tailored specifically to the needs of women. Emphasizing the importance of prevention, the commission noted:

> AIDS prevention programs remain the single most effective strategy for slowing the spread of HIV infection. Inmates, like others in our society, have the right to be protected from life-threatening illnesses. For legal, moral and public health reasons, correctional and health officials should develop effective and comprehensive AIDS prevention programs in correctional settings. (National Commission on AIDS, 1991, p. 21)

Despite this emphasis the importance of prevention approaches, the report was surprisingly silent about the kind of content to include in these programs. When the concept of "risk reduction" was raised, it was also left unspecified and undefined. The report came closest to exposing the difficulty of balancing public health knowledge and pragmatism against the prohibition of illegal and "deviant" behaviors within the criminal justice system in the following recommendation, stressing the importance of skills-based competence:

> Inmates need to learn skills that will protect them against HIV infection both inside and outside the correctional system. Whether to distribute condoms in prison and whether to teach inmates how to sterilize needles and works have proven to be controversial questions for correctional officers. Both these questions have important political, social and moral dimensions. From a public health perspective, however, it is clear that where unprotected sexual and drug behavior are known to occur, the availability of condoms and bleach and water can reduce the risk. Prison officials need to decide whether it is more ethical to acknowledge the existence of illegal behavior or to withhold life-saving equipment or skills.
>
> For inmates who are about to be released, providing condoms and teaching how to sterilize needles can protect them and their sexual and drug partners as well as their future children from potential infection. A pre-release counseling session and prevention kit can achieve this goal. (National Commission on AIDS, 1991, p. 20)

Although it openly declared the importance of skills, the report carefully acknowledged the commission's difficulty in making clear recommendations for implementing effective preventive strategies, and instead left it up to prison officials to resolve the ethical dilemma. An explicit recommendation for the distribution of the "life-saving" prevention kits was made only for inmates upon their release. The irony here, of course, was that preventive materials could only be made available once these individuals had direct access to them on their own through the usual means.

The Glenochil Jail Incident: A Case Study

In 1988, between 350 and 500 of the 50,000 prisoners in England and Wales were seropositive. Highly critical of prison authorities for an inadequate response to the high rates of HIV infection among inmates, the Prison Reform Trust (see Christie, 1993) recommended that prompt and pragmatic measures be implemented to prevent an outbreak of HIV infection within the corrections system. Recommendations included distributing condoms to male prisoners, abolishing segregation of seropositive prisoners, and conducting a full evaluation of drug treatment provisions for drug-abusing inmates (McMillan, 1988). Despite this call to action, U.K. prison reform for the prevention of HIV infection became snarled in an unresolved net of political and public health obstacles.

Nearly 5 years later, an outbreak of HIV infection was reported in the Glenochil jail in Glasgow, Scotland, where at least 15 prisoners were found to be infected with hepatitis B and a number were believed to be infected with HIV after sharing contaminated injecting equipment (Christie, 1993). Ironically, this incident coincided with the Ninth International Conference on AIDS in Berlin. As a result, news of the outbreak spread quickly and increased international awareness of the problem of HIV infection in prisons (Emslie, 1993).

In an effort to provide an adequate response to the crisis and to prevent future spread of infection, numerous recommendations were again generated by various government groups. As the Prison Reform Trust had done in 1988, the House of Commons Committee on Scottish Affairs argued for harm reduction actions to prevent such situations from occurring in the future, including the exchange of needles and syringes (Christie, 1993). In the end, the Scottish Prison Department (with a record of opposing such strategies) ignored the committee's recommendations and instead resorted to less controversial actions. Prison officials appealed to prisoners to turn over all "works" to prevent additional spread of infection, and an "amnesty" period was created to allow prisoners the opportunity to turn over drug-injecting equipment without penalty. Confidential HIV counseling and testing services were extended (Gore & Bird, 1993; Christie, 1993).

The amnesty solution quickly came under attack by public health professionals, who described it as shortsighted, ineffectual, and potentially very damaging. Some criticized the plan for its focus on "the surrender of needles" in the absence of a needle exchange scheme and efforts to reduce injection drug use (Riley, 1993; Dunn et al., 1993). Riley (1993) observed, for example, that the simple removal of needles from the pool of available equipment without reducing the number of IDUs in the end functioned to increase needle sharing, thereby increasing the risk of spreading hepatitis B and HIV infection. Citing recommendations from the 1988 and 1989 reports of the government's Advisory Committee on the Misuse of Drugs (Dunn et al., 1993), and data from a community-wide, multisite study of HIV risk behaviors in prison (Taylor et al., 1993), others balked at the amnesty solution and argued instead for a comprehensive intervention that could include replacement drug therapy (e.g., methadone), full access to cleaning agents to sterilize needles, and distribution of condoms.

Regrettably, the only unique aspect of the HIV outbreak at the Glenochil jail was its location. This case nonetheless illustrates the enormous difficulty involved in bridging the gap between pragmatic harm reduction approaches to reduce rates of infection and a correctional institution's duties of serving the law, decreasing illegal behavior, and maintaining social order. In this case, the Scottish prison administrators were well aware of effective strategies to reduce the risks of HIV infection, as well as of the fact that prison inmates were at considerable risk for infection. Preventive actions, however, were not taken until after a crisis emerged. In the end, the response by prison officials seems to have been more of an effort to present a public face of concern and responsiveness than a real effort to reduce the actual risk of HIV spread.

HIV/AIDS Risks in Correctional Facilities

Concern about HIV infection and AIDS in correctional facilities in the United States and abroad are typically centered in three broad areas: (1) transmission of HIV infection within prisons; (2) transmission of HIV once inmates are released from prison; and (3) quality of health care and quality of life while in prison for seropositive inmates and inmates with AIDS.

Transmission of HIV within Prisons

Transmission of HIV within prisons typically occurs through unprotected and high-risk sex, both consensual and nonconsensual (e.g., rape), between male inmates; sharing of contaminated needles and syringes to inject drugs; and sharing of contaminated needles for tattooing. Noting the bleak and boring prison environment, Curran, McHugh, and Nooney (1989) observed that many inmates will engage in these high-risk behaviors for the first time while in prison. In an epidemiological and preventive policy review of AIDS in prison, Brewer and Derrickson (1992) estimated that up to 25% of inmates inject drugs and up to 33% engage in homosexual sex while in prison, with the probability of these behaviors increasing over the period of incarceration.

McMillan (1988) notes that although it is difficult to assess the actual prevalence of high-risk sex between male inmates, the anecdotal evidence of genitourinary physicians who have treated rectal gonorrhea in male prisoners is proof of unprotected anal sex between male inmates. He further observes that because the prison population is generally young in age and likely to be sexually active, in the absence of women sexual urges are likely to be relieved either by self-masturbation or homosexually. In a study of 50 incarcerated inmates (Carvell & Hart, 1990), one woman and four men reported that they had had sex while in custody. Subjects were selected for participation on the basis of their history of injecting drugs prior to incarceration. Three of the four men reported having both oral and anal sex, and the four men indicated having had a mean of 7 male partners (range = 2–16) while in custody. Inmates in this sample who reported having sex while in custody served shorter prison sentences than those who denied engaging in sexual behaviors while incarcerated.

The prevalence of injection drug use in prisons constitutes another significant risk factor for the transmission of HIV. Whereas many drugs are easily concealed and are therefore reasonably easy to smuggle into prisons, drug equipment (e.g., needles and syringes) is more difficult both to acquire and to dispose of. In one study, researchers nevertheless estimated a ratio of one needle for every 10–15 prisoners, or one needle for every 4–6 IDUs, in prisons in South Australia (Gaughwin et al., 1991).

In a study of IDUs in central London, 47 out of 50 inmates surveyed reported use of illicit drugs while in custody, and 33 reported drug injection; of these 33, 26 reported sharing equipment (Carvell & Hart, 1990). Gaughwin et al. (1991) estimated that 36% of South Australian prison inmates had injected themselves with drugs at least once while incarcerated. Fifty of the men who had previously been incarcerated since 1985, and who had a history of injection drug use, were interviewed. Of these, 26 (52%) reported that they had injected drugs at least once while in prison. Among Scottish inmates, Power et al. (1992) found that 27.5% were involved in injection drug use prior to imprisonment, and 7.7% reported such use on at least one occasion during imprisonment; 5.7% reported use of shared needles while incarcerated. Over half of those who reported sharing needles made some effort to sterilize the equipment before use, with use of bleach as the most common method. In an anonymous survey of high-risk drug-using behaviors in two prison sites in Glasgow and Alberdeen, Bird and colleagues (1997) found that 41% and 37%, respectively, of the inmates surveyed reported a history of IDU. Of the combined injector inmates ($n = 112$) who had been in prison for more than 4 weeks, 57 had injected in the previous 4 weeks.

Between 1990 and 1992, Taylor et al. (1993) conducted 1,553 interviews with IDUs in Glasgow about HIV risk behaviors. Ninety percent of those interviewed reported injecting on a daily basis. Of the total, 51.2% reported having been incarcerated in the past 6 months for approximately 1 month. Overall, only a minority of IDUs injected drugs while incarcerated (8.9% for men, compared to 4.9% for women), and many attempted to clean their works before shooting: Of the total of 67 who reported sharing works while in custody, 22 used hot water, 17 used bleach, 9 used cold water, 4 boiled water, and 15 used other methods. Results from this study indicate that IDUs do make efforts to clean works prior to shooting drugs while incarcerated. What is not known, of course, is how successful their attempts are in thoroughly disinfecting the equipment prior to use.

Given the prevalence of injection drug use and high-risk sex between male inmates while in prison, one would expect to find more HIV outbreaks such as the one reported at the Glenochil jail. Surprisingly, documented cases of seroconversion, and the rates of HIV transmission, are quite low among inmates. In a study of over 98,000 HIV tests administered to inmates within the United States, only 14 demonstrated seroconversion (National Commission on AIDS, 1991). In a smaller and more controlled study of 3,837 inmates in a state prison where 2.4% of the inmates were seropositive, seroconversion occurred in only two inmates while in prison (Horsburgh, Jarvis, McArther, Ignacio, & Stock, 1990). Similar findings were observed in Rome, prompting the investigators there to conclude that imprisonment does not necessarily result in HIV infection (Scano et al., 1991).

The Florida State Department of Corrections recently conducted a study of inmates who had been continuously incarcerated since 1977, to further assess rates of seroconversion in prisons. Only 15% of the 556 inmates eligible to participate agreed to do so, resulting in a significant compromise of the investigation's internal validity. Of all inmates tested, 21% tested seropositive. Although these results must be viewed with a cautious eye in light of the low recruitment rate, the results nonetheless indicate that rates of seroconversion may be somewhat higher than previously documented. Indeed, the actual number of seroconversion cases may have been higher than documented in this study, in light of the small sample size. But even when the total of these testing seropositive is compared to all 556 inmates eligible to participate, the minimum seroconversion rate is still higher than previously documented in other studies at 3%.

Transmission of HIV outside Prisons

Although the jury remains out in terms of the actual prevalence of seroconversion within prisons and jails, there is little disagreement about the extent to which prison populations as a group are at high risk for contracting and transmitting HIV by virtue of extensive drug use. Despite this widespread agreement, few studies to date have examined the high-risk behaviors of inmates following their release.

O'Mahony and Barry (1992) conducted a study of past risk behaviors and intentions with respect to future risk behavior among known seropositive inmates within the Irish prison system. Of the 42 inmates identified, 38 agreed to participate. Of those, 30 (81%) reported having unprotected sex while on leave from prison, despite knowledge of their HIV status. Of the 37 inmates who had gone on leave during their prison sentence, only 6 (16%) reported *not* injecting drugs while outside prison; 70% reported sharing needles during these periods. Overall, 65% of those surveyed acknowledged having put others at risk for HIV infection, through either risky sex or sharing of injection drug equipment. Each inmate averaged 7 sexual partners and 9.5 needle-sharing partners since being diagnosed with HIV, resulting in the potential direct transmission of infection to 517 individuals among those involved with these men. With respect to future behavioral intentions, only 16% of the sample reported that they would never share works again; only 32% said that they would inform future sexual partners of their HIV status. Thirty-four percent of the sample said they planned never to wear a condom.

Quality of Health Care and Standard of Living for Seropositive Inmates and Inmates with AIDS

Following an investigation of the conditions faced in prison by inmates with HIV and AIDS, the National Commission on AIDS (1991) described its findings with grave concern. Inmates with AIDS in 1990 were dying at twice the rate of nonprisoners with AIDS; the median period from the time an inmate received an AIDS diagnosis and his or her death was 159 days, compared to 318 days for nonprisoners with AIDS. Moreover, physicians and dentists often refuse to treat inmates with AIDS. Many prisoners are refused access to AIDS specialists, and distribution of medications is unreliable. For example, whereas 90% of all state and federal prisons offered zidovudine to seropositive inmates in 1989, only 77% of county and city jails did (Hammett & Dubler, 1990). Other drugs that treat AIDS symptoms are also less available to needy inmates; for example, aerosolized pentamidine, a drug prescribed for *Pneumocystis carinii* pneumonia, was available in 1989 at only 75% of state and federal prisons and at 45% of county and city jails (Hammett & Dubler, 1990). The National Commission on AIDS (1991) found that AIDS inmates were more susceptible to air-borne diseases (e.g., tuberculosis) because of problematic environmental factors, such as overcrowding and poor ventilation. Rates of tuberculosis in 29 state prisons in 1990 were three times higher than for age-matched nonprison control subjects.

Incarcerated Women: A Special At-Risk Population

A number of researchers have described the extent to which imprisoned women, particularly women of color, have special needs and risk factors for HIV that gave been insufficiently recognized and addressed (Polonsky,

Kerr, Harria, Gaiter, et al., 1994; Wellisch, Anglin, & Prendergast, 1993). In addition to the lack of general health care services afforded to women inmates in comparison to men, little attention is given to the risk of pregnant female inmates' infecting their infants. Both in prisons and in general, because the largest percentage of illicit drug use by women occurs among women of childbearing years, their use increases not only their own risk of HIV infection, but also their children's risks of infection or drug exposure. For example, the CDC (1992) has estimated that approximately 375,000 babies are born each year in the United States to drug-using mothers. Harm reduction strategies are therefore needed to improve the health of these women and their children; such strategies are notably absent in correctional settings.

Approximately 9% of U.S. women of childbearing years (between the ages of 15 and 44) are currently drug users (NIDA, 1992). Unlike other illicit drugs (whose use has remained steady over the past two decades), cocaine abuse has increased dramatically, particularly among women of childbearing age; indeed, the majority of female cocaine abusers are between the ages of 16 and 35 (Deschenes, 1988). Illicit drug use among women in federal prisons has been estimated at 63.2% (National Institute of Justice, 1990). Women arrestees test positive for drugs at the time of arrest more frequently than men arrestees do (Wellisch et al., 1993). From 1982 to 1991, the number of women arrested for drug offenses (e.g., possession, manufacturing, and sales) increased by 89%, nearly twice the increase found for men during the same period (Federal Bureau of Investigation, 1992). In various cities, between 26% and 70% of all women arrested in 1989 tested positive for at least one drug; about 20% across all cities assessed tested positive for two or more drugs at the time of arrest (National Institute of Justice, 1990). Of those testing positive, 83% had been arrested for sales and possession of drugs, and 82% for prostitution. In contrast to male offenders, women offenders are less likely to commit violent crimes and are more likely to commit crimes with an economic motive (Wellisch et al., 1993).

Wellisch et al. (1993) conclude that women inmates have even greater problems than men. Whereas nearly 80% of incarcerated women are mothers, and two-thirds have children under the age of 18 (Bureau of Justice Statistics, 1990), few institutions provide the facilities and child care services needed for visitation. Most facilities provide male-biased vocational training in low-paying occupations traditionally held by women, despite the fact that the majority of these women are single parents who receive little to no assistance from their children's fathers. With respect to drug abuse treatment, a survey of more than 85% of state correctional institutions for women reported that over 40% of their inmates required substance abuse treatment at the initial intake (American Correctional Association, 1990). As of 1987, however, only 11% (51,500) of all inmates in need of such treatment were actually participating in a prison-based drug treatment program (Chaiken, 1989). In light of the general shortage of programs for women, it is likely that much fewer than 11% of women in prisons received treatment.

Mapping the Implications and Terrain for Harm Reduction in Prisons

The Glenochil jail incident in Glasgow provides a small-scale illustration of the enormous barriers faced by public health officials in the fight against HIV transmission and AIDS. Despite undeniable and objective evidence of the realities of HIV transmission in prisons, public health recommendations from numerous committees and officials, and the palpable consequences of superficial HIV/AIDS prevention efforts that fail, the best solution following the HIV outbreak at Glenochil was the "amnesty solution." At best a damage control bandage to prevent public perception of failure to respond, the solution in reality served only to increase the probability of additional spread by collecting injection needles and syringes from inmates without penalty. The failure to address drug dependence and to distribute bleach and/or clean needles to those who refused to surrender their works could only function to increase the ratio of users to works, with more people having to share a more limited resource.

As described by the National Commission on AIDS (1991), political, social, and moral dimensions continue to restrict the adequate implementation of pragmatic and effective harm reduction strategies in prisons. As a result, well-intentioned and well-informed commissions and committees are significantly handicapped in their ability to recommend such prevention approaches. Harm reduction strategies are thereby relegated to postimprisonment planning in the form of distributing "safety kits" once prisoners are released.

Perhaps the biggest obstacle to effective prevention of HIV transmission and AIDS in prison settings is the fact that it would require official institutional acknowledgment of illegal behaviors in the very institutions set up to punish violators of the law. A host of other complicated questions would also undoubtedly emerge if these realities were to be addressed. For example, is it ethically feasible to distribute bleach and clean needles without providing drug treatment to those wishing to "kick" drug dependence? Furthermore, how ready is society to accept and finance nonabstinence drug treatment programs, such as methadone maintenance or drug-tapering programs? These obstacles become even greater in proportion when one considers the scarcity of drug treatment programs for drug-addicted people outside prisons. From an ethical perspective, can society ethically restrict access to harm-reducing products shown to effectively limit the risk of HIV infection, such as bleach and condoms, that are readily and legally available outside prisons?

Although the risk of contracting HIV inside prisons appears reasonably low at the present time, prison inmates are nevertheless a high-risk population for contracting HIV. This is particularly true for IDUs, and non-injection-drug-using inmates, and male inmates who engage in sex with other male inmates. In this sense, prison populations are indeed a captive audience to receive HIV/AIDS prevention education and skills training to reduce risky behaviors. However, the implementation of harm reduction and other preventive intervention strategies in the prison setting lags dramatically behind both the need for such approaches and the scientific evidence for their effectiveness.

CONCLUSION

As we have seen, HIV brings with it its own unique set of challenges, affecting populations that are often already stigmatized, and involving critical issues of health risk and potentially life-threatening harm. From the beginning of the HIV epidemic, harm reduction (whether or not it has been called by that name) has informed and offered salient approaches to the prevention of HIV/AIDS. In this chapter we have reviewed applications of harm reduction concepts and interventions to the problem of HIV/AIDS within five populations at elevated risk: IDUs, MSM, women, adolescents, and prisoners. In each instance, the goal of harm reduction approaches has been the same—to reduce the risk of harm by reducing the risk of HIV infection.

NEPs exemplify harm reduction. NEPs use a variety of strategies to provide services to IDUs, and the locations of these services range from storefronts to vans to card tables on street corners. Typically, clients can exchange used syringes for new, clean ones with a minimum of effort. Some NEPs also offer other related services, such as primary care, STD screening, and referrals to social services. Although the number of such programs is growing, many remain under the cloud of operating in violation of state or local laws. Yet, increasingly, NEPs appear to be part of the spectrum of harm reduction efforts for those using injection drugs. A critical reason for this shift is the evidence that NEPs work in reaching drug-using populations and in reducing the spread of HIV and other diseases transmitted through the use of unclean needles.

NEPs appear to be particularly successful when they address the special needs of the groups they target. Examples include programs that target women, or those that target special drug-using populations (e.g., methamphetamine users, as has been done in Seattle). Such programs recognize that IDUs are not all the same, but in fact are consumers of services that relate to their own particular patterns of use. Our recommendations for the further development of NEPs include the following:

1. NEPs need to be developed in areas of the United States that have not yet had the opportunity to do so. This recommendation entails working closely with local law enforcement officials and with community, treatment,

and harm reduction advocates, so that such programs can be given a chance.

2. Experimentation with new types of NEPs—including those that target women, ethnic minorities, migrants, the gay homeless, bisexuals, lesbians, and transgendered individuals—should be continued. NEPs appropriate for rural areas also need to be developed and disseminated.

3. Several NEPs provide harm reduction information for drug users that goes beyond HIV prevention and addresses other health concerns facing this population. NEPs should consider expanding their services further by conducting brief motivational enhancement interventions, to take advantage of the window of opportunity the contact provides.

In regard to MSM, we have explored the history of early HIV prevention/education and have noted that although they may not have been conceived of as "harm reduction" efforts, such programs as STOP AIDS, the GMHC, and other approaches (e.g., Roffman et al.'s innovative phone counseling, Kelly et al.'s peer-mediated interventions) have embraced a philosophy that can be described as harm reduction. By refusing to pathologize male–male sexual behavior and by working alongside gay/bisexual men to reduce risk, as opposed to insisting on eliminating it, such programs have helped create a new paradigm of prevention imbued with compassionate pragmatism. These programs have featured low-threshold access to services and information, and in many cases have been developed from the "bottom up" (i.e., the community itself), instead of being delivered in a "top-down" fashion by public health or other authorities. Moreover, these programs have rejected moral judgments of homosexuality as well as of HIV/AIDS. Most importantly, sexual abstinence has not been typically deemed reasonable or appropriate.

In the case of MSM who are also IDUs, harm reduction philosophies have predominated as well. The 1990s have seen the evolution of gay-identified drug and alcohol treatment alternatives, such as GMHC's SUCE program and San Francisco's Operation Recovery, which have been imbued with the harm reduction philosophy. Our recommendations for the further development of harm reduction efforts for MSM are as follows:

1. Barriers to access need to be further reduced for various groups of MSM, including those who are transgendered, those who are members of ethnic minorities, those who may still be leading hidden lives, and those who live outside major metropolitan centers.

2. Efforts to develop new and innovative treatment programs, including programs targeted to dual-risk populations (e.g., MSM who are also IDUs or methamphetamine users), should continue.

Many of the same harm reduction strategies described for IDUs and MSM are appropriate for women as well. However, the contextual factors that facilitate and constrain women's behavioral choices need to be understood and addressed in harm reduction interventions. Many women at risk for HIV are also subject to conditions of poverty and power imbalance in their relationships. Barriers to HIV risk reduction for such women thus include few resources, limited access, and a lack of power.

A population of women at particularly elevated risk of HIV consists of those who use crack; they are at the intersection of sexual and drug-related risk. Similarly at risk are the female partners of IDUs and women who work in the sex industry. In all of these populations (some of which overlap), consistent use of male or female condoms is essential yet often difficult to achieve, given the complications of negotiating condom use with male sexual partners.

In general, three key issues have to be addressed in implementing programs for women. First, optimally reaching women requires casting a broader net to a multitude of sites (e.g., welfare offices), as well as locating outreach and needle exchange sites in areas more private than street corners. Second, drug treatment programs need to be tailored to the specific barriers experienced by women, particularly with respect to histories of abuse, domestic violence, and the need for child care. A third issue to be considered when designing harm reduction programs for women is the impact of economic dependence and unequal power relationships as obstacles to maintaining or even adopting risk reduction strategies. One possible advancement in this area is the development of the female condom, which, while perhaps not applicable in all situations, provides a greater measure of control.

An example of a harm reduction program targeted to heterosexual women is the Women's Health Project conducted under the auspices of the University of Washington. A hallmark of this innovative program is its use of a relapse prevention model in collaboration with an advisory board of community members and high-risk women. Our recommendations for the further development of harm reduction efforts for women include the following:

1. Programs need to do everything possible to meet women where they are (e.g., ease of access, safe and nonthreatening settings). In addition, more outreach programs targeted to homeless women and to women who sell sex for money or drugs should be developed.

2. More innovative treatment programs like the Women's Health Project are needed—programs that are sensitive to the specific challenges faced by women, and informed by both the values and actual involvement of those women served.

In the case of adolescents, an understanding of and sensitivity to the developmental challenges facing this population are particularly important. Ideally, adolescents should be engaged and involved in the development and implementation of their own programs. This may be crucial to establishing the credibility and encouraging the acceptance of adolescent HIV prevention programs. Moreover, providing low-threshold access to this population is critical.

One of the most outspoken defenders of pragmatic harm reduction efforts is former U.S. Surgeon General Joycelyn Elders, who spoke out candidly about the need for pragmatic sex education for young people. The NYPAEC is a very innovative program targeting youth. A defining characteristic of this program is the involvement of youth at all levels of decision making; in fact, program participants appear to be improving this experience on an ongoing basis by providing constructive feedback to peer educators. Our suggestions for the further development of harm reduction efforts for adolescents are as follows:

1. Society at large needs to move beyond the abstinence versus nonabstinence debate as it applies to adolescent prevention programs. The real need is to establish and evaluate youth-oriented, low-threshold services and programs that empower youth to make informed decisions about their lives, and that help them develop the skills and access the resources to reduce their risk for harm.

2. More harm reduction programs that target youth at highest risk of HIV infection are needed; these groups currently include street youth, urban minority youth, and gay/bisexual male youth.

The HIV-related issues facing prison populations represent a particularly challenging opportunity for the development of harm reduction efforts. Both men and women in prison are at risk for HIV infection because of several factors: high-risk sexual behavior, the use of drugs, and especially the lack of access to preventive measures.

Although there is some debate concerning the actual incidence of seroconversion within prisons, prison populations are at elevated risk for HIV. Women in prisons may represent an especially high-risk population, due to the combination of drug-related behaviors and the lack of prevention efforts targeted to them. Despite these data, prisons do not presently offer compelling examples of harm reduction programs, and in this regard they represent a fertile field for the development of innovative programs. Our recommendations include the following:

1. A harm reduction program should be developed in a prison setting and evaluated with respect to its effects on such outcomes as knowledge, attitudes and beliefs about HIV/AIDS, condom usage, and rates of seroconversion and STDs. Such a program might include the provision of informational kits and possibly educational and/or treatment vouchers for inmates. Particular attention should be paid to both incoming inmates and those leaving the prison system. Intervening at such critical transition points may be particularly effective in terms of reaching people who might not otherwise hear the message.

2. A working group of HIV education, prevention, and drug treatment experts should be convened to address the concerns of prison officials and state and federal legislators about harm reduction approaches. An explicit goal of this group should be closing the gap between what is known to exist in the real world of prisons in terms of sexual and drug-using behaviors, and the belief systems about such behaviors (i.e., how they are thought to be).

3. Treatment opportunities should be created for all prisoners who need or want them, including use of opiate substitution for those who need it (e.g., methadone and LAAM). With more drug-dependent individuals entering the prison system than ever before, significant opportunities to intervene exist.

In conclusion, we reiterate the importance of both compassion and pragmatism in adapting harm reduction efforts to HIV-affected populations. Keeping both of these in mind will make us better able to meet clients and those at risk where they are, and to be of assistance to them in reducing harm in their lives.

ACKNOWLEDGMENTS

Several people reviewed earlier drafts of this chapter, and their efforts are greatly appreciated. We would like to thank Sharon Baker, Chilly Clay, Michael Hanarahan, Roger Roffman, and Brent Whitteker for taking the time to read the chapter and providing is with thoughtful, helpful suggestions. We would also like to thank Elizabeth Hawkins for the hard work and many hours she contributed editing the final version of the chapter and locating missing references.

REFERENCES

Ajzen, I., & Fishbein, M. (1980). *Understanding attitudes and predicting social behavior.* Englewood Cliffs, NJ: Prentice-Hall.

Allen, D. M., Lehman, J. S., Green, T. A., Lindegren, M. L., Onorato, I. M., Forrester, W., & Field Services Branch. (1994). HIV infection among homeless adults and runaway youth, United States, 1989–1992. *AIDS, 8,* 1593–1598.

Allen, K. (1994). Female drug abusers and the context of their HIV transmission risk behaviors. In R. J. Battjes, Z. Sloboda, & W. C. Grace (Eds.), *The context of HIV risk among drug users and their sexual partners* (NIDA Research Monograph No. 143, pp. 48–63). Rockville, MD: U.S. Department of Health and Human Services.

Amaro, H. (1995). Love, sex, power: Considering women's realities in HIV prevention. *American Psychologist, 50,* 437–438.

Amaro, H., Zuckerman, B., & Cabral, H. (1989). Drug use among adolescent mothers: Profile of risk. *Pediatrics, 84,* 144–151.

American Correctional Association. (1990). *The female offender: What does the future hold?* Washington, DC: St. Mary's Press.

Anglin, M. D., Hser, Y. I., & McGlothlin, W. H. (1987). Sex differences in addict careers: Becoming addicted. *American Journal of Drug and Alcohol Abuse, 13,* 59–71.

Aral, S. O., & Holmes, K. K. (1991). Sexually transmitted diseases in the AIDS era. *Scientific American, 264,* 62–69.

Baker, A., Kochan, N., Dixon, J., Wodak, A., & Heather, N. (1995). HIV risk-taking behavior among injection drug users currently, previously and never enrolled in methadone treatment. *Addiction, 90,* 545–555.

Barnard, M. A. (1993). Needle sharing in context: Patterns of sharing among men and women injectors and HIV risks. *Addiction, 88,* 805–812.

Battjes, R. J. (1994). Drug use and HIV risk among gay and bisexual men: An overview. In R. J. Battjes, Z. Sloboda, & W. C. Grace (Eds.), *The context of HIV risk among drug users and their sexual partners* (NIDA Research Monograph No. 143, pp. 82–86). Rockville, MD: U.S. Department of Health and Human Services.

Battjes, R. J., Leukefeld, C. G., & Pickens, R. W. (1992). Age at first injection and HIV risk among intravenous drug users. *American Journal of Drug and Alcohol Abuse, 18,* 263–273.

Beadnell, B. A., Baker, S., Gordon, J., Collier, C., & Ryan, R. (1997). Preventing STD and HIV in women: Using multiple sources of data to inform intervention design. *Cognitive and Behavioral Practice, 4,* 325–347.

Becker, M. H., & Joseph, J. G. (1988). AIDS and behavioral change to reduce risk: A review. *American Journal of Public Health, 78,* 394–410.

Bell, T. A., & Hein, K. (1984). Adolescents and sexually transmitted diseases. In K. Holmes, P. Mardh, P. F. Sparling, & P. J. Wiesner (Eds.), *Sexually transmitted diseases* (pp. 73–84). New York: McGraw-Hill.

Bird, A. G., Gore, S. M., Hutchinson, S. J., Lewis, S. C., Cameron, S., & Burns, S. (1997). The European Commission Network on HIV Infection and Hepatitis in Prison. Harm reduction measures and injecting inside prison versus mandatory drug testing: Results of a cross-sectional anonymous questionnaire survey. *British Medical Journal, 315,* 21–24.

Braine, N. (1994, October). Women, drugs, and harm reduction. *People with AIDS Coalition Newsline,* pp. 16–21.

Brettle, R. P. (1991). HIV and harm reduction for injection drug users. *AIDS, 5,* 125–136.

Brewer, T. F., & Derrickson, J. (1992). AIDS in prison: A review of epidemiology and prevention policy. *AIDS, 6,* 623–628.

Broadhead, R. S. (1991). Social constructions of bleach in combating AIDS among injection drug users. *Journal of Drug Issues, 21,* 713–737.

Broadhead, R. S., Heckathorn, D. D., Grund, J. P. C., Stern, L. S., & Anthony, D. L. (1995). Drug users versus outreach workers in combating AIDS: Preliminary results of a peer-driven intervention. *Journal of Drug Issues, 25,* 531–564.

Brown, L. K., DiClemente, R. J., & Beausoleil, N. I. (1992). Comparison of human immunodeficiency virus related knowledge, attitudes, intentions, and behaviors among sexually active and abstinent young adolescents. *Journal of Adolescent Health, 13,* 140–145.

Brown, L. K., DiClemente, R. J., & Park, T. (1992). Predictors of condom use in sexually active adolescents. *Journal of Adolescent Health, 13,* 651–657.

Brown, L. K., Fritz, G. K., & Barone, V. J. (1989). The impact of AIDS education on junior and senior high school students: A pilot study. *Journal of Adolescent Health Care, 10,* 386–392.

Brownell, K. D., Marlatt, G. A., Lichtenstein, E., & Wilson, G. T. (1986). Understanding and preventing relapse. *American Psychologist, 41,* 765–782.

Buning, E. C. (1991). Effects of Amsterdam needle and syringe exchange. *International Journal of the Addictions, 26,* 1303–1311.

Bureau of Justice Statistics. (1990). *Women in prison: A special report.* Washington, DC: U.S. Department of Justice.

Bureau of Justice Statistics. (1997). *HIV in prisons and jails, 1995.* Washington, DC: U.S. Department of Justice.

Bye, L. L. (1990). Moving beyond counseling and knowledge-enhancing interventions: A plea for community-level AIDS prevention strategies. In D. G. Ostrow (Ed.), *Behavioral aspects of AIDS* (pp. 157–167). New York: Plenum Press.

Calsyn, D. A., Saxon, A. J., Freeman, G., & Whittaker, S. (1991). Needle-use practices among intravenous drug users in an area where needle purchase is legal. *AIDS, 5,* 187–193.

Campbell, C. A. (1991). Prostitution, AIDS and preventive health behaviors. *Social Science and Medicine, 32,* 1367–1378.

Carlin, L., & Wagner, L. S. (1995). *Project P.I.E. program evaluation, time 2 analyses.* Unpublished manuscript, University of Washington.

Carvell, A. L. M., & Hart, G. H. (1990). Risk behaviours for HIV infection among drug users in prison. *British Medical Journal, 300,* 1383–1384.

Catania, J., Coates, T., & Kegeles, T. (1992). Towards an understanding of risk behavior: An AIDS risk reduction model. *Health Education Quarterly, 17,* 53–72.

Catania, J. A., Coates, T. J., Stall, R., Turner, H., Peterson, J., Hearst, N., Colcini, M. M., Hudes, E., Gagno, J., Wiley, J., & Groves, R. (1992). Prevalence of AIDS-related risk factors and condom use in the United States. *Science, 258,* 1101–1106.

Catania, J. A., Dolcini, M. M., Coates, T. J., Kegeles, S. M., Greenblatt, R. M., Pucket, S., Corman, M., & Miller, J. (1989). Predictors of condom use and multiple partnered sex among sexually active adolescent women: Implications for AIDS-related health interventions. *Journal of Sex Research, 26,* 514–524.

Cates, W. J. (1991). Teenagers and sexual risk taking: The best of times and the worst of times. *Journal of Adolescent Health, 12,* 84–94.

Centers for Disease Control and Prevention (CDC). (1987). Antibody to human immunodeficiency virus in female prostitutes. *Morbidity and Mortality Weekly Report, 36,* 267–282.

Centers for Disease Control and Prevention (CDC). (1992). HIV prevention in the U.S. correctional system, 1991. *Morbidity and Mortality Weekly Report, 41,* 389–391.

Centers for Disease Control and Prevention (CDC). (1994). Health risk behaviors among adolescents who do and do not attend school—United States, 1992. *Morbidity and Mortality Weekly Report, 43*(8), 1–4.

Centers for Disease Control and Prevention (CDC). (1995a). Updates: AIDS among women—United States, 1994. *Morbidity and Mortality Weekly Report, 44*(5), 81–84.

Centers for Disease Control and Prevention (CDC). (1995b). Trends in sexual behavior among high school students—United States, 1990, 1991, 1993. *Morbidity and Mortality Weekly Report, 44*(7), 124–125, 131–132.

Centers for Disease Control and Prevention (CDC). (1996). Update: Mortality attributable to HIV infection among persons aged 25–44 years—United States, 1994. *Morbidity and Mortality Weekly Report, 46*(8), 121–124.

Centers for Disease Control and Prevention (CDC). (1997a). *HIV/AIDS Surveillance Report, 9*(2), 1–43.

Centers for Disease Control and Prevention (CDC). (1997b). Update: Syringe-exchange programs—United States, 1996. *Morbidity and Mortality Weekly Report, 46*(24), 565–568.

Centers for Disease Control and Prevention (CDC). (1997c). Update: Trends in AIDS incidence, death, and prevalence—United States, 1996. *Morbidity and Mortality Weekly Report, 45*(6), 165–172.

Chaiken, M. R. (1989). *In-prison program for drug-involved offenders.* Washington, DC: National Institute of Justice, U.S. Department of Justice.

Chiasson, M. A., Stoneburner, R. L., Lifson, A. R., Hildebrandt, D., & Jaffe, H. W. (1988, June). *No association between HIV-1 seropositivity and prostitute contact in New York City.* Paper presented at the Fourth International Conference on AIDS, Stockholm.

Christensson, B., & Ljungberg, B. (1991). Syringe exchange for prevention of HIV infection in Sweden: Practical experiences and community reactions. *International Journal of the Addictions, 26,* 1293–1302.

Christie, B. (1993). HIV outbreak investigated in Scottish jail. *British Medical Journal, 307,* 151–152.

Christopher, F. S., & Roosa, M. W. (1990). An evaluation of an adolescent pregnancy prevention program: Is "just say no" enough? *Family Relations, 39,* 68–72.

Coates, R. A., Calzavara, L. M., Read, S. E., Fanning, M. M., Shepherd, F. A., Klein, M. H., Johnson, J. K., & Soskolne, C. L. (1988). Risk factors for HIV infection in male contacts of men with AIDS or an AIDS-related condition. *American Journal of Epidemiology, 128,* 729–739.

Coates, T. J. (1990). Strategies for modifying sexual behavior for primary and secondary prevention of HIV disease. *Journal of Consulting and Clinical Psychology, 58,* 57–69.

Cohen, E., Mackenzie, R. G., & Yates, G. L. (1991). HEADSS, a psychosocial risk assessment instrument: Implications for designing effective intervention programs for runaway youth. *Journal of Adolescent Health, 12,* 539–544.

Cohen, E., Navaline, H., & Metzger, D. (1994). High-risk behaviors for HIV: A comparison between crack-abusing and opioid-abusing African-American women. *Journal of Psychoactive Drugs, 26,* 233–241.

Cohen, J. B., Lyons, C. A., Lockett, G. J., McConnell, P. A., Sanchez, L. R., & Wofsy, C. B. (1989, July). *Emerging patterns of drug use, sexual behavior, HIV infection and STDs in high-risk San Francisco areas from 1986–1989.* Paper presented at the Fifth International Conference on AIDS, Montreal.

Compton, W. M., III, Cottler, L. B., Decker, S. H., Mager, D., & Stringfellow, R. (1992). Legal needle buying in St. Louis. *American Journal of Public Health, 82,* 595–596.

Corby, N. H., Wolitski, R. J., Thornton-Johnson, S., & Tanner, W. M. (1991). AIDS knowledge, perception of risk, and behaviors among female sex partners of injection drug users. *AIDS Education and Prevention, 3,* 353–366.

Coutinho, R. A. (1990). Epidemiology and prevention of AIDS among intravenous drug users. *Journal of Acquired Immune Deficiency Syndromes, 3,* 413–416.

Curran, L., McHugh, M., & Nooney, K. (1989). HIV counseling in prisons. *AIDS Care, 1,* 11–25.

Day, S., Ward, H., & Harris, J. R. W. (1988). Prostitute women and public health. *British Medical Journal, 297,* 1585.

DeCarlo, P. (1994). *What are women's HIV prevention needs? HIV prevention: Looking back, looking ahead.* San Francisco: Center for AIDS Prevention Studies (CAPS), University of California at San Francisco.

DePhilippis, D., & Metzger, D. S. (1993). *Needle acquisition difficulty is associated with needle-sharing, not drug use.* Paper presented at the annual convention of the American Psychological Society, Chicago.

D'Eramo, J. E. (1988). Report from Stockholm: The enemy within. *Christopher Street, 126,* 16–29.

D'Eramo, J. E., Quadland, M. D., Shatts, W., Schuman, R., & Jacobs, R. (1988, June). *The "800 men" project: A systematic evaluation of AIDS prevention programs demonstrating the efficacy of erotic, sexually explicit safer sex education on gay and bisexual men at risk for AIDS.* Paper presented at the Fourth International Conference on AIDS, Stockholm.

Department of Health, State of Hawaii. (1992, January). *Needle exchange evaluation report.* Honolulu: Author.

Des Jarlais, D. C., & Friedman, S. R. (1990). The epidemic of HIV infection among injecting drug users in New York City: The first decade and possible future direction. In J. Strang & G. V. Stimson (Eds.), *AIDS and drug misuse* (pp. 86–94). London: Tavistock/Routledge.

Des Jarlais, D. C., & Friedman, S. R. (1992). AIDS and legal access to sterile drug injection equipment. *Annals of the American Academy of Political and Social Science, 52,* 42–65.

Des Jarlais, D. C., Marmor, M., Paone, D., Titus, S., Shi, Q., Perlis, T., Jose, B., & Friedman, S. R. (1996). HIV incidence among injecting drug users in New York City syringe-exchange programmes. *Lancet, 348,* 987–991.

Des Jarlais, D. C., & Maynard, H. (1992, January 3). *Evaluation of needle exchange program on HIV risk behavior: Final report.* New York: American Foundation for AIDS Research.

Des Jarlais, D. C., Paone, D., Marmor, M., Titus, S., Sotheran, J. L., & Friedman, S. (1994, November). *The New York City syringe exchange program: Evaluation of a public health intervention.* Paper presented at the annual convention of the American Public Health Association, Washington, DC.

Des Jarlais, D. C., Marmor, M., Paone, D., Titus, S., Shi, Q., Perlis, T., Jose, B., & Friedman, S. R. (1996). HIV incidence among injecting drug users in new York City syringe–exchange programmes. *Lancet, 348,* 987–991.

Detels, R., English, P., Visscher, V. R., Jacobson, L., Kingsley, L. A., Chmiel, J. S., Dudley, J. P., Eldred, L. J., & Ginzburg, H. M. (1989). Seroconversion, sexual activity, and condom use among 2915 HIV seronegative men followed for up to 2 years. *Journal of Acquired Immune Deficiency Syndromes, 2,* 77–83.

DeWitt, C. B. (1992, July). *Drug use forecasting: Third quarter, 1992*. Washington, DC: National Institute of Justice.

Diaz, T., Chu, S. Y., Byers, R. H., Hersh, B. S., Conti, L., Rietmeijer, C., Mokotoff, E., Fann, A., Boyd, D., Iglesias, L., Checko, P., Frederick, M., Hermann, P., Herr, M., & Samuel, M. (1994). Types of drugs used by injection drug users with HIV/AIDs in a multisite surveillance project: Implications for intervention. *American Journal of Public Health, 84,* 1971–1975.

DiClemente, R. J., Durbin, M., Siegel, D., Krasnovsky, F., Lazarus, N., & Comacho, T. (1992). Determinants of condom use among junior high school students in a minority, inner-city school district. *Pediatrics, 89,* 197–202.

DiClemente, R. J., Pies, C. A., Stoller, E., Straits, C., Olivia, G. E., Haskin, J., & Rutherford, G. W. (1989). Evaluation of school-based AIDS education curricula in San Francisco. *Journal of Sex Research, 26,* 188–198.

Dolan, K., Donoghoe, M., Jones, S., & Stimson, G. (1991, April). *A cohort study of syringe exchange clients and other drug injectors in England*. London: Centre for Research on Drugs and Health Behaviour.

Donoghoe, M. C. (1992). Sex, HIV and the injecting drug user. *British Journal of Addiction, 87,* 405–416.

Dorfman, L. E., Derish, P. A., & Cohen, J. B. (1992). Hey girlfriend: An evaluation of AIDS prevention among women in the sex industry. *Health Education Quarterly, 19,* 25–40.

Drug Abuse Warning Network. (1989). *Data from the Drug Abuse Warning Network (DAWN): 1988 annual data*. Rockville, MD: U.S. Department of Health and Human Services.

Dryfoos, J. G. (1990). *Adolescents at risk: Prevalence and prevention*. New York: Oxford University Press.

Dunn, J., Riley, A., Emslie, J., Taylor, A., Goldberg, D., Frischer, M., & Emslie, J. (1993). Transmission of HIV in prison. *British Medical Journal, 307,* 622–623.

Dwyer, R., Richardson, D., Ross, M. W., Wodak, A., Miller, M. E., & Gold, J. (1994). A comparison of HIV risk between women and men who inject drugs. *AIDS Education and Prevention, 6,* 379–389.

Edlin, B. R., Irwin, K. L., Faruque, S., McCoy, C. B., Word, C., Serrano, Y., Inciardi, J. A., Bowser, B. P., Schilling, R. F., Holmberg, S. D., & the Multicenter Crack Cocaine and HIV Infection Study Team. (1994). Intersecting epidemics: Crack cocaine use and HIV infection among inner-city young adults. *New England Journal of Medicine, 331,* 1422–1427.

Edlin, B. R., Irwin, K. L., Ludwig, D. D., McCoy, V. H., Serrano, Y., Word, C., Bowser, B. P., Faruque, S., McCoy, C. B., Schilling, R. F., Holmberg, S. D., & the Multicenter Crack Cocaine and HIV Infection Study Team. (1992). High-risk sex behavior among young street-recruited crack cocaine smokers in three American cities: An interim report. *Journal of Psychoactive Drugs, 24,* 363–371.

Ekstrand, M. L., & Coates, T. J. (1990). Maintenance of safer sexual behaviors and predictors of risky sex: The San Francisco Men's Health Study. *American Journal of Public Health, 80,* 973–977.

Elders, J. (1994, December 20). Someone had to speak up. *The New York Times,* p. A19.

Ellickson, P. L., & Bell, R. M. (1990). Drug prevention in junior high: A multi-site longitudinal test. *Science, 247,* 1299–1305.

Emslie, J. A. (1993). Transmission of HIV in prisons: Different aims, different strategies [Letter]. *British Medical Journal, 307*, 622–623.

Espinoza, P., Bouchard, I., & Ballian, P. (1988). Has the open sale of syringes modified the syringe exchanging habits of drug addicts? In *Final program and abstracts of the IV International Conference on AIDS, 1988, Stockholm* (Abstract No. 8522). Frederick, MD: University Publishers Group.

Estebanez, P., Fitch, K., & Najera, R. (1993). HIV and female sex workers. *Bulletin of the World Health Organization, 71*, 397–412.

Farrow, J. A., Deisher, R. W., Brown, R., Kulig, J. W., & Kipke, M. D. (1992). Health and health needs of homeless and runaway youth. *Journal of Adolescent Health, 13*, 717–727.

Federal Bureau of Investigation. (1988). *Uniform crime reports.* Washington, DC: Author.

Federal Bureau of Investigation. (1992). *Crime in the United States in 1991.* Washington, DC: U.S. Department of Justice.

Federal Bureau of Prisons. (1998). *Quick facts, March 28, 1998.* Washington, DC: U.S. Department of Justice.

Feldman, L., & Elovich, R. (1989, June). *Staying negative—it's not automatic.* Paper presented at the Fifth International Conference on AIDS, Montreal.

Firlik, A. D., & Schreiber, K. (1992). AIDS prevention by needle exchange. *New York State Journal of Medicine, 92*, 426–430.

Fisher, J. D. (1988). Possible effects of reference group-based social influence on AIDS-risk behavior and AIDS prevention. *American Psychologist, 43*, 914–920.

Fisher, J. D., & Fisher, W. A. (1992). Changing AIDS-risk behavior. *Psychological Bulletin, 111*, 455–474.

Fisher, J. D., & Misovich, S. J. (1990). Social influence and AIDS-preventive behavior. In E. J. Tinsdale, L. Health, & E. J. Posavac (Eds.), *Social influence processes and prevention* (pp. 36–69). New York: Plenum Press.

Fleming, P. (1996). *Youth and HIV/AIDS: An American agenda—A report to the President.* Washington, DC: White House National AIDS Policy Office.

Flowers, J. V., Booraem, C., Miller, T. E., Iverson, A. E., Copeland, J., & Furtado, K. (1991). Comparison of the results of a standardized AIDS prevention program in three geographic locations. *AIDS Education and Prevention, 3*, 189–196.

Flynn, N., Jain, S., Keddie, E. M., Carlson, J. R., Jennings, M. B., Haverkos, H. W., Nassar, N., Anderson, R., Cohen, S., & Goldberg, D. (1994). In vitro activity of readily available household materials against HIV-1: Is bleach enough? *Journal of Acquired Immune Deficiency Syndromes, 7*, 747–753.

Gaughwin, M. D., Douglas, R. M., Liew, C., Davies, L., Mylvaganam, A., Treffke, H., Edwards, J., & Ali, R. (1991). HIV prevalence and risk behaviours for HIV transmission in South Australian prisons. *AIDS, 5*, 845–851.

Gibbs, N. (1993, May 24). How should we teach our children about sex? *Time*, pp. 60–66.

Gleghorn, A. A. (1994). Use of bleach by injection drug users. In Institute of Medicine (Ed.), *Proceedings: Workshop on needle exchange and bleach distribution programs.* Washington, DC: National Academy Press.

Gleghorn, A. A., Doherty, M. C., Vlahov, D., Celentano, D. D., & Jones, T. S. (1994). Inadequate bleach contact times during syringe cleaning among injection drug users. *Journal of Acquired Immune Deficiency Syndromes, 7,* 767–772.

Goldberg, D., Watson, H., Stuart, F., Millar, M., Gruer, L., & Follett, E. (1988). Pharmacy supply of needles and syringes: The effect on spread of HIV in intravenous drug misusers. In *Final program and abstracts of the IV International Conference on AIDS, 1988, Stockholm* (Abstract No. 8521). Frederick, MD: University Publisher Group.

Goldsmith, B. (1993, April 26). A reporter at large: Women on the edge. *The New Yorker,* pp. 64–81.

Gostin, L. O., Lazzarini, Z., Jones, S., & Flaherty, K. (1997). Prevention of HIV/AIDS and other blood-borne diseases among injection drug users. *Journal of the American Medical Association, 277,* 53–62.

Gore, S. M., & Bird, A. G. (1993). No escape: HIV transmission in jail. Prisons need protocols for HIV outbreaks. *British Medical Journal, 307,* 147–148.

Gorman, E. M. (1996). Speed use and HIV transmission. *Focus, 11*(7), 4–6.

Gorman, E. M., Morgan, P., & Lambert, E. Y. (1995). Qualitative research considerations and other issues in the study of methamphetamine use among men who have sex with other men. In E. Y. Lambert, R. S. Ashery, & R. H. Needle (Eds.), *Qualitative methods in drug abuse and HIV research* (NIDA Research Monograph No. 157, pp. 156–181). Rockville, MD: U.S. Department of Health and Human Services.

Green, J. M., Ennett, S. T., & Ringwalt, C. L. (1997). Substance use among runaway and homeless youth in three national samples. *American Journal of Public Health, 87,* 229–235.

Green, S. T., Goldberg, D. J., Christie, P. R., Frischer, M., Thomson, A., Carr, S. V., & Taylor, A. (1993). Female streetworker–prostitutes in Glasgow: A descriptive study of their lifestyle. *AIDS Care, 5,* 321–335.

Hagan, H., Des Jarlais, D. C., Friedman, S. R., Purchase, D., & Alter, M. J. (1995). Reduced risk of hepatitis B and hepatitis C among injection drug users in the Tacoma syringe exchange program. *American Journal of Public Health, 85,* 1531–1537.

Hagan, H., Des Jarlais, D. C., Friedman, S. R., Purchase, D., & Reid, T. R. (1992). Multiple outcome measures of the impact of the Tacoma syringe exchange. In *Final program and abstracts of the VIII International Conference on AIDS, 1992, Amsterdam* (Abstract No. 4283). Amsterdam: CONGREX Holland B.V.

Hagan, H., Des Jarlais, D. C., Purchase, D., Friedman, S. R., & Bell, T. A. (1991). The incidence of HBV and syringe exchange programs. *Journal of the American Medical Association, 266,* 1646–1647.

Hagan, H., Des Jarlais, D. C., Purchase, D., Reid, T., & Friedman, S. R. (1991). The Tacoma syringe exchange. *Journal of Addictive Diseases, 10,* 81–88.

Hammett, T. M., & Dubler, N. N. (1990). Clinical and epidemiological research on HIV infection and AIDS among correctional inmates: Regulations, ethics and procedures. *Evaluation Review, 14,* 482–501.

Hando, J., & Hall, W. (1994). HIV risk-taking behaviour among amphetamine users in Sydney, Australia. *Addiction, 89,* 79–85.

Hankins, C., Gendron, S., Rouah, F., & Lepine, D. (1993). Rising prevalence? Declining incidence? Montreal's needle exchange: A successful verdict or is the jury still out? In *Final program and abstracts of the IX International confer-*

ence on AIDS, 1993, Berlin (Abstract No. PO-C24-3182). London: Wellcome Foundation.

Hart, G. J., Carvell, A. L. M., Woodward, N., Johnson, A. M., Williams, P., & Parry, J. V. (1989). Evaluation of needle exchange in central London: Behaviour change and anti-HIV status over one year. *AIDS, 3,* 261–265.

Hart, G. J., Woodward, N., Johnson, A. M., Tighe, J., Parry, J. V., & Adler, M. W. (1991). Prevalence of HIV, hepatitis B and associated risk behaviours in clients of a needle-exchange in central London. *AIDS, 5,* 543–547.

Hartel, D. (1994). Context of HIV risk behavior among female injecting drug users and female sexual partners of injecting drug use. In R. J. Battjes, Z. Sloboda, & W. C. Grace (Eds.), *The context of HIV risk among drug users and their sexual partners* (NIDA Research Monograph No. 143, pp. 41–47). Rockville, MD: U.S. Department of Health and Human Services.

Haverkos, H., & Jones, T. S. (1994). HIV, drug-use paraphernalia, and bleach. *Journal of Acquired Immune Deficiency Syndrome, 7,* 741–742.

Hayes, L. D. (1987). Trends in adolescent sexuality and fertility. In L. D. Hayes (Ed.), *Risking the future: Adolescent sexuality, pregnancy and childbearing* (Vol. 1, pp. 33–74). Washington, DC: National Academy Press.

Hays, R., Kegeles, S., & Coates, T. (1990). High risk taking among young gay men. *AIDS, 4,* 901–907.

Heimer, R., Kaplan, E. H., Khoshnood, K., Jariwala, B., & Cadman, E. C. (1993). Needle exchange decreases the prevalence of HIV-1 proviral DNA in returned syringes in New Haven, Connecticut. *American Journal of Medicine, 95,* 214–220.

Hellinger, F. (1993). The lifetime cost of treating a person with HIV. *Journal of the American Medical Association, 270,* 474–478.

Hingson, R., Strunin, L., & Berlin, B. (1990). Acquired immunodeficiency syndrome transmission: Changes in knowledge and behaviors among teenagers, Massachusetts statewide surveys, 1986 to 1988. *Pediatrics, 85,* 24–29.

Holland, J., Ramazanoglu, C., Scott, S., Sharpe, S., & Rhomson, R. (1992). Risk, power and the possibility of pleasure: Young women and safer sex. *AIDS Care, 3,* 273–283.

Holmberg, S. D. (1996). The estimated prevalance and indicidence of HIV in 96 large U.S. metropolitan areas. *American Journal of Public Health, 86,* 642–654.

Home Office. (1992, March). *Statistics of drug addicts notified to the home office, United Kingdom, 1991.* London: Government Statistical Service.

Hooykaas, C., van der Pligt, J., van Doornum, G. J., van der Linden, M. M., & Coutinho, R. A. (1989). Heterosexuals at risk for HIV: Differences between private and commercial partners in sexual behavior and condom use. *AIDS, 3,* 525–532.

Horsburgh, C. R. Jr., Jarvis, J. Q., McArther, T., Ignacio, T., & Stock, P. (1990). Seroconversion to human immunodeficiency virus in prison inmates. *American Journal of Public Health, 80,* 209–210.

Hornung, R., Alvo, K., Fuchs, W., & Grob, P. (1994). Lifestyle oriented AIDS-prevention and health promotion in the drug subculture. In J. Dauwalder (Ed.), *Swiss monographs in psychology: Vol. 2. Psychology and promotion of health* (pp. 35–40). Bern: Hogrefe & Huber.

Hsia, D. C., Fleishman, J. A., East, J. A., & Hellinger, F. J. (1995). Pediatric human immunodeficiency virus infection. Recent evidence on the utilization and costs of health services. *Archives of Pediatrics and Adolescent Medicine, 149,* 489–496.

Hurley, S. F., Jolley, D. J., & Kaldor, J. M. (1997). Effectiveness of needle-exchange programmes for prevention of HIV infection. *Lancet, 349,* 1797–1800.

Ickovics, J. R., & Rodin, J. (1992). Women and AIDS in the United States: Epidemiology, natural history, and mediating mechanisms. *Health Psychology, 11,* 1–16.

Inciardi, J. A. (1994). HIV/AIDS risks among male, heterosexual noninjecting drug users who exchange crack for sex. In R. J. Battjes, Z. Sloboda, & W. C. Grace (Eds.), *The context of HIV risk among drug users and their sexual partners* (NIDA Research Monograph No. 143, pp. 26–40). Rockville, MD: U.S. Department of Health and Human Services.

Ingold, F. R., & Ingold, S. (1989). The effects of the liberalization of syringe sales on the behaviour of intravenous drug users in France. *Bulletin on Narcotics, 41,* 67–81.

Institute of Medicine. (Ed.). (1994). *Proceedings: Workshop on needle exchange and bleach distribution programs.* Washington, DC: National Academy Press.

Irwin, C. E., & Millstein, S. G. (1986). Biopsychosocial correlates of risk-taking behaviors during adolescence: Can the physician intervene? *Journal of Adolescent Health Care, 7,* 82S–96S.

Jackson, L., Highcrest, A., & Coates, R. A. (1992). Varied potential risks of HIV infections among prostitutes. *Social Science Medicine, 35,* 281–286.

Janz, N. K., & Becker, M. H. (1984). The health belief model: A decade later. *Health Education Quarterly, 11,* 1–47.

Jeffrey, R. W. (1989). Risk behaviors and health. *American Psychologist, 44,* 1194–1202.

Jemmott, J. B., III, Jemmott, L. S., & Fong, G. T. (1992). Reductions in HIV risk-associated sexual behaviors among black male adolescents: Effects of an AIDS prevention intervention. *American Journal of Public Health, 82,* 372–377.

Jones, T. S., Allen, D. M., Onorato, I. M., Petersen, L. R., Dondero, T. J. J., & Pappaionou, M. (1990). HIV seroprevalence surveys in drug treatment enters. *Public Health Reports, 106,* 280–292.

Joseph, J., Montgomery, S. B., Kessler, R. C., Ostrow, D. G., & Wortman, C. B. (1988, June). *Determinants of high risk behavior and recidivism among gay men.* Paper presented at the Fourth International Conference on AIDS, Stockholm.

Joseph, J. G., Montgomery, S. B., Kirscht, J., Kessler, R. C., Ostrow, D. G., Emmmons, C. A., & Phair, J. P. (1987, June). *Behavioral risk reduction in a cohort of homosexual men: Two year follow-up.* Paper presented at the Third International Conference on AIDS, Washington, DC.

Kaplan, E. (1993). *Back-of-the-envelope estimates of needle exchange effectiveness.* Unpublished manuscript.

Kaplan, E. H., Khoshnood, K., & Heimer, R. (1994). A decline in HIV-infected needles returned to New Haven's needle exchange program: Client shift or needle exchange? *American Journal of Public Health, 84,* 1991–1994.

Kaplan, E. H., & O'Keefe, E. (1993). Let the needles do the talking!: Evaluating the New Haven needle exchange. *Interfaces, 23,* 7–26.

Kaplan, E. H., O'Keefe, E., & Heimer, R. (1991, June). *Evaluating the New Haven needle exchange program.* Paper presented at the meeting of the Seventh International Conference on AIDS, Florence, Italy.

Katoff, L., & Dunne, R. (1988) Supporting people with AIDS: The Gay Men's Health Crisis model. *Journal of Palliative Care, 4,* 88–95.

Kelly, J. A., Kalichman, S. C., Kauth, M. R., Kilgore, H. G., Hood, H. V., Campos, P. E., Rao, S. M., Brasfield, T. L., & St. Lawrence, J. S. (1991). Situational factors associated with AIDS risk behavior lapses and coping strategies used by gay men who successfully avoid relapses. *American Journal of Public Health, 81,* 1335–1338.

Kelly, J. A., Murphy, D., & Roffman, R. (1992). AIDS risk behavior among gay men in small cities: Findings of a 16-city national sample. *Archives of Internal Medicine, 15,* 2293–2297.

Kelly, J. A., & St. Lawrence, J. S. (1988). AIDS prevention and treatment: Psychology's role in the health crisis. *Clinical Psychology Review, 8,* 255–284.

Kelly, J. A., St. Lawrence, J. S., Betts, R., Brasfield, T. L., & Hood, H. V. (1990). A skills training group intervention model to assist persons in reducing risk behaviors for HIV infection. *AIDS Education and Prevention, 2,* 24–35.

Kelly, J. A., St. Lawrence, J. S., & Brasfield, T. L. (1991). Predictors of vulnerability to AIDS risk behavior relapse. *Journal of Consulting and Clinical Psychology, 59,* 163–166.

Kelly, J. A., St. Lawrence, J. S., Diaz, Y. E., Stevenson, L. Y., Hauth, A. C., Brasfield, T. L., Kalichman, S. C., Smith, J. E., & Andrew, M. E. (1991). HIV risk behavior reduction following intervention with key opinion leaders of a population: An experimental analysis. *American Journal of Public Health, 81,* 168–171.

Kelly, J. A., St. Lawrence, J. S., Hood, H.V., & Brasfield, T. L. (1989). Behavioral intervention to reduce AIDS risk activities. *Journal of Consulting and Clinical Psychology, 57,* 60–67.

Kelly, J. A., St. Lawrence, J. S., Stevenson, L. Y., Hauth, A. C., Kalichman, S. C., Diaz, Y. E., Brasfield, T. L., Koob, J. J., & Morgan, M. G. (1992). Community AIDS/HIV risk reduction: The effects of endorsements by popular people in three cities. *American Journal of Public Health, 82,* 1483–1489.

Kennedy, M. R. (1991). Homeless and runaway youth mental health issues: No access to the system. *Journal of Adolescent Health, 12,* 576–579.

Kingsley, L. A., Detels, R., Kaslow, R., Polk, B. F., Rinaldo, C. R., Chmiel, J., Detre, K., Kelsey, S. F., Odaka, N., Ostrow, D., van Raden, M., & Visscher, B. (1987). Risk factors for seroconversion to human immunodeficiency virus among male homosexuals: Results from the Multicenter AIDS Cohort Study. *Lancet, i,* 345–349.

Kirby, D., Short, L., Collins, J., Rugg, D., Kolbe, L., Howard, M., Miller, B., Sonenstein, F., & Zabin, L. S. (1994). School-based programs to reduce sexual risk behaviors: A review of effectiveness. *Public Health Reports, 109,* 339–360.

Kochems, L. M., Paone, D., Des Jarlais, D. C., Ness, I., Clark, J., & Friedman, S. R. (1996). The transition from underground to legal syringe exchange: The New York City experience. *AIDS Education and Prevention, 8,* 471–489.

Kolata, G. (1995, February 28). New picture of who will get AIDS is crammed with addicts. *The New York Times,* p. B6.

Koopman, C., Rosario, M., & Rotheram-Borus, M. J. (1994). Alcohol and drug use and sexual behaviors placing runaways at risk for HIV infection. *Addictive Behaviors, 19,* 95–103.

Krepcho, M. A., Fernandez-Esquer, M. E., Freeman, A. C., Magee, E., & McAlister, A. (1993). Predictors of bleach use among current African-American injecting drug users: A community study. *Journal of Psychoactive Drugs, 25,* 135–41.

Lart, R., & Stimson, G. V. (1990). National survey of syringe exchange schemes in England. *British Journal of Addiction, 85,* 1433–1443.

Leigh, B. C., Morrison, D. M., Trocki, K., & Temple, M. T. (1994). Sexual behavior of American adolescents: Results from a U.S. national survey. *Journal of Adolescent Health, 15,* 117–125.

Lemp, G., Hirozawa, A., Givertz, D., Nieri, G., Bishop, J., Fuqua, V., Hernandez, M., Goni, L., Militante, W., Ramos, E., Nguyen, S., Jones, M., Anderson, L., Jsansses, R., Lindegren, M., & Katz, M. (1993). *HIV seroprevalence and risk factors among young gay and bisexual men: The San Francisco/Berkeley Young Men's Survey.* Paper presented at the Ninth International Conference on AIDS, Berlin.

Ljungberg, B., & Christensson, B. (1991). Still no HIV epidemic among local drug users at four year follow-up of the first Swedish syringe exchange program. In *Final program and abstracts of the VII International Conference on AIDS, 1991, Florence* (Abstract No. WC 3290). Rome: Conference Organizing Committee.

Lloyd, L. S., O'Shea, D. J., & the Injection Drug Use Study Group. (1994). *Injection drug use in San Diego County: A needs assessment.* San Diego, CA: Alliance Healthcare Foundation.

Luna, G. C. (1991). Street youth: Adaptation and survival in the AIDS decade. *Journal of Adolescent Health, 12,* 511–514.

Lurie, P., Reingold, A. L., Lee, P. R., Bowser, B., Chen, D., Foley, J., Guydish, J., Kahn, J. G., Lane, S., & Sorenson, J. (1993, October). *The public health impact of needle exchange programs in the United States and abroad* (2 vols.). Atlanta, GA: Centers for Disease Control and Prevention (CDC).

Magura, S., Grossman, J. I., Lipton, D. S., Siddiqi, Q., Shapiro, J., Marion, I., & Amann, K. R. (1989). Determinants of needle sharing among intravenous drug users. *American Journal of Public Health, 79,* 459–462.

Marlatt, G. A., & Gordon, J. R. (Eds.). (1985). *Relapse prevention: Maintenance strategies in the treatment of addictive behaviors.* New York: Guilford Press.

Martin, J. L. (1987). The impact of AIDS on gay male sexual behavior patterns in New York City. *American Journal of Public Health, 77,* 578–581.

Maticka-Tyndale, E. (1991). Modification of sexual activities in the era of AIDS: A trend analysis of adolescent sexual activities. *Youth and Society, 23,* 31–49.

McCoy, C. B., Rivers, J. E., McCoy, H. V., Shapshak, P., Weatherby, N. L., Chitwood, D. D., Page, J. B., Inciardi, J. A., & McBride, D. C. (1994). Compliance to bleach disinfection protocols among injecting drug users in Miami. *Journal of Acquired Immune Deficiency Syndromes, 7,* 773–776.

McCusker, J., Stoddard, A. M., Koblin, B. A. Sullivan, J., Lewis, B. F., & Sereti, S. M. (1992). Time trends in high-risk injection practices in a multi-site study in Massachusetts: Effects of enrollment site and residence. *AIDS Education and Prevention, 4,* 108–119.

McKeganey, N., & Barnard, M. (1992). Selling sex: Female street prostitution and HIV risk behaviour in Glasgow. *AIDS Care, 4,* 395–407.

McKusick, L., Coates, T. J., Morin, S. F., Pollack, L., & Hoff, C. (1990). Longitudinal predictors of reductions in unprotected anal intercourse among gay men in San Francisco: The AIDS Behavioral Research Project. *American Journal of Public Health, 80,* 978–983.

McMillan, A. (1988). HIV in prisons. *British Medical Journal, 297,* 873–874.

Miller, H. G., Turner, C. F., & Moses, L. E. (Eds.). (1990). *AIDS: The second decade.* Washington, DC: National Academy Press.

Miller, T. E., Booraem, C. D., Flowers, J. V., & Iversen, A. E. (1990). Changes in knowledge, attitudes, and behavior as a result of a community AIDS outreach educational program. *AIDS Education and Prevention, 2,* 12–23.

Millson, P., Myers, T., Rankin, J., McLaughlin, B., Major, C., Mindell, W., Coates R., Rigby, J., & Strathdee, S. (1993). Trends in HIV seroprevalence and risk behavior in IDUs in Toronto, Canada. In *Final program and abstracts of the IX International Conference on AIDS, 1993, Berlin* (Abstract No. PO-C15-2936). London: Wellcome Foundation.

Morgan, D. L. (1992). Intravenous injection of household bleach. *Annals of Emergency Medicine, 21,* 1394–1395.

Morgan, P., Beck, J., Joe, K., McDonnell, D., & Gutierrez, R. (1994, September). *Ice and other methamphetamine use: An exploratory study* (Final Report to the National Institute on Drug Abuse, No. RO-1DA6853).

Morgan, P., McDonnell, D., Beck, J., Joe, K., & Gutierrez, R. (1993). Ice and other methamphetamine use: Preliminary findings from three sites. In B. Sowder & G. Beschner (Eds.), *Methamphetamine: An illicit drug with high abuse potential.* Rockville, MD: T. Head.

Morrison, D. M., Gillmore, M. R., & Baker, S. A. (1995). Determinants of condom use among high-risk heterosexual adults: A test of the theory of reasoned action. *Journal of Applied Social Psychology, 25,* 651–676.

Moss, A. R., Vranizan, K., Gorter, R., Bacchetti, P., Watters, J., & Osmond, D. (1994). HIV seroconversion in intravenous drug users in San Francisco, 1985–1990. *AIDS, 8,* 223–231.

National Commission on AIDS. (1991). *HIV disease in correctional facilities* (Report No. 4). Washington, DC: Author.

National Institute of Justice. (1990). *Drug use forecasting annual report 1989.* Washington, DC: U.S. Department of Justice.

National Institute on Drug Abuse (NIDA). (1992). *National Household Survey on Drug Abuse: Main findings 1991* (DHHS Publication No. ADM 91-1788). Rockville, MD: U.S. Department of Health and Human Services.

Nelson, K. E., Vlahov, D., Cohn, S., Lindsay, A., Solomon, L., & Anthony, J. C. (1991). Human immunodeficiency virus infection in diabetic intravenous drug users. *Journal of the American Medical Association, 266,* 2259–2261.

Newcombe, R. (1990, November). The first conference of European cities at the centre of illegal trade in drugs. *Drug use and drug policy in Merseyside.*

Office of National Drug Control Policy. (1990, June). *White paper: Understanding drug treatment.* Washington, DC: Author.

O'Keefe, E., Kaplan, E., & Khoshnood, K. (1991, July 31). *Preliminary report: City of New Haven needle exchange program.* New Haven, CT: City of New Haven.

O'Leary, A. (1994). Factors associated with sexual risk or AIDS in women. In R. J. Battjes, Z. Sloboda, & W. C. Grace (Eds.), *The context of HIV risk among drug users and their sexual partners* (NIDA Research Monograph No. 143, pp. 64–81). Rockville, MD: U.S. Department of Health and Human Services.

O'Mahony, P., & Barry, M. (1992). HIV risk of transmission behaviour amongst HIV-infected prisoners and its correlates. *British Journal of Addiction, 87,* 1555–1560.

Osmond, D., Page, K., Wiley, J., Garrett, K., Sheppard, H. W., Moss, A. R., Schrager, L., & Winkelstein, W. (1994). Human immunodeficiency virus infection in homosexual/bisexual men, ages 18–29: The San Francisco Young Men's Health Study. *American Journal of Public Health, 84,* 933–937.

Ostrow, D. G. (1996). Substance use, HIV, and gay men. *Focus, 11,* 1–3.

Overby, K. J., & Kegeles, S. M. (1994). The impact of AIDS on an urban population of high-risk female minority adolescents: Implications for intervention. *Journal of Adolescent Health, 15,* 216–227.

Padian, N. S. (1988). Prostitute women and AIDS: Epidemiology. *AIDS, 2,* 413–419.

Padian, N. S., Shiboski, S. C., & Jewell, N. P. (1990). The effect of number of exposures on the risk of heterosexual HIV transmission. *Journal of Infectious Diseases, 161,* 883–887.

Paone, D., Des Jarlais, D. C., Caloir, S., & Friedman, P. (1993). AIDS risk reduction behaviors among participants of syringe exchange programs in New York City, USA. In *Final program and abstracts of the IX International Conference on AIDS, Berlin.* London: Wellcome Foundation.

Paone, D., Des Jarlais, D. C., Gangloff, R., Milliken, J., & Friedman, S. R. (1995). Syringe exchange: HIV prevention, key findings, and future directions. *International Journal of the Addictions, 30*(12), 1647–1683.

Paul, P., Stall, R., & Davis, F. (1993). Sexual risk for HIV transmission among gay/bisexual men in substance abuse treatment. *AIDS Education and Prevention, 5,* 11–24.

Peterson, J. L., & Marin, G. (1988). Issues in the prevention of AIDS among black and Hispanic men. *American Psychologist, 43,* 871–877.

Peterson, J. L., Coates, T. J., Catania, J. A., Middleton, B. A., Hilliard, B., & Hearst, N. (1992). High-risk sexual behavior and condom use among gay and bisexual African-American men. *American Journal of Public Health, 82,* 1490–1494.

Petty, R. E., & Cacioppo, J. T. (1981). *Attitudes and persuasion: Classic and contemporary approaches.* Dubuque, IA: William C. Brown.

Polosky, S., Kerr, S., Harris, B., & Gaiter, J. (1994). HIV prevention in prisons and jails: Obstacles and opportunities. *Public Health Reports, 109,* 615–626.

Power, K. G., Markova, I., Rowlands, A., McKee, K. J., Anslow, P. J., & Kilfedder, C. (1992). Intravenous drug use and HIV transmission amongst inmates in Scottish prisons. *British Journal of Addiction, 87,* 35–45.

Reinfield, M. (1994, Spring). Harm reduction theory in practice: An update on AmFAR's syringe exchange program. *The AmFAR Report,* pp. 6–8.

Resnick, L., Veren, K., & Salahuddin, S. A. (1986). Stability and inactivation of HTLV/LAV under clinical and laboratory environments. *Journal of the American Medical Association, 255,* 1887–1891.

Rhodes, T., Donoghoe, M., Hunter, G., & Stimson, G. V. (1994). HIV prevalence no higher among female drug injectors also involved in prostitution. *AIDS Care, 6,* 267–268.

Riley, A. (1993). Transmission of HIV in prison: Prevention depends on enlightened approach [Letter]. *British Medical Journal, 307,* 622.

Roffman, R. A., Beadnell, B. A., Gordon, J. R., Stern, M. J., & Siever, M. D. (1991, August). *Relapse prevention counseling by telephone as a means of reducing AIDS risk in men who have sex with other men.* Paper presented at the annual convention of the American Psychological Association, San Francisco.

Roffman, R. A., Downey, L., Beadnell, B., Gordon, J. R., Craver, J. N., & Stephens, R. S. (1997). Cognitive-behavioral group counseling to prevent HIV transmission in gay and bisexual men: Factors contributing to successful risk reduction. *Research on Social Work Practice, 7,* 165–186.

Roffman, R. A., Gordon, J. R., Beadnell, B. A., Stern, M. J., Craver, J. N., Simpson, D., & Stephens, R. S. (1989, November). *Reaching gay and bisexual men who continue to engage in unsafe sexual activity: A comparison of subjects recruited for in-person or telephone counseling formats.* Paper presented at the annual convention of the Association for Advancement of Behavior Therapy, Washington, DC.

Rogers, E. M. (1973). *Communication strategies for family planning.* New York: Free Press.

Rotheram-Borus, M. J., Koopman, C., Haignere, C., & Davies, M. (1991). Reducing HIV sexual risk behaviors among runaway adolescents. *Journal of the American Medical Association, 266,* 1237–1241.

Sadownick, D. (1994, January). Kneeling at the crystal cathedral: The alarming new epidemic of methamphetamine use in the gay community. *Genre, 15,* 40–45.

Scano, G., Luzi, G., Mezzaroma, I., Aiuti, F., Vellucci, A., Guastini, L., Lepri, F., & Starnini, G. (1991). One year follow up of a HIV seropositive jail population. *Allergologia et Immunopathologia* (Madrid), *19,* 165–166.

Schilling, R. F., El-Bassel, N., Gilbert, L., & Schinke, S. P. (1991). Correlates of drug use, sexual behavior, and attitudes toward safer sex among African-American and Hispanic women in methadone maintenance. *Journal of Drug Issues, 21,* 685–698.

Schilling, R. F., Schnicke, S. P., Nichols, S. E., Zayas, L. H., Miller, S. O., Orlandi, M. A., & Botvin, G. L. (1989). Developing strategies for AIDS prevention research with black and Hispanic drug users. *Public Health Reports, 104,* 2–11.

Sellers, D. E., McGraw, S. A., & McKinlay, J. B. (1994). Does the promotion and distribution of condoms increase teen sexual activity?: Evidence from an HIV prevention program for Latino youth. *American Journal of Public Health, 84,* 1952–1959.

Shilts, R. (1987). *And the band played on: Politics, people, and the AIDS epidemic.* New York: St. Martin's Press.

Siegel, J. E., Weinstein, M. C., & Fineberg, H. V. (1991). Bleach programs for preventing AIDS among i.v. drug users. *American Journal of Public Health, 81,* 1273–1279.

Smith, G. L., & Smith, K. F. (1986). Lack of HIV infection and condom use in licensed prostitutes [Letter]. *Lancet, ii,* 1392.

Sonenstein, F. L., Pleck, J. H., & Ku, L. C. (1989). Sexual activity, condom use and AIDS awareness among adolescent males. *Family Planning Perspectives, 21,* 152–158.

Sorge, R. (1990, Fall). A thousand points: Needle exchange around the country. *Health PAC Bulletin,* pp. 16–22.

Springer, E. (1992). *Peer AIDS education with street youth: Reaching the unreachable.* Unpublished manuscript, New York Peer AIDS Education Coalition.

Stall, R., Barrett, D., Bye, L., Catania, J., Fritchey, C., Henne, J., Lemp, G., & Paul, J. (1992). A comparison of younger and older gay men's HIV risk-taking behaviors: The Community Technologies 1989 Cross-Sectional Survey. *Journal of Acquired Immune Deficiency Syndromes, 5,* 682–687.

Stall, R. D., Coates, T. J., & Hoff, C. (1988). Behavioral risk reduction for HIV infection among gay and bisexual men: A review of results from the United States. *American Psychologist, 43,* 878–885.

Stall, R. D., Ekstrand, M., Pollack, L., McKusick, L., & Coates, T. J. (1990). Relapse from safer sex: The next challenge for AIDS prevention efforts. *Journal of Acquired Immune Deficiency Syndromes, 3,* 1181–1187.

Stimson, G. V. (1992). Drug injecting and HIV infection: New directions for social science research. *International Journal of the Addictions, 27,* 147–163.

Stricof, R. L., Kennedy, J. T., Nattell, T. C., Weisfuse, I. B., & Novick, L. F. (1991). HIV seroprevalence in a facility for runaway and homeless adolescents. *American Journal of Public Health, 81*(Suppl.), 50–53.

Strunin, L., & Hingson, R. (1992). Alcohol, drugs, and adolescent sexual behavior. *International Journal of the Addictions, 27,* 129–146.

Substance Abuse and Mental Health Services Administration (SAHMSA). (1997). *National Household Survey on Drug Abuse: Population estimates, 1996.* Rockville, MD: U.S. Department of Health and Human Services.

Taylor, A., Goldberg, D., Frischer, M., Emslie, J., Green, S., & McKeganey, N. (1993). Transmission of HIV in prison: Evidence of risk. *British Medical Journal, 307,* 623.

Tellado, I., Moran, N., Vargas Vidot, J., & Yamamura, Y. (1997). Pattern of injecting drug uses and HIV-I infection: Analysis from needle exchange program. *Cellular and Molecular Biology, 43,* 1091–1096.

Tirelli, U., De Mercato, R., Caprilli, F., Guiliani, M., Saracco, A., Rezza, G. (1989, June). *HIV seropositivity and risk behaviours of Italian prostitutes.* Paper presented at the Fifth International Conference on AIDS, Montreal.

Tortu, S., Beardsley, M., Deren, S., & Davis, W. R. (1994). The risk of HIV infection in a national sample of women with injection drug-using partners. *American Journal of Public Health, 84,* 1243–1249.

Tsai, R., Goh, E. H., Webeck, P., & Mullins, J. (1988). Prevention of human immunodeficiency virus infection among intravenous drug users in New South Wales, Australia: The needles and syringe distribution programme through retail pharmacies. *Asia–Pacific Journal of Public Health, 2,* 245–251.

Turner, C. F., Miller, H. G., & Moses, L. E. (Eds.). (1989). *AIDS: Sexual behavior and intravenous drug use.* Washington, DC: National Academy Press.

U.S. Department of Justice. (1993). *Survey of state prison inmates, 1991.* Washington, DC: Author.

U.S. General Accounting Office. (1993, March 23). *Needle exchange programs: Research suggests promise as an AIDS prevention strategy.* Gaithersburg, MD: Author.

U.S. Preventive Services Task Force. (1996). *Guide to clinical preventive services* (2nd ed.). Baltimore, MD: Williams & Wilkins.

Valdiserri, R. O., Lyter, D. W., Leviton, L. C., Callahan, C. M., Kingsley, L. A., & Rinaldo, C. R. (1989). AIDS prevention in homosexual and bisexual men:

Results of a randomized trial evaluating two risk reduction interventions. *AIDS, 3,* 21–26.

Valleroy, L., Weinstein, B., Groseclose, S., Kassler, W., & Jones, S. (1993). Evaluating the impact of a new needle/syringe law: Surveillance of needle/syringe sales at Connecticut pharmacies. In *Final program and abstracts of the VI International Conference on AIDS, 1993, Berlin* (Abstract No. PO-C24-3189). London: Wellcome Foundation.

Vlahov, D., Brewer, F., Castro, K. G., Narkunas, J. P., Salive, M. E., Ullrich, J., & Munoz, A. (1991). Prevalence of antibody to HIV-1 among entrants to U.S. correctional facilities. *Journal of the American Medical Association, 265,* 1129–1132.

Wallace, J. I., Mann, J., & Beatrice, S. (1988, June). *HIV-1 exposure among clients of prostitutes.* Paper presented at the Fourth International Conference on AIDS, Stockholm.

Walter, H. J., Vaughan, R. D., Gladis, M. M., Ragin, D. F., Kasen, S., & Cohall, A. T. (1992). Factors associated with AIDS risk behavior among high school students in an AIDS epicenter. *American Journal of Public Health, 82,* 528–532.

Ward, H., Day, S., Mezzone, J., Dunlop, L., Donegan, C., Farrar, S., Whitaker, L., Harris, J. R. W., & Miller, D. L. (1993). Prostitution and risk of HIV: Female prostitutes in London. *British Medical Journal, 307,* 356–358.

Watters, J. K., Cheng, Y. T., Clark, G. L., & Lorvick, J. (1991, June). *Syringe exchange in San Francisco: Preliminary findings.* Paper presented at the Ninth International Conference on AIDS, Florence, Italy.

Watters, J. K., Cheng, Y. T., Segal, M., Lorvick, J., Case, P., & Carlson, J. (1990). Epidemiology and prevention of HIV in intravenous drug users in San Francisco, 1986–1989. In *Final program and abstracts of the VI International Conference on AIDS, 1990, San Francisco* (Abstract No. FC 106). San Francisco: Conference Organizing Committee.

Weatherby, N. L., Schultz, J. M., Chitwood, D. D., McCoy, H. V., McCoy, C. B., Ludwig, D. D., & Edlin, B. R. (1992). Crack cocaine use and sexual activity in Miami, Florida. *Journal of Psychoactive Drugs, 24,* 373–380.

Weissman, G., & the National AIDS Research Consortium (NARC). (1991). AIDS prevention for women at risk: Experience from a national demonstration research program. *Journal of Primary Prevention, 12,* 49–63.

Wellisch, J., Anglin, M. D., & Prendergast, M. L. (1993). Numbers and characteristics of drug-using women in the criminal justice system: Implication for treatment. *Journal of Drug Issues, 23,* 7–30.

Wenger, L. D., & Murphy, S. (1994, November). *They are not just giving out needles: The impact of needle exchange on the San Francisco drug using community.* Paper presented at the annual convention of the American Public Health Association, Washington, DC.

Wexler, H. W. (1994). Progress in prison substance abuse treatment: A five year report. *Journal of Drug Issues, 24*(2), 349–360.

Wight, D. (1992). Impediments to safer heterosexual sex: A review of research with young people. *AIDS Care, 4,* 11–21.

Wilsnack, R. W., Wilsnack, S. C., & Klassen, A. D. (1984). Women's drinking and drinking problems: Patterns from a 1981 survey. *American Journal of Public Health, 74,* 1231–1238.

Winkelstein, W. W., Lyman, D., Padian, N., Grant, R., Samuel, M., Wiley, J., Anderson, R., Lang, W., Riggs, J., & Levy, J. (1987). Sexual practices and risk of infection by the human immunodeficiency virus: The San Francisco Men's Health Study. *Journal of the American Medical Association, 257,* 321–325.

Wolk, J., Wodak, A., Guinan, J. J., Macaskill, P., & Simpson, J. M. (1990). The effect of a needle and syringe exchange on a methadone maintenance unit. *British Journal of Addiction, 85,* 1445–1450.

Wormser, G. P., Krupp, L. B., Hanrahan, J. P., Gavis, G., Spira, T. J., & Cunningham-Rundles, S. (1983). Acquired immunodeficiency syndrome in male prisoners: New insights into an emerging syndrome. *Annals of Internal Medicine, 98,* 297–303.

Yates, G. L., MacKenzie, R., Pennbridge, J., & Cohen, E. (1988). A risk profile comparison of runaway and non-runaway youth. *American Journal of Public Health, 78,* 820–821.

Yates, G. L., MacKenzie, R. G., Pennbridge, J., & Swofford, A. (1991). A risk profile comparison of homeless youth involved in prostitution and homeless youth not involved. *Journal of Adolescent Health, 12,* 545–548.

PART THREE

MATCHING STRATEGIES TO DIVERSE ETHNIC COMMUNITIES

CHAPTER EIGHT

Bringing Harm Reduction to the Black Community

There's a Fire in My House and You're
Telling Me to Rearrange My Furniture?

IMANI P. WOODS

PERSONAL HISTORY:
HOW I CAME TO SUPPORT HARM REDUCTION

People look at me like I'm crazy when I go to the black community to explain harm reduction. I am accused of supporting a policy that makes peace with genocide. How can one talk about "reducing harm" to a people under siege? The scourge must be lifted; the villain must be vanquished. Harm reduction is seen as settling, giving up, accepting failure, and bargaining with the devil. The comments come fast and furious:

"Who's going to pay for my stolen TV?"
"I've been taking care of my little grandbaby for 8 years. Don't you know my son and his woman in jail because of that mess?"
"We're being robbed and knocked down in the street for drugs, and you want to talk about giving out needles and keeping people alive?!"

Invariably, comparisons are made:

"White folks' kids get jobs even after they do all that!"

And, finally:

> "Who are those white folks trying to come in our neighborhood with
> needles? They just trying to kill us. And you missin' it!"

It's difficult for me to defend my position when all around us is the
wreckage of lives damaged by the use of illicit drugs. The high unemployment of community members results in a greater use of these drugs, as well
as an increased participation in the drug economy. The presence of
numerous addicted individuals leads to an increase in crime as they attempt
to secure the outlawed substances. The criminal acts perpetrated upon the
community by those who profit from the sale of these substances are
legendary. The mass media attest to their real and imagined brutality.
Merchants are preyed upon; mothers are beaten; schools become battle-
grounds. Prisons bulge with community members accused and convicted,
rightly or wrongly, of countless offenses. Children lose their parents to jail,
addiction, violence, and premature death. Families lose their houses due to
the activities of one of their tribe. Young drug-addicted mothers lose their
children and end up in shelters for the homeless or in transient hotels.
Children are born addicted and, try as they might, have trouble keeping
up with their classmates or calming their jitters. And if that were not
enough, drug-related HIV disease disproportionately affects the black
community.

"There's a fire in my house and you're telling me to rearrange my
furniture?" The fact that I am African American and have lived and worked
in the community all of my life does not win me any converts or even any
ready listeners. As Derrick Bell (1994) writes in *Confronting Authority:
Reflections of an Ardent Protester*, "The hostile response of friends and
associates is complex, unexpected and far more devastating than enemies'
predictable attacks" (p. 133). I have found this to be true as, over the years,
I have become an "ardent protester" in support of harm reduction.

It was not always so, however. I first heard of the concept of harm
reduction during my training at the Narcotic and Drug Research Institute
in New York in 1986 (the term "harm reduction" would not be used
regularly until 1988, when Alan Perry of Liverpool began sharing what was
being done in parts of England). I met Edith Springer at the institute. Edith,
a trainer who taught a variety of workshops, motivated me through her
obvious dedication to issues related to the association of HIV/AIDS and
substance abuse. I took every class Edith offered. I was impressed with
Edith's training style. Her unadulterated manner conveys an integrity and
a sense of "oneness" that she easily transfers to her students. During her
workshop on AIDS and substance abuse, Edith introduced the idea of harm
reduction. Constrained by the then-current political and professional climate, Edith delivered a compelling harm reduction proposition. During this
time Edith spoke more of harm reduction in theory rather than actual

practice. Also, she was training counselors and needed to insure that certain counselor training specifications were met. In 1986 I was a card-carrying abstinence proponent! Fortunately, Edith and I would meet again.

In 1987, the Association for Drug Abuse Prevention and Treatment (ADAPT), a nonprofit organization founded by Edith Springer and other drug treatment specialists, received a grant (service contract) from the New York City Health Department. A colleague had recruited me to apply for the newly created position of ADAPT's director of education. To my understanding, this was the first project of this kind in the United States. I was very enthusiastic and longed to become involved in any effort that would address the problems of injection drug users (IDUs) in New York City. In her capacity as ADAPT's board secretary, Edith Springer was one of my interviewers for this position. My educational experiences regarding the associations between HIV and substance abuse, coupled with 5 years of direct services to homeless persons, served me well. During the interview I demonstrated my program design skills, specifically regarding the topics of outreach and intervention. As a result, I was offered the position. I decided to accept the position, but as fate would have it, there were contractual disagreements that could not be resolved so I remained with the Human Resources Administration, hesitant to leave the security of civil service employment for what appeared to be a precarious undertaking. ADAPT went on to be recognized nationally for its outreach efforts. Throughout my tenure at the Human Resources Administration, I continued to be a vocal opponent of needle exchange and other harm reduction strategies. Things would soon change, however.

November 1989 marked a very significant occurrence: I was moving to Seattle, Washington. I had watched my soul brother, Keith, a former IDU, succumb to a 5-year battle with HIV, never relenting in his opposition to needle exchange. The two of us would laugh about what a ridiculous idea giving clean needles to addicts was—ineffective, immoral, crazy, ridiculous. I sought escape after Keith died on August 7, 1989, and visited Seattle. Because Seattle had just been voted "America's most livable city," I figured this would be a good place to rest and to grieve.

As I always do whenever I visit a new city, I quickly made my way downtown. I wanted to see where the action was. Standing on the corner of Second and Pike—one block from the famous Pike Place Market, Seattle's number one tourist attraction—I was shocked to see a man set up a table and display needles. I started to move away, not wanting to be associated with such a shady operation. I hadn't come 3,000 miles to get arrested, I reasoned, and I was sure this man would be handcuffed and carted off at any moment. But something quite different happened. People I deemed to be career addicts approached the table and dropped contaminated needles into a sharps disposal. They began talking to the man, Carlton Clay (known as "Chilly"), and taking literature from his table along with bleach packets, condoms, and clean needles. I was stunned. I was standing there dumbfounded when something inside me clicked. "That's effective outreach," I thought, "and that's harm reduction." Back in New York, I had heard harm reduction ridiculed as ineffective—indeed, I had participated in the ridicule—and vilified as genocidal, but I had never actually seen it in action. I went over to the table and talked to Chilly. He worked for the health department. I was impressed. We exchanged information. He told me that there was a job opening in a nationally funded AIDS education and prevention outreach demonstration project. I applied for and got the job. This was the beginning of my conversion from being an outspoken opponent of needle exchange to being a firm supporter.

In New York City in 1989, a scenario similar to the one I have described above played out on a grand level, only with a different outcome. New York's fledgling needle exchange program was under attack, and many of its most prominent opponents were African American. The city's needle exchange program was operating out of a government building in downtown Manhattan commonly known as 125 Worth Street. The program was not successful, as addicts were not likely to seek help in a government building. This did not remove the controversy, however. I had then, as I do now, tremendous admiration and respect for the many renowned black addiction specialists living and working in New York. The Black Leadership Commission on AIDS was composed of my heroes. They considered needle exchange to be a flawed strategy in working with people addicted to drugs, and characterized the program as evidence of the city's unwillingness to allocate the kind of resources necessary to support drug treatment programs. Drug treatment in New York City, as in all major U.S. cities, is sorely underfunded. Culturally relevant services are extremely scarce in our communities. Needle exchange was seen as a quick fix—a bandage approach, a service by default, Novocain for the irretrievable.

Shortly after becoming Mayor, David Dinkins, under pressure from New York African American leadership (including the Black Leadership Commission on AIDS), ordered the New York City needle exchange program dismantled. I should have felt vindicated. However, by now I had too much information about needle exchange. The consequences would compromise the lives of the very persons the black leadership hoped to save! I knew that thousands of drug users would needlessly get infected with HIV. I had been a very vocal opponent of needle exchange during my tenure with the Human Resources Administration. "They're trying to kill us" was not only a phrase I had heard others use, but one I employed myself whenever the occasion warranted it. I had now come full circle. I was a firm supporter of and advocate for harm reduction.

This chapter illustrates the importance of sensitivity and community involvement in approaching the black community in regard to harm reduction. In addition, I emphasize the need to be mindful of the complexities involved in individual responses to the problems associated with substance abuse. I explore the realities of substance abuse in African American communities—the realities that make this topic such a difficult one. I also take a look at the unreality of many expectations regarding substance users. And I demonstrate how harm reduction can help an individual user by "breaking the fall" into self-destruction. Along the way, and especially at the end of this chapter, I suggest strategies I consider invaluable if harm reduction is to become a viable and widespread option in the black community.

HISTORICAL BARRIERS TO HARM REDUCTION IN THE BLACK COMMUNITY

The Effects of Slavery and Its Aftermath

What are the realities that cause many people in the African American community to reject the concept of harm reduction and to renounce the suggestion that anything other than full eradication of drug use, drug activity, and drug availability might be acceptable as a goal or strategy? To begin with, the very real history of slavery, and black Americans' consequent distrust of white Americans' strategies, play a very big role.

The "peculiar institution" of slavery involved the most brutal and ongoing massive torture, killing, family dislocation, degradation, and terror ever known; it was quite similar, in fact, to the history of American Indians after European contact and colonization. Many Africans arrived in the "free" America, packed side by side in the bowels of a slave ship and then sold as animals branded and belonging to other human beings. After decades of this, almost all traces of our languages disappeared. Families were separated to ensure the negation of kinship, and our ancestors were forced to depend on the white "massa" for food, clothing, and shelter—all of which were discarded, the throwaways and garbage of white households. We were forbidden education and the right to worship. These restrictions carried on until legislation was enacted in an attempt to protect some small portion of the liberties of African Americans.

After the Emancipation Proclamation, a concerted effort was made by the white majority to damage our self-concept, self-image, and self-esteem. This was planned in anticipation of any self-sufficiency blacks might ponder. This effort was effected through the mass media and by all forms of propaganda. African Americans were, and too often still are, characterized as lazy, ignorant, sex-hungry, ugly, and animal-like. The societal consensus imposed on all Americans who were not black resulted in a desire to distance themselves from the designated demons. So began the struggles of Black folks among black folks; many of us are not sure whether we want to be black folks. Drug use is seen by the majority culture as one characteristic of those who are a disgrace to the race, without a deeper understanding of why some black Americans use drugs.

Earl Ofari Hutchinson (1990) writes in *The Mugging of Black America*:

> The drug plague is the single greatest cause of the escalation of crime and violence among African Americans during the past decade. Blacks, like white Americans, often take drugs to escape personal pain, problems and pressures of daily life. Unlike the white middle and upper classes, they also take drugs to escape the stress of racial and class oppression. (p. 99)

To Hutchinson's remarks, I would add that drug users of African descent suffer disproportionately from an array of drug-related adverse effects: unemployment; substandard housing; homelessness; family dislocation; police brutality; incarceration and recidivism; poor educational outcome; inadequate health care in response to disproportionate incidence of disease; and high rates of mortality and morbidity. These disparities can create a barrier of mistrust that prevents the African American community from even considering, much less embracing, programs seen as imposed on it by the majority culture. Before I discuss these factors, however, one specific aspect of African American history needs to be described: the fact that the African American community has been the target of some misguided, highly unethical treatment in public health programs.

The Black Community's Victimization by Public Health Programs

Among the most significant realities remain the appalling early interventions and programs of the U.S. Public Health Service (PHS). The best-known of these is the PHS's syphilis experiment at Tuskegee, Alabama—a shameful part of U.S. history. In 1928 the PHS, with the support of black church and community leaders, plantation owners, and the Tuskegee Institute (an institution with a history of service to African Americans), began a prospective study on the effects of untreated syphilis. African American men were offered much-needed medical care, food, and transportation in return for participating in the study. However, none of the men were told that they were infected with syphilis. The participants were either treated or not treated. During World War II, the draft board agreed to exclude study participants from the traditional requirement for treatment for syphilis. This study continued until the 1970s, and local health departments continued to work with the PHS to keep study subjects from receiving treatment. This study was finally brought to a halt when a venereal disease interviewer and investigator for the PHS told the story to an Associated Press reporter.

The syphilis study at Tuskegee remains an outrageous example of disregard for basic ethical principles, not to mention absolute lack of compassion and humane behavior. The suspicion and fear resulting from this study are still apparent today. Many African Americans do not trust hospitals or other community health care service providers. The Southern Christian Leadership Conference surveyed 1,056 African American church members in five cities in an AIDS awareness project; 35% of the respondents believed that AIDS is a form of genocide, and 44% believed that the government is not telling the truth about AIDS (Jones, 1981). Is there any wonder why the African American community remains highly suspicious of services offered to them from agencies outside the black community?

Brothas and sistas in the neighborhood caution me:

> "You say harm reduction is a public health model! This public health system here in the U.S.! Those are the same people that used us for 40 years!"
>
> "Imani, think about it, they used us to find out how to keep themselves *alive*! They didn't want us to have penicillin, so why *now* do they want to give us clean needles?"

My passionate pleas fall on the ears of skeptics. And why should they believe me? I could be the Nurse Rivers of harm reduction. (Nurse Rivers was an African American nurse affiliated with the Tuskegee study, who went to black communities to conduct study procedures. She is believed to have been convinced of a long-term benefit to African Americans, despite the unethical nature of the project.)

UNEMPLOYMENT AS AN ISSUE IN THE BLACK COMMUNITY

Unemployment as a Key Factor in Drug Abuse

According to Farai Chideya (1995) in *Don't Believe the Hype*:

> Socioeconomic and neighborhood type are a much better predictor of drug use than race. Poverty, despair and drug use go hand and hand. For both blacks and whites, unemployed people are over twice as likely to be current drug users as individuals with jobs. Fully 28 percent of unemployed African Americans and 23 percent of unemployed whites use drugs. (p. 211)

Unemployment rates among African Americans of all educational levels are disproportionately high (Hacker, 1992, pp. 232–233). Drug use in poor black communities is a persistent problem. I would further argue that drug use among the unemployed is more likely to be excessive and therefore problematic; by contrast, many employed drug users function well on the job. Drug use poses a problem only when random drug screenings occur. An individual's use or nonuse of substances, however, should not be investigated unless and until drug use begins to interfere with job performance in a noticeable way. Many companies now offer confidential counseling and/or treatment for employees with a substance abuse problem. The goal of these offerings, however, is to stop all drug use, not to reduce or maintain use or to use drugs more safely. Sadly, U.S. mainstream society has skillfully used propaganda to develop unreasonable standards for what may be considered successful treatment. In addition, access to these confidential programs is contingent on employment. This is one more loop that the unemployed are left out of.

One practical component of harm reduction is that it allows some people to remain employed. An employed addict typically does less harm—to himself or herself and to others—than an unemployed one. To illustrate this point, I present an excerpt from Charles Faupel's 1991 book *Shooting Dope*:

Following is a typical day as recalled by an addict known as Little Italy for a period quite early in his drug-using career. During this time, he was working as a salesman at a men's clothing store, dealing drugs, pimping on a small-time basis.

Typical Day for Little Italy While Working at the Clothing Store

(CAPITALIZED ITEMS INDICATE DRUG/CRIME-RELATED ACTIVITIES)
7:30 am Get out of bed
SHOOT UP ("wake-up shot"—3 bags)
Get ready for work
SELL DRUGS
8:30 am Leave for work
9:00 am Begin work
1:00 PM Off for lunch
SHOOT UP (3 bags)
SELL DRUGS (most sales during this time)
2:00 PM Back to work
5:00 PM Off work
Eat dinner
6:00 PM SHOOT UP (after-dinner shot—3 bags)
Relax around the house
7:30 PM Hit the streets
SELL DRUGS
Party, gamble, etc.
SPEND TIME WITH PROSTITUTES
11:00 PM Back home
SHOOT UP (3 bags)
11:30 PM Go to bed

Contrast this with a Typical Day for Little Italy After Losing His Job at the Clothing Store

9:00 am Get up (no breakfast)
Stay at home playing cards

Wait for drug customers
SHOOT UP (5 bags)
12:00 PM Eat lunch
SHOOT UP (5 bags)
Hit the streets
SPEND TIME WITH PROSTITUTES
6:00 PM SHOOT UP (5 bags)
Hit the streets
SPEND TIME WITH PROSTITUTES
SHOOT UP (5 bags)
11:00 PM Go to bed

It is not difficult to understand how Little Italy's drug consumption nearly doubled (from about 12 bags to 20 bags per day) after he lost his job at the clothing store. He suddenly had more unstructured time, making it much more difficult to regulate his consumption behavior. Just as cigarette smokers and coffee drinkers rely on regularly scheduled coffee breaks to gauge their consumption of nicotine and caffeine, a highly structured daily routine is essential in regulating drug-consumption behaviors of heroin users as well. (Faupel, 1991, pp. 43–47)

As your moral deity dictates, you may consider Little Italy a saint or an imp. Employed or unemployed, he represents a certain reality that it makes no sense to deny—and I, for one, prefer Little Italy working and using clean needles and condoms. The sheer numbers of people that he alone would be capable of infecting with HIV through the practice of unprotected sex and the use of dirty needles is horrifying. Black communities across America have experienced the impact that one Little Italy who is not "staying safe" can have upon a whole community for generations to come.

From Unemployment to Alternative Employment: The Rise of the Illegal Drug Trade

The interaction between unemployment and substance use, and the impact of this interaction upon African American communities, are critical because our communities have become the "distribution grounds" for all manner of illegal substances. As long as there have been black communities in the United States, whites have "crossed the tracks" to partake of every kind of "vice"—from prostitution to gambling to illegal substances. *The Autobiography of Malcolm X* relates Malcolm's stories of arranging for white men to visit prostitutes in Harlem to satisfy their sexual and sadomasochistic fantasies (Haley & X, 1965/1989). It is still common to find whites in "all-black" inner-city neighborhoods cruising in search of "sin." Young, wealthy whites are often seen and arrested in these neighborhoods while buying drugs, mostly heroin and cocaine (Brisbane & Womple, 1985, p. 175).

This arrangement seems to serve a practical purpose in the white U.S. psyche, allowing white Americans to associate blacks with illicit activities and desires, and causing blacks to bear the brunt of this stigma along with the consequences of being "peddlers." Hence, these very activities, particularly the tasks associated with the drug trade, come to be viewed by some in the black community as the most lucrative and therefore attractive employment available. And the fact that illegal drugs are so often filtered through black neighborhoods into the larger society causes these same communities to feel in a most direct and painful way the ill effects that some community members then attribute to the mere presence of drugs.

Legalization of currently illicit substances is seen by many black people as a plot to destroy them and their communities. This is a widely held belief and a justifiable concern. Why give us needles when we can't get an education? Is it a coincidence that throughout the United States the retail, street-level distribution of drugs is the burden of the urban poor neighborhoods? Regardless of the validity of our conspiracy worries, we are justified in our suspicions of legalization. The history and outcome of the legalization of alcohol serve as but one reminder. African Americans are now the targets of over 40% of the entire alcohol advertisement budget. We are victimized excessively by the day-to-day consequences of too much ethanol and not enough jobs, too much ethanol and no Head Start, too much ethanol and no affirmative action, and too much ethanol and too little compassion.

Ironically, as James DeVidts (1990) states, "It is interesting to note that enforcement of modern drug laws appears to target the Black population rather than the white majority[, which] is by far the larger consumer" (p. 98). This seems especially true in urban areas.

EFFECTS OF THE PRESENCE OF ILLEGAL SUBSTANCES IN BLACK COMMUNITIES

Dislocation and Disruption of Families

The presence of crack houses has a devastating effect on black communities, and heavy substance abusers are more likely than any other group to be thrown out of their homes by landlords and family members alike. Sometimes users are asked to leave because all their resources, both emotional and monetary, are exhausted in the daily routine. The nature of the presence of drugs in "the hood" dictates a compromised existence—one devoid of any reasonable positive expectations.

The presence of illegal drug activity can jeopardize an entire family's safety. U.S. President Bill Clinton recently signed a measure mandating the removal of families who are directly or indirectly involved in drug activity from public housing. This kind of random dislocation of families defeats its purpose. These days, it is not uncommon in black communities across the nation to hear of hard-working parents and grandparents who have been put out of their homes as a result of the illegal activities of their offspring.

The violence that accompanies the illegal drug trade is another disruptive factor that many black families are forced to live with. In *Deadly Consequences*, Deborah Prothrow-Stith (1991) declares:

> Drug trafficking violence does not originate with the inability to handle anger and other emotions. It may be unrelated to the model describing a "typical" homicide—two people who knew drinking, who argue, one of whom has a gun. This form of violence is calculated rather than spontaneous and premeditated. (p. 119)

Public officials are reacting against this violence with punitive measures. Many states and municipalities now have "drug abatement" laws allowing for the seizure of property used in the manufacture or distribution of illegal drugs. Police use "battering rams" in Los Angeles to destroy the homes of purported drug dealers. Meanwhile, landlords aware of illegal activities related to drugs taking place on their property prosper. The residents, however, must live surrounded by the violence and instability often associated with heavy substance abuse. And, of course, children follow their parents into shelters, emergency housing, and homelessness.

Severe substance abuse also leads to a general breakdown in adults' ability to parent offspring. Substance abuse can result in the breakup of families, with one or both parents in drug treatment, in prison, dead, or on the streets. Children are placed in foster care or are farmed out to relatives. It is often members of these drug-addicted families who meet me with the most drastic criticism when I talk about harm reduction. They have witnessed the suffering of children as a result of parents' substance abuse; they are often the ones who have taken their grandchildren in. To these overburdened grandparents, it's difficult to justify reducing drug use rather than eliminating it. Minkler, Roe, and Robertson-Beckley (1994) stated, "The mental and emotional health consequences of caring for grandchildren whose parents have been lost to the crack-cocaine epidemic, and the role of social support and social networks in mediating or buffering the stresses associated with such caregiving, deserve special attention" (p. 27). Lives end up in shambles. A mother may have been using while she was pregnant; the children may have been born addicted, premature, disabled, and disadvantaged from the start. According to 1990 census data, more than 20% of black adults are taking care of youngsters other than their own (Hacker, 1992, p. 72). Too often, drug use on the part of one or both parents has led to this reconfiguration of families.

The majority of black families living in communities pay an exorbitant price for the substance use of a few individuals. The ill effects of media stereotyping are felt by all. Yet another factor disrupting black families is that every state in the union has skyrocketing rates of blacks in prison. blacks in Nebraska are more than 15 times as likely to be imprisoned as their white neighbors; the ratio is 13.4 in Pennsylvania and 9.5 in Michigan (Hacker, 1992, p. 236). For many in black communities, the "war on drugs" is really a "war on black people," an excuse to incarcerate increasing numbers of black men and women. The penitentiary system, which rationalizes indentured servitude and recognizes free labor as reha- bilitation, benefits from the pain of black folks. A harm reduction advocate who is unaware of these statistics marches before a black audience naked. "How can you talk about helping addicts shoot up safely? This stuff is killing us!"

Health-Related Consequences

Indeed, "this stuff is killing us," literally: An epidemic of diseases associated with substance abuse plagues America's black communities. According to Dawn Day (1995),

> At one time a person injecting illicit drugs was at risk of dying from overdose, from a reaction to the substance used to cut the drug, or from hepatitis B. Those risks continue. In addition, a person injecting drugs is now also at risk for HIV/AIDS. (p. 2)

In many African American communities, a majority of residents lack access to adequate, affordable health care, with substance abusers having the least access of any group. Since both African Americans and substance users are more likely to be unemployed, and since health care for most people in the United States is tied to employment, African American substance users are more likely to be uninsured, less likely to seek care, more apt to receive inadequate care when they do seek it (i.e., to be treated as criminals first and patients second), and far more likely to die as a result of prolonged substance abuse. By 1994, over 73,400 African Americans had drug-related AIDS or had died from it (Day, 1995, p. 1). For the most recent year that data were available, among persons who injected drugs, African Americans were almost five times as likely as whites to be diagnosed as having AIDS; in her discussion, Day (1995 p. 1) ties this fact directly to the lack of access to clean needles.

Other Effects and Interactions of Effects

Beny J. Primm (a leading expert on substance abuse in the black commu- nity) and James E. Wesley, in their discussion of the barriers to treating multiply addicted black alcoholics, have much to say about the adverse effects of substance abuse in the black community. Some of these factors have already been discussed in this chapter, and others are discussed later, but their list is worth quoting in full:

> A partial list of socio-political and cultural factors that [affect] the multiply addicted Black alcoholic [includes] (a) the history of racism in the United States and the psychological handicap it imposes on an individual's self-esteem; (b) poverty, unemployment, lack of job and career opportunities; (c) failure of police to rid communities of drug pushers, hence easy availability of drugs in Black communities; (d) use of the lucrative economic rewards from selling drugs as alternative careers; (e) hopelessness of ghetto life; (f) life styles that reject menial or subsistence jobs in favor of hustling and the drama of drug dealing; (g) peer pressure; (h) culture and class conflicts; (i) inadequate educational preparation and the dropout syndrome; (j) rising material, social and success aspirations; (k) breakdown of family life and welfare policies that encourage single-parent households; (l) frustration from continuing discrimination and rejection; (m) constant or occasional use of alcohol by drug-addicted individuals as though alcohol is not a drug; and (n) stress. (Primm & Wesley, 1985, p. 157)

If I attempt to expand this list further, I find that I run out of letters before I run out of barriers: (o) lack of access to health care, as noted above; (p) miseducation about substance abuse; (q) increased risk for and incidence of numerous diseases, especially again as noted above; (r) isolation from family; (s) lack of support systems; (t) lack of transportation; (u) depression; (v) lack of discipline and inability to act in one's own behalf; (w) lack of culturally appropriate treatment options; (x) view of drug abuse as a moral as opposed to a public health problem; (y) the demonization of the addict in the media, community, and larger society; and (z) excess mortality. These are the realities that black communities are facing all over the United States. And this is the context in which the idea of harm reduction will be received.

UNREALISTIC EXPECTATIONS
AND UNFULFILLED DREAMS

Once we in the harm reduction community have acknowledged the acute suffering caused by substance abuse in the African American community, including the reality of devastation that substance abuse has wrought upon the users, their families, and the community at large, our work has only begun. We must then embark on an education program—not only to counter misperceptions about harm reduction, but to deal with the community's (as well as the larger society's) miseducation about substance use and substance users. This miseducation is U.S. government policy, as manifested in the "war on drugs" and the "just say no" campaign which treat substance abuse as a political, moral, and criminal justice issue instead of a public health issue. I maintain that it is this policy, *not harm reduction,* that is crippling the ability of the black community and the nation as a whole to deal effectively with substance abuse. Because government policies and media propaganda regarding substance abuse are steeped in a racism particularly suited to political purposes, it is the black community that bears the brunt of these misperceptions, in addition to the burden of the aforementioned realities. So harm reductionists in the black community must be willing to design and implement effective drug use education programs if we wish to get past "Go" (or, in this case, "Go away!") with such projects as needle exchange programs. Any such education programs must demonstrate the limits of the abstinence model and the need for other treatment options. They must also address the unrealistic expectations black people hold of substance users, which stem from the following:

- Denial, including the denial of multigenerational substance abuse.
- Our culture as Americans, which encourages us to see everything in terms of good or evil, all or nothing.
- The need *not* to play into stereotypes of drug abuse as a black, inner-city problem.
- The strong moral ethic and deep faith of black Christians.

I briefly define how each of these factors contributes to the idea that complete abstinence and the elimination of substance use are the only ways to treat the problem of substance abuse. As long as this idea holds sway (even if it doesn't hold water), advocates of harm reduction will not make strides within the black community.

Denial and the Disease Model

Addicts seek treatment and start down the road to recovery, only to fall off the path and begin using again. Family members who live with this pattern recognize its impact but deny its implications. Some view an addict as a sinner who must be brought into the light. Others see the addict as one who is sick, who must take his or her medicine and be cured, once and for all. Both of these views, which are sometimes directly related (e.g., "God visits disease upon the sinner"), protect family members from the unthinkable: Suppose this person is always going to have this condition? Suppose his or her substance abuse is chronic and recurring, something we have to learn to live with? Suppose this child's problem is tied to generations of substance use, centering on the abuse of legal substances such as alcohol, prescription drugs, and cigarettes—problems the family has tolerated even as beloved relatives have succumbed to them? Might not programs such as needle exchange and methadone maintenance reduce some of the adverse effects of substance abuse, particularly in regard to the spread of AIDS in the black community? Even the harshest of judges who might condemn the "sinners" to die for their transgressions would not condemn their own children, their spouses, and everyone they sleep with.

All-or-Nothing View of the World

Like other Americans, black Americans have been brainwashed into seeing the world in terms of good or evil, all or nothing. In *The Tyranny of the Majority*, Lani Guinier (1994, p. 79) has characterized ours as a "winner take all" democracy. This tendency to think in terms of extremes and polarities does not win any converts to harm reduction and contributes heavily to the view that addicts need to "hit bottom" or "ride it till the wheels fall off." In our all-or-nothing culture, it is hard for people to embrace the ideas of moderation and mitigation. It is particularly difficult for many black Americans to accept moderation and temperance as good options, because our problems are and have always been so overwhelming, and our government and fellow citizens have rarely seen fit to move with anything other than all due moderation and temperance in alleviating them. To these skeptics, harm reduction seems like one more in a long line of insincere, half-hearted, unrealistic, and racist attempts to convince us to lower our expectations and accept our abasement. Such critics do not see it as a way to stem the tide of death and disease resulting from unsafe drug use and sexual practices.

Resistance to the View of Drugs as a Black, Inner-City Problem

Although African Americans account for only 12% of United States substance users (roughly proportional to our percentage in the population), the image persists that drugs are a black, inner-city problem (Chideya, 1995, p. 210). To counter this stereotype, community members often reject the notion that African Americans must shoulder the burden of the "war on drugs": "Why do you people always want to come up here talking about drugs? Like we're all some kind of junkies? Take those needles over to the other side of town!" When asked why he didn't take his "get tough on crime" message to black communities, Boston University President John Silber, a contender in the Democratic primary of the 1990 Massachusetts governor's race, replied, "There is no point in making a speech on crime control to a bunch of addicts" (quoted in Chideya, 1995, p. 209). How does one possibly respond to these kind of allegations, which are presented daily for political gain or entertainment value? Most people become defensive. It's a matter of pride.

Americans of African descent are cast as losers by mainstream U.S. society. Sadly, it is unlikely that this unjust characterization will ever be reversed. Y. N. Kly's 1990 book, *International Law and the Black Minority in the US*, is an in-depth discussion of the realities of inequality. Kly asserts: "There are no known examples since 'The Rise of Ethnic Awareness,' whereby two ethnic groups starting their relationship as slave and slave master were able to create an environment of equality and assimilation" (1990, p. 63). In the light of this harsh reality, black abusers of drugs are accused of living up (or, more accurately, down) to racist expectations. Such expectations require substance users to be criminals, sinners, crack mothers and deadbeat dads. Under these circumstances, it is difficult for those who choose responsible drug use to select other profiles.

The Moral Ethic of Black Christians

"Jesus will set you free." This simple but powerful statement represents the beliefs of many in the black community. The failure of the addict to "come clean" is a failure of faith. And for the community to call for harm reduction instead of the total eradication of drugs would represent a failure of faith on the community's part—a betrayal and sacrificing of our loved ones by aiding and abetting their pact with the devil. As black Christians see it, there can be no moderation in matters of morals. Would one talk about reducing slavery, reducing racism, reducing police brutality? Is one content to reduce evil? It would be foolish to suppose that black believers will ever agree to "help somebody sin." Only when harm reduction can be presented as a useful step toward eradication, and not only as an end in and of itself, can we expect to gain credence among churchgoers. Needle exchange is to drugs what condoms are to sex: Both are a hard sell when "you're not supposed to be doing it in the first place."

In summary, it is necessary to present an education program that treats substance abuse as a public health matter, and not as a criminal justice or moral issue. We can find encouragement in the gains made by Deborah Prothrow-Stith (1991, p. 38) toward recasting violence in this manner. "Stop the violence!" is still a far more common rallying call than "Reduce the violence!", but many people are willing to concede that reducing violence and its devastating effects may be a more realistic short-term goal, and that this goal may perhaps be accomplished if we approach the problem as a public health one. Perhaps these same people will also concede that reducing the harm associated with substance use may be a more realistic short-term goal, which may be accomplished by approaching the problem as a public health issue rather than a moral or criminal one. Still, we have a long way to go among the African American community.

PHILOSOPHICAL DIFFERENCES AMONG AFRICAN AMERICAN LEADERS

Kurt Schmoke, the present mayor of Baltimore, is a courageous and fascinating African American leader. Admittedly, the first time I heard him

I thought he must be crazy. However, what he says is pure common sense: "Unfortunately, our current national drug policy remains heavily oriented towards the criminal law and is mired in failure" (Schmoke, 1993, pp. xiii–xvi). Mayor Schmoke serves Baltimore residents with an integrity few politicians can muster. By speaking out in favor of needle exchange programs, by forcing debate on current drug policy, and by connecting prohibition with the inevitable creation of a profitable illegal market, Mayor Schmoke stands for social justice!

Where are the others? Colin Powell, Jesse Jackson, Carol Moseley Braun? We need more pundits of African American descent to speak out! Admittedly, speaking out is risky. I was honored to be present at the speech former U.S. Surgeon General Joycelyn Elders delivered at the Drug Policy Foundation Awards Banquet in November 1995. Elders was honored for her courage in speaking out on the need to "examine" the legalization of drugs and to provide young people with realistic education about safer sex practices. In 1994, Elders was forced to resign as Surgeon General—in everyday terms, she was "kicked to the curb"—just for asking folks to think!

The unfortunate truth is that black leaders' political tenure is fragile; thus, they will probably be the last political envoys to bring the drug policy discussion to the table. Ironically, a consequence of this reticence will be a polarization between drug users and nonusers in the black community. As the harm reduction movement gains favor in the United States, drug users will affiliate themselves with the harm reduction activists. As it was in the 1960s during the civil rights movement, harm reduction activists, primarily of European descent, will promote safe use to communities of color. Drug users will welcome their aid, while other community folk will feel insulted and put upon. At day's end, the enthusiastic reformers will go home to their own neighborhoods, while the drug users—now abandoned both by their neighbors and by the reformers—are left behind until the next benevolent exercise. We need black leadership to explore options and alternatives. We need leadership from within!

ISSUES IN DEVELOPING HARM REDUCTION EFFORTS FOR THE BLACK COMMUNITY

The value of harm reduction to the black community lies largely in its potential to encourage a number of characteristics and attitudes. Primm and Wesley (1985) outline some such characteristics:

> Some characteristics, attitudes, and achievements of Blacks who do not become substance addicts or self-destructive individuals are: (a) a realistic perception of the "American dream"—material possessions alone do not insure happiness; (b) the ability to solve problems rather than trying to forget them; (c) feelings

of self-worth emanating from a positive acceptance of oneself as a Black person; (d) models of physical, emotional and career fulfillment; (e) opportunities for alternative forms of relaxation or entertainment; (f) experience of success or mastery which develops confidence to overcome environmental handicaps; (g) a sense of identification with a larger group, in whose accomplishments one can take pride; (h) achievable short-range goals; (i) sources of help; (j) un-glamorized picture of drug effects and drug life-style; (k) a perception of self by standards other than normative. (p. 160)

If an addict is not stigmatized or viewed judgmentally, he or she can be seen as a person making decisions rather than a demon reacting to substances. In Primm and Wesley's terms, a user who makes securing clean needles a priority is already dealing with "(h) achievable short-range goals" (by reducing the risk of disease) and has accessed at least one "(i) source of help." The more normalized and less vilified the experience of using becomes for the drug user, the more he or she is inclined to gain a more "(j) un-glamorized picture of drug effects and drug life-styles." And the more the user is valued and accepted by those close to him or her, the more the user is likely to maintain "(c) feelings of self-worth emanating from a positive acceptance of oneself as a Black person" and to find "(d) models of physical, emotional and career fulfillment" and "(e) opportunities for alternative forms of relaxation or entertainment." In particular, those who are able to moderate their use of substances are more likely to gain and retain employment and to gain access to treatment programs.

Adopting a Shared Definition of "Harm Reduction"

How, then, can harm reduction be brought to America's black communities and not just to the few African American addicts who currently exchange their needles? How can we support the drug users in our neighborhoods? To begin with we need to adopt a workable, shared definition of "harm reduction." So many different definitions and ideas presently exist in the harm reduction movement that this lack of consistency is a problem in itself. African Americans will scrutinize and examine harm reduction efforts, searching for uniformity. In the black community, we've all got to be "on the same page" when we consider what's at stake. G. Alan Marlatt and Susan Tapert (1993) provide us with a workable definition:

Harm reduction methods can be employed in three main areas: (a) AIDS prevention (e.g. safe sex and condom use programs, needle exchange for IDU's); (b) treatment of ongoing, active addictive behaviors (e.g. methadone maintenance for opiate addiction, nicotine replacement therapy for tobacco smokers); and (c) prevention of harmful addictive or excessive behaviors (e.g. controlled drinking, moderation of excessive food intake). (p. 258)

Designing Projects within a Culturally Specific Framework

Once a definition of "harm reduction" has been agreed upon, two further prerequisites must be met if harm reduction is to become a viable option in African American communities:

1. Harm reduction advocates must acknowledge and accept the reality of disproportionate adverse effects of illicit substances on black communities.
2. Harm reduction projects must be designed within a culturally specific framework—one that acknowledges the natural talents already present in the black community.

I have already explored the first of these prerequisites in some detail in this chapter; I now address the second.

The Need for Black Self-Determination in Harm Reduction Efforts

Harm reduction programs for black communities must, of course, explore the nature of addiction, demonstrate the limits as well as the applicability of the abstinence model, and identify a full range of treatment options. Over and above this, however, such programs *must* be the creations of black communities themselves. For all the reasons I have discussed above, efforts by well-meaning harm reductionists of European descent to design programs for and introduce them into African American communities will be regarded with suspicion and distrust by the members of those communities. Moreover, I have found that despite (or in some cases as a result of) their good intentions, white harm reductionists tend to reenact patterns of white dominance–black submission in their attempts to work with their black counterparts. U.S. society as a whole is being forced to reevaluate us black folks, and the harm reduction movement is no exception.

Black people and white people are not the same; we experience the world through two different sets of eyes. This is as true in the harm reduction movement as it is in any other aspect of society. My experience has been that those of us black folks who are involved in the harm reduction movement are constantly taken to task, as white folks grow impatient with our prudence and caution. Our racial authenticity is challenged as we seek the normality that transcends cultural commitment and allows for independent thinking. Our actions in proceeding prudently and thoughtfully serve not only ourselves, but the members of our community, who catch hell every day.

Meanwhile, our white counterparts require and demand the full benefit of our symbolic participation. We experience our "two-ness" as our white counterparts' expectations become overbearing. Almost 100 years ago, W. E. B. DuBois (1903) wrote: "One ever feels his two-ness—an American; a Negro; two souls, two thoughts, two unreconciled strivings; two warring ideals in one dark body, whose dogged strength alone keeps it from being torn asunder" (DuBois, 1903, p. 3). We are constantly aware that we are not just harm reduction advocates; we are *black* harm reduction advocates—a rare but powerful commodity!

Nonacademic white harm reductionists, who are often associated with a countercultural identity, have a tendency to include transracial solidarity as a part of their image. As long as there are no shifts in power, all is well. But when black folks begin to develop their own priorities, these people begin to feel threatened. Unconsciously, some of these advocates experience and demonstrate a type of behavior that I characterize as "New Age white guilt." Convinced of their capacity to relate to the "brothers and sisters," they approach the black community with a cumbersome, patronizing, and intrusive attitude that is easily identified by persons of African descent, who have a lifetime of experience with such conduct. New Age white guilt, however, does not allow any retreat from those individuals who, because of their racial identification and experience, are the most obvious problem solvers. Those with New Age white guilt, because of their perceived familiarity with our circumstances, confront us black folks and are not afraid to take us on. They are unable, however, to forgo their tradition of setting standards that create unfriendly environments for black people. I would suggest, with all due courtesy and respect, that we black folks may have a better sense of our communities' needs and the best ways of addressing these than harm reductionsists suffering from New Age white guilt may have.

The Need to Incorporate African American Characteristics into Harm Reduction Efforts

Naim Akbar (1981, pp. 6–16) has described six major characteristics of African American communicative and behavioral patterns. These six characteristics must be incorporated and interwoven into harm reduction efforts for the black community:

> 1. African American Language. African American language is at best a symbolic expression of the mental contents of the group. Our language has evolved based upon certain shared experiences and agreed upon symbols for the expression of these experiences. It is because of the many subtle patterns of African American language and body language that African Americans are often misunderstood when communicating with unfamiliar persons.

Harm reductionists tend to use either very technical language or a loose "Euro-slang" kind of talk that often does not translate multiculturally. Our rhythmic self-expression looks for its harmonious match. Harm reduction as it presently exists is primarily a "white thing," often lacking in the expression of emotions and often responding to the heartfelt emotions of black folks with threatening behavior. Standard American English is sometimes (but by all means not always) a second language for urban blacks. Moreover, the European composure that can camouflage anger and distress is not our instinctive response. We convey our message as we "feel it."

> 2. Oral Patterns. Oral communication remains the predominant means of information transmission within the African American community. While Euro-American people demonstrate a highly developed visual orientation as is evidenced by the heavy emphasis on written material that characterizes American culture, African Americans rely much more on the spoken word than the written word. (Akbar, 1981)

A competent harm reduction effort designed for African Americans must, at the very least, allow for oral communication as a primary means of delivering the "411" (information). We Africans love to tell stories; thus, stories will be a natural context for harm reduction concepts and practices, and harm reductionists will need proficiency in speech and storytelling. The heady expression of people of African descent also requires developing a taste for direct experience and familiarity, unaccompanied by judgment and standards.

> 3. People Orientation. One very important element of the African American oral tradition which distinguished it from the visual tradition of the Euro-American culture is the centrality of a speaker in the former case and his dispensability in the latter. The crucial difference indicates another significant characteristic of the African American cultural experience. Effective communication in the African American tradition consists of a correlation between the rhythm and content of a message or the message and the medium. (Akbar, 1981)

Harm reduction efforts must be therefore transmitted in a clear and understandable format. In addition, the harm reductionist must have a sense of self and realize the potential of the message. We can't "disconnect" and teach harm reduction in the black community.

> 4. Interaction vs. Reaction. Another pattern of considerable prominence found in the African American life experience is the interaction patter of call-and-response. The spontaneous reactions and supportive statements of encouragement involve the speaker and listeners in a dialogue of interaction. This stands in contrast to the traditional Euro-American speaker/audience setting in which the speaker or expert dispenses wisdom and the audience listens attentively and reacts only at appropriately defined moments. (Akbar, 1981)

In the African American community, there is no such thing as a "captive audience." It is my job to deliver a harm reduction message that arouses kinship and recognizes oneness! I try to recreate and expand on everyday urban life in particular, while romancing the complex African American experience influenced by class differences. My advice, therefore, is to talk harm reduction last—address the basic, everyday issues first, and you are guaranteed to get an "Amen!"

> 5. African Thought. Another distinctive characteristic of African Americans is the form of thinking and problem solving that they have gained from the conditioning of their cultural and life experience. This characteristic is a strong reliance on internal cues and reactions as a means of problem solving in contrast to the reliance on external cues. There is a cultural respect for internal cues and "hunches" as a means of acquiring information and knowledge. (Akbar, 1981)

As we begin to create a harm reduction agenda for black people, those outside of our community must relax some of their rigid rituals that are presumed to present their genius. Sometimes these rituals and actions are the reasons why intervention efforts fails. African Americans trust internal cues and hunches, allowing for us to do what is right and fair in a particular situation.

> 6. Spontaneity. Another highly distinguishing characteristic of African Americans is the capacity to be spontaneous—the facility for easy, rapid adaptation to different situations. The capacity to respond quickly and appropriately to environmental changes is one of the African American's most remarkable strengths. It facilitates his/her basic comfort in most settings, where there are positive interpersonal relations. (Akbar, 1981)

Harm reduction will be a spontaneous response. When we are aware of our predicament, those of us involved will be ready to change. We have to feel it!

In summary, without a working knowledge of African American culture, respect for the black agenda, and appreciation of the complexities involved, any harm reduction endeavor targeting the black community will fail.

Advocating for Changes in U.S. Drug Policy

Decriminalization of Drug Use

Even as harm reduction becomes recognized in the United States, its detractors will use the plight of users from the urban ghettos to rally opposition against it. The fact that the use of most street drugs is illegal makes it extremely difficult to "undemonize" drug users. African Americans need to consider the radical notion that decriminalization of drug use and drug-seeking behaviors could serve to unclog the criminal justice system and to halt the cottage industry of prison construction.

The notion that all drug users are pernicious demons determined to convert our children into criminals or "lazy bums" must be examined and confronted. Many an alcoholic held a job until cirrhosis of the liver took its toll. Our society encourages changes in mood and enlightening experiences. Why, then, should the government dictate which pleasures are acceptable and which should be prohibited? The parallels between drug policy reform and the civil rights struggle are based in the same law-creating processes. Drugs will never be eliminated from the international society. Ethyl alcohol was legalized in the United States after a failed attempt at prohibition in the 1920s and 1930s. Nicotine is so powerful a drug that state governments are filing suit against tobacco industries in an effort to recoup revenue spent addressing morbidity and mortality among their cigarette-smoking constituents.

In Seattle, Washington, home of the coffee craze, I meet my other drug-using buddies each morning at the drug house. Our local Starbucks coffee shop is a respectable drug den. Prior to 1990, I had never heard of a latte. By the end of that year, I was drinking a short (one-shot) latte a few times a week. By 1991, I had a real coffee habit; too little coffee resulted in headaches. From 1992 to mid-1993, I managed to quit coffee drinking. I missed the buzz, however, and despite the warnings of my physicians, I returned to my coffee, just a little bit each day. Now every day I have a grande latte, 2%, warm—not hot! I'm clear about it: I drink for effect! I "go cop" everyday, just like my illicit-drug-using sistas. It makes me feel good. My point is that drugs are here and they are here to stay, and the choice to use drugs should be an individual one.

The illegal aspect of drug use is what hurts us as black folks the most—the fact that users have to commit a crime to obtain the substance that sustains their spirit. How do drugs get to the black community? We don't manufacture them. We don't own the high-tech vehicles necessary to transport drugs. We know where the drugs are and who sells them; yet the Coast Guard can't stop drugs from coming ashore. This fact is unsettling when we ponder it: We don't control the drugs, but we go to jail for possession of the drugs. Drug availability also supports the economy in poor neighborhoods, and the government, through prohibition, offers a profitable venture for young entrepreneurs. These entrepreneurs are then incarcerated for grabbing the bait!

Legalization deserves its day in black court. We just need to examine it. Bruce Wright points out in his 1987 classic *Black Robes, White Justice* that "for those of the inner cities, the judges are the assembly line feeders of the prison system" (p. 13). Even judges are frustrated with this system; some are actually refusing to adhere to seemingly arbitrary guidelines such as mandatory minimum sentencing.

Other Changes

Most drug treatment programs are privately funded and unavailable to blacks because of prohibitive costs. Both private and public funding must be made available to finance programs in black neighborhoods, and neighbors must be lobbied to support such programs. Moreover, these programs should not be limited to offering abstinence-based treatment only. As Dawn Day (1995) writes,

> Drug treatment is vital and necessary. But not all people are ready for treatment. Having a needle exchange program is like having lifeguards at the beach. We need to get clean needles to persons who inject drugs so that they will not become infected with HIV/AIDS. Then, when they are ready to stop using drugs, as many will, they will have their whole lives ahead of them, not just a series of painful, expensive illnesses ending in death. (p. 5)

And if we are serious about keeping our youth off drugs, we will need to develop and fund many more programs that encourage them to develop the characteristics of blacks who do not become addicted, as outlined above in the passage I have quoted from Primm and Wesley (1985).

Approaching drug use as a public health problem would also eliminate the need for random drug testing. Only employees whose drug use results in a failure to perform their jobs would be at risk. Many substance abusers, be they alcoholics and/or drug users, are legally employed. It is unfair to target and penalize low-income and blue collar workers for drug use, provided that it does not interfere with job performance.

Educational opportunities that examine the numerous theories, styles, and opinions of the many addiction pundits should be available to drug counselors, trainers, and administrators. Prior to my exposure to harm reduction, I was ignorant of the wide array of approaches to treatment and prevention. As a trained chemical dependence specialist, I regret the biases my previous education instilled in me. My approach was often based on illusion and fantasy; I saw all attempts to examine other possible approaches as deceptions. The simple acknowledgment that there are numerous ways to treat addiction does not mean that those efforts not demanding abstinence will encourage the user to continue, or to increase, use.

Norman Zinberg's 1984 book *Drug, Set and Setting* is a recent addition to my library. Zinberg wrote: "Our culture does not yet fully recognize, much less support, controlled use of most illicit drugs. Users are declared deviant, a threat to society, or 'sick' and in need of help or 'criminal' and deserving punishment" (1984, p. 15). Back when I supported abstinence, these observations would have challenged me. I had to get real. I was not meeting the needs of the people. Rather, I was preaching and recruiting. Heroin clinics such as the experimental ones tested recently in Switzerland (see Chapter 2) may be an alternative to methadone maintenance programs. All I am saying is we must enter the debate. Imagine what our society would be like if drug addicts who currently depend on expensive, illegal street heroin of uncertain quality could sustain themselves on legal regulated, safer, and less expensive heroin. Turf wars would diminish. Addicts would not have to use all their mental and physical resources to stay "normal." With training and support, black men could hold jobs instead of jail cell bars.

We must explore the strategies used in other countries, such as Switzerland (as noted above) and the Netherlands. The Dutch emphasize treatment and risk minimization. Communities and drug users are both priorities. Dutch drug policy provides users with medical and social services, ensures their access to treatment programs, promotes health education for both users and communities, and works to rehabilitate users regardless of their willingness to cease using drugs. The United Kingdom, Canada, and Australia are also going far beyond the U.S. model and treating substance abuse more effectively by recognizing it as a public health issue. Perhaps we in the black community, who are so plagued by the problems associated with substance abuse, could become leaders in the U.S. efforts to bring these problems under control. Harm reduction can be an important first step.

REFERENCES

Akbar, N. (1981). Cultural expressions of the African-American child. *Child Journal, 2*(2), 6–16.

Bell, D. (1994). *Confronting authority: Reflections of an ardent protester.* Boston: Beacon Press.

Brisbane, F. L., & Womble, M. (Eds.). (1985). *Treatment of black alcoholics.* New York: Hawoth Press.

Butler, J. P. (1997). Of kindred minds: The ties that bind. In M. A. Orlandi (Ed.), *Cultural competence for evaluators.* Rockville, MD: U.S. Department of Health and Human Services.

Chideya, F. (1995). *Don't believe the hype: Fighting cultural misinformation about African-Americans.* New York: Penguin.

Day, D. (1995). *Health emergency 1995: The spread of drug-related AIDS among African-Americans and Latinos.* Princeton, NJ: Dogwood Center.

DeVidts, J. (1990). Laws and racial discrimination in the United States: A historical overview. In A. S. Trebach & K. B. Zeese (Eds.), *The great issues of drug policy.* Drug Policy Foundation.

DuBois, W. E. B. (1903). *The souls of black folk: Essays and sketches.* Chicago: A. C. McClurg.

Faupel, C. E. (1991). *Shooting dope: Career patterns of hard-core heroin users.* Gainesville: University of Florida Press.

Guinier, L. (1994). *The tyranny of the majority: Fundamental fairness in representative democracy.* New York: Free Press.

Hacker, A. (1992). *Two nations: Black and white, separate, hostile, unequal.* New York: Scribner.

Haley, A., & X., Malcolm. (1965/1989). *The autobiography of Malcolm X*. New York: Ballantine Books.

Hutchinson, E. O. (1990). *The mugging of black America*. Chicago: African American Images.

Jones, J. H. (1993). *Bad blood: The Tuskegee syphilis experiment*. New York: MacMillan.

Kly, Y. N. (1990). *International law and the black minority in the US*. Atlanta, GA: Clarity Press.

Lusane, C. (1991). *Pipeline dream blues: Racism and the war on drugs*. Boston: South End Press.

Marlatt, G. A., & Tapert, S. F. (1993). Harm reduction: Reducing the risks of addictive behaviors. In J. S. Baer, G. A. Marlatt, & R. J. McMahon (Eds.), *Addictive behaviors across the lifespan* (pp. 243–273). Newbury Park, CA: Sage.

Minkler, M., Roe, K. M., & Robertson-Beckley, R. J. (1994). Raising grandchildren from crack cocaine households: Effects on family and friendship ties of African-American women. *American Journal of Orthopsychiatry, 64*(1), 20–29.

Primm, B. J., Cook, D. R., & Drew, J. (1981). *The problem of addiction in the black community: Clinical problems and perspectives*. Baltimore: Williams & Wilkins.

Primm, B. J., & Wesley, J. E. (1985). Treating the multiply addicted black alcoholic. Special issue: Treatment of black alcoholics. *Alcoholism Treatment Quarterly, 2*(3–4), 155–178.

Prothrow-Stith, D. (1991). *Deadly consequences*. New York: Harper.

Schmoke, K. L. (1993). Foreword. In S. Staley, *Drug policy and the decline of American cities*. New Brunswick, NJ: Transaction.

Wright, B. (1987). *Black robes, white justice*. New York: Carol.

Zinberg, N. (1984). *Drug, set and setting: The basis for controlled intoxicant use*. New Haven, CT: Yale University Press.

CHAPTER NINE

Alcohol Use and Harm Reduction within the Native Community

FRANSING DAISY
LISA R. THOMAS
CHARLENE WORLEY

> Let me explain it this way. Today, Indians are like a man
> who got up early in the morning and looked out his
> door and saw something shining in the road a little
> ways away. It was something he wanted and he walked
> over and picked it up and when he was done picking it
> up, he saw something further along that he also wanted.
> Then, all of a sudden, he turned around and he couldn't
> find his way back home again.
> —MEKETON (1983, pp. 110–111)

The application of the harm reduction model with Native (American Indian, Indian, First Nation, Aboriginal) substance users—particularly alcohol consumers, since we emphasize alcohol abuse in this chapter, calls for a community consensus approach to substance abuse problems. Such an approach includes readily available health care, community and family support, a stable living environment, and a reconnection with spirituality for those who use alcohol or other drugs. It does not relegate behavioral change to one path focused solely upon the medical model of substance elimination. Within a harm reduction model, Native substance abusers are perceived by their families and communities as having the potential to alter their lifestyle and to minimize the negative consequences of their consumption.

The current high morbidity/mortality rates associated with substance abuse among Native groups, and the minimal effectiveness of current treatment programs, have provided an incentive for Native communities to initiate not only a community dialogue regarding the use of substances, but an investigation of alternative approaches for altering substance use (Indian Health Service, 1996a; Swinomish Tribal Mental Health Project, 1991). Current Native alcohol treatment programs generally take the standard position that any consumption of alcohol, regardless of amount, is too much. Conversely, many Native prevention programs are focused primarily on ensuring that the amount of alcohol consumed by the individual is controlled in a manner acceptable to her or his family and community—a principle consistent with harm reduction—rather than imposing a complete elimination of the substance.

Due to sovereignty rights legislation (which is unavailable for non-Native communities), tribes have the potential to regulate, legislate, and control the advertisement of alcohol, as well as to clarify their position on consumption and/or use of other substances (May, 1992; Norman, 1992). Tribal self-determination and local decision making are relatively new phenomena in Indian country. In the last two decades, self-determination has resulted in tribal groups taking greater ownership of health service delivery (articulated in the form of tribal compacting and contracting) and greater control over the direction and goals of health programs. Increasing tribal self-determination and self-governance has allowed for initial change in business endeavors and education, as well as in health service models. With time and patience, the principle of self-determination may bring about significant change in Native communities' perceptions and control of substance use. Harm reduction aligns well with sovereign self-determination. The harm reduction model offers elements of community determination, individual goal setting, self-empowerment, and personal choice regarding change-related decisions—all of which may be helpful to Indian tribes and urban groups who are restructuring their health programs around community-determined mission statements and associated goals. Thus, a harm reduction approach is one viable option for tribal and urban Native groups who are seeking sound, innovative methods for reducing substance use.

HISTORICAL ANTECEDENTS

The history of the relationship between Native tribes and the U.S. government has been a disruptive and stressful one. As a result of this experience, many Native people today have developed inadequate coping skills, which hinder the successful implementation of community change.

During the last two centuries, both germ warfare (smallpox and influenza) and chemical warfare (alcohol) were effectively used by the U.S. government to weaken and eradicate the Native population of North

America, so as to gain access to Native land and resources (K. LaFountaine, personal communication, 1997; Mail, 1985). The initial relationship between the U.S. government and the tribes consisted of uneasy nation-to-nation business interactions, with tribal political alliances with various federal officials, depending upon particular political issues and wars. The federal government subsequently solidified its power base and expanded the objective of land acquisition for its multiplying non-Native, immigrant population, primarily through relocation of and/or war with tribes. Wars and the trauma of wars physically and psychologically weakened tribal groups, creating significant gaps in both population and cultural continuity (Napoleon, 1991).

Alcohol became a formidable weapon in treaty negotiations with which to sway the odds and weaken the articulate. The use of alcohol as a bargaining method in the hands of the U.S. government subsequently became a method by which tribal members themselves could mask the sorrow of losses, the deaths of leaders and spiritual guides, and the passing of traditional ways of life—and, for those who remained, the onset of reservations, the rise of colonial government, and the elimination of spiritual freedom.

The process of treaty negotiations began prior to the establishment of the U.S. government and continued until the late 1800s. The early 20th century saw the implementation of such colonial policies as the General Allotment Act of 1887, the Indian Citizenship Act of 1924, and the Indian Reorganization Act of 1934. These acts established federal control over Indian land, Indian resources, and Indian lives, resulting in tribal struggles to maintain sovereignty in relation to the federal government (Jaimes, 1992). No longer able to exert power and erect barriers to colonial expansion and settlement, Native people moved from being the government's problem to having the problem of alcohol abuse (Lowery, 1994).

By 1832, furthermore, colonial laws had been enacted that prohibited the use of alcohol by Native people. These laws of prohibition were not rescinded until 1953, yielding 150 years of federal prohibition, which in many cases has continued in tribal statutes and ordinances. These laws have resulted in a pattern of drinking referred to as "bingeing." This stereotyped Native drinking pattern, which includes large quantities consumed in a rapid fashion (known as "partying"), remains a common mode of consumption within Native communities.

THE DIRECT IMPACT OF ALCOHOL UPON NATIVE HEALTH

During the last 30 years, alcohol abuse has been perceived as a serious health and social problem within many Native communities. Numerous data illustrate the far-reaching impact of alcohol abuse. Despite the fact that the age-adjusted alcoholism death rate for Native peoples has decreased 37% since 1979–1981, in 1990–1992, it was 37.2 deaths per 100,000, or 5.5 times the U.S. all-races rate of 6.8 in 1991 (Indian Health Service, 1995). This astronomical rate includes deaths due to alcohol dependence syndrome, alcoholic psychosis, and alcoholic cirrhosis among Natives served by the Indian Health Service; it does not include alcohol-related mortality from accidents, suicide, or homicide, which are often alcohol-related (Indian Health Service, 1995). May and Hymbaugh (1989) report that within certain tribes, the prevalence of fetal alcohol syndrome and of fetal alcohol effects is much higher than in the non-Native population. Similarly for the same time period, Chavez, Cordero, and Becerra (1989) recount a fetal alcohol syndrome rate 33 times higher for Native peoples than for non-Indians.

Alcohol also serves as an exacerbating factor in a number of illness conditions prevalent in Native communities, including high blood pressure, diabetes, gastritis, cardiomyopathy, HIV/AIDS, and accidental alcohol poisoning (Bouey, 1997; Indian Health Service, 1995; National Native American AIDS Prevention Center, 1996). Alcohol-induced behavior often results in violence (Kuklinski & Buchanan, 1997; Mail & Johnson, 1993, Support Services International, 1996a)—particularly domestic violence, incest and other sexual abuse, and inner-city group altercations (Beiser, 1984; Trimble, 1984). Finally, reduced inhibitions in situations involving sexual decision making (Rowell, 1990; Rowell & Bouey, 1997), intergenerational family dysfunction, and homelessness also contribute substantially to poor health status indicators among alcohol abusers within tribal communities.

DIVERSITY OF FACTORS AFFECTING ALCOHOL/OTHER SUBSTANCE USE

Great diversity is found among Native people in tribal membership, cultural identity, preservation of traditions, and living circumstances. As of 1996, the United States formally recognized 550 tribes (Indian Health Service, 1996b). Numerous other tribes, bands, and Native villages are not formally recognized by the government; consequently, these groups are more dependent upon alliances with non-Native communities and have more limited access to culturally sensitive services. Until recently, the limited ability to control and allocate tribal resources has resulted in lower academic attainment (with a median of ninth-grade education), as well as high unemployment (80% on some reservations) (Gurnee, Virgil, Krill-Smith, & Crowley, 1990). Recent changes in tribal resource development have resulted in some positive developments in Native communities, such as expanded health care. Within the last 20 years there have accordingly been some changes in the treatment of alcohol dependence, although the primary mode of service delivery has continued to be based on variations of the medical model, with an emphasis on biological antecedents.

Studies have suggested that alcohol and other substance abuse among Native people is influenced by many factors, including genetic predisposition (Bennion & Li, 1976; Fenna, Mix, Schaefer, & Gilbert, 1971; Reed, Kalant, Gibbons, Kapur, & Rankin, 1976; Schaefer, 1981); sociocultural factors (Beauvais & LaBoueff, 1985; Ferguson, 1976; Leland, 1981; May, 1992; Medicine, 1982), including intergenerational trauma (Napoleon, 1991); and psychological components (Bach & Bornstein, 1981; Cockerham, 1977; Daisy & Marlatt, 1997; Escalante, 1980; Forslund, 1978; Hughes & Dodder, 1984; Oetting, Beauvais, & Edwards, 1988; Trimble, 1984). These varying antecedents have provided some understanding of alcohol and other substance use within the general Native community. Collectively, this plethora of potential causal variables suggests that a wide variety of prevention and treatment modalities may be necessary to address the many factors contributing to substance use.

ALCOHOL/OTHER SUBSTANCE USE AMONG NATIVE YOUTH

Since 1976, annual surveys of high school seniors conducted by the National Institute on Drug Abuse have reported that Native adolescents consistently have the highest rates for use of alcohol, cigarettes, and some illicit drugs than any other racial/ethnic group (Beauvais, 1992; Bachman et al., 1991; Oetting et al., 1988). For some young adults heavy alcohol consumption is the norm, with variability occurring in preferred type and dose. Young adult substance abuse generally involves polydrug use. Substances ranging from black tar heroin to "designer drugs," often used intravenously, have become more common on many reservations and commonplace within cities (Gregory, 1992).

Research conducted by Beauvais (1996) suggests that substance use initiation among some Native people occurs between 10 and 13 years of age, with the onset among some individuals occurring as early as 5 or 6 years of age. Notably, Beauvais found that among Native adolescents, frequency of drunkenness was a better indicator of problem drinking than frequent consumption. Beauvais (1996) reported that 15% of Native adolescents had consumed alcohol or used drugs at least once by 12 years of age, and that 62% had been intoxicated at least once by 15 years of age. This finding was supported in another study (Moncher, Holden, & Trimble, 1990), which indicated among fourth- and fifth-grade Native youth in the Pacific Northwest and Oklahoma (mean age = 10.27, 48.1% female), alcohol was the most prevalent substance used by the sample, with 44% indicating use. Marijuana had been tried by over 10% of the sample, and inhalants and cocaine by 7% and 3%, respectively.

Early-onset drinking and problem drinking among youth, particularly heavy consumption per occasion, appear to be related to later problems with substance abuse (May & Moran, 1995). Modeling variables in operation during youth provide a basis for handling difficult situations that arise in later life; some of the variables shown to be correlated include peer pressure, experimental substance use as an expression of adolescent rebelliousness, tension reduction and coping, and a sense of alienation from the larger culture (Moncher et al., 1990). During adult phases of drinking, peer reinforcement and reliance upon alcohol use as a coping mechanism combine with increasing social stressors, such as occupational, spousal, parental, and extended familial demands, to produce day-to-day living conditions that encourage continued dependence upon alcohol for various purposes: to overcome powerlessness (Mohatt & Blue, 1982); to overcome inhibitions and to be more assertive (Levy & Kunitz, 1974); and to diffuse feelings of anxiety, low self-esteem, and frustration (Mail, 1985). According to studies of alcohol-related outcome expectancies, this medley of circumstances thus results in the perception of alcohol as a mechanism for attaining increased social assertiveness, aggressiveness, and other emotional expression (Daisy & Marlatt, 1998), as well as improvement in the ability to sustain family responsibilities (Lowery, 1994).

EFFECTS OF GENDER AND RESIDENCE

Research has suggested that there are significant age- and gender-based differences (Beauvais, 1996; Leland, 1981; Leung, Kinzie, Boehnlein, & Shore, 1993), as well as important residence-based and tribal differences (Weibel-Orlando, 1986–1987; May, 1992; Mail & Johnson, 1993), in substance use attitudes and behavior. Leung et al. (1993) found in a replication study that fewer women than men in one Native village drank, and that when they did drink, they consumed a lesser amount and suffered from less social and vocational impairment than men did. Hussong, Bird, and Murphy (1994) reported that a majority of their sample of Native women (55%) used alcohol to socialize with friends, their partners, and/or their families. Other research has also reported that rural reservation women use substances to increase socialization and to maintain interpersonal relationships (Leland, 1981). Weibel-Orlando, Weisner, and Long (1984) found that urban residence increased consumption for some women and had minimal influence on consumption for other women. Similarly, research investigating tribal differences and residence (rural areas/reservations vs. cities) has found that some city-based Native people appear to consume more substances than rural-based residents, and that members of some tribes abuse substances heavily, regardless of residence or gender (Weibel-Orlando et al., 1984).

Because of the relocation of families (which may or may not have been dependent upon earlier legislation), 56% of the Native population in 1990 resided in urban environments (i.e., areas with populations of 2,500 or more; U.S. Bureau of the Census, 1992). The Native community is characterized by tribal differences, residential differences, and (last but not least) variations in tribal identity (see below). Without a clear understanding and acceptance of tribal self—an identity integrally linked to gender and residence factors—an individual often feels disconnected and becomes vulnerable to alcohol or other substance abuse.

For Native people readjusting to changes in residence and resultant social norms, particularly in the context of relocation from reservations to urban areas, gender differences in health status are quite remarkable. Some have attributed these differences to degrees of acculturation/assimilation. Han et al. (1992) found in their study of the Cheyenne River Sioux that the healthiest women were the most traditional and least acculturated, whereas the healthiest men were the least traditional and most acculturated. Price (1972) found Navajo men to be less acculturated than women, and Martin (1974) indicated that Navajo men were less well adjusted than Navajo women. The apparent gender variation by level of acculturation is not well explained, but is nevertheless important to attend to when one is addressing alcohol use as a coping skill for changing circumstances.

THE IMPORTANCE OF NATIVE IDENTITY

Depending upon individuals' assessment of their tribal identification and families connectedness with traditional tribal value systems, there appear to be wide variations in individual identification either with specific tribal communities or with the general category of Native (or American Indian), independent of enrollment status with a particular tribe. Identification with a biological or nonbiological extended family, acceptance by a tribal community, knowledge of tribal values and language, and capability of understanding (as well as comfort with) the norms of tribal-specific communication are all some of the basic factors characteristic of a traditional tribal individual. Self-identification becomes increasingly complicated for Native people who reside in urban areas, particularly in regard to language and value acquisition. Whether a person lives on a reservation or in a city, the availability of an extended family facilitates the development of an effective tribal-specific communication style.

With the increasing interchange between tribes and non-Native society, LaFromboise and Rowe (1983) have suggested that for a Native individual, developing effective communication skills means "making one's desires or preferences known both in a Native and non-Native setting" (p. 592). Many individuals find the process of developing and applying bicultural communication skills difficult and often threatening, because arriving at a reasonable middle ground of interpretation and redirected conversation takes an inordinate amount of time and practice. Invariably, this action requires switching back and forth between non-Native and Native traditional values and rules for communication. Unfortunately, in cases where this capability is lacking, it becomes even more difficult to have a positive sense of self. For others, regardless of their cross-cultural capacity, some Native individuals will experience significant stress, resulting in adverse psychiatric conditions such as anxiety and depression; in severe cases, the outcome may be suicide (Shore, Manson, Bloom, Keepers, & Neligh, 1987; Neligh, 1990).

PREVENTION

The issue of alcohol and other substance abuse within tribes can be perceived as a community problem, regardless of the existence of individuals both on reservations and within urban Native communities who use substances only moderately or infrequently (May, 1992). Consequently, investment in substance abuse prevention efforts is in the best interest of both tribal and urban communities. Alcohol misuse on the part of some individuals becomes the concern of the entire community as a collective, because traditional Native values suggest that the well-being of the community takes precedence over the well-being of select individuals. The diffusion of problems caused by the alcohol abuse of some heavier consumers (assaults, accidents, suicides, health issues, and family disruption) points to the need for prevention and control by Native communities.

It has been suggested that a dualistic public health approach to alcohol prevention and treatment services allows for education of the community as a whole, while simultaneously targeting those high-risk individuals who demonstrate such problems as heavy, prolonged drinking; driving while intoxicated; and/or increased numbers of assaults, accidents, or misdemeanors (Indian Health Service, 1996a). It has also been suggested that those individuals experiencing major drinking problems be worked with in the least restrictive environment possible (Indian Health Service, 1996a). This suggestion indicates prevention efforts should adopt a flexible approach that accommodates or allows for variation in causal and contributing factors to alcohol use. Similarly, given the diversity in tribal values and lifeways, prevention efforts call for multifaceted approaches that recognize tribal differences, because programs designed for one tribe or group of tribes may have limited relevance for other tribes (May, 1986).

Although many Native community members display moderate to infrequent alcohol consumption patterns, most also experience regular, indirect repercussions from the problematic patterns of a few. To alter these phenomena, it has been suggested that a community consensus should be formulated regarding acceptable patterns of alcohol consumption, and that this consensus should become part of formal tribal policy. This self-determined policy should include a community definition of safe drinking, as well as definition and promotion of specific safe policies (e.g., not drinking while driving or having a designated nondrinking driver). The policy should also address the development of community support for a comprehensive prevention plan, including regulation of alcohol, taxation, reconsideration of the tribal prohibition found on many reservations, shaping of drinking practices of consumers, and other major prevention efforts by all aspects of the community (May, 1992).

The Aberdeen area office of the Indian Health Service in South Dakota in collaboration with local tribal communities has been actively investigating ways to implement such a prevention project with the adolescent population in that area. The Indian Health Service has suggested the use of screening tools, particularly the Personal Experience Screening Questionnaire, to distinguish moderate drinkers from heavier drinkers (Indian Health Service, 1996a). A subsequent evaluation of problem drinkers would be followed by the application of an intensive secondary prevention program targeting reduction in consumption. Prevention efforts would also include a primary prevention component for those ascertained to be less frequent drinkers or nondrinkers, synchronous with a more broad-based community-level effort.

Prevention programs also have the potential to work with the entire community even when less frequent drinkers have progressed to problem drinkers. If this is the case, the Institute of Medicine (IOM) (1990) suggests targeting high-risk individuals for intense early identification and intervention. For those who have developed alcohol dependence, relapse prevention or tertiary prevention is a viable option; at this juncture, efforts need to be focused on the individuals whose substantial and/or severe drinking will limit their capacity for achieving sobriety unless they are given coping skill choices and personal and provider resources are reestablished. For some of these individuals, intervention might include limited outpatient treatment in combination with counseling and educational/vocational interventions. For others, intervention might include treatment in an inpatient setting, with a health care and social services component providing direct and referral services. Regardless of the type of prevention required to address the level of drinking in a community, it is clear that a broad spectrum of services and interventions developed by the local tribal community is necessary to ensure a full range of comprehensive and tailored services to meet the needs of those with no alcohol use, mild to moderate use, and substantial to severe use.

CURRENT TREATMENT APPROACHES

Treatment programs targeting the Native population have been providing direct services since the 1970s, but few investigations of treatment outcome have been carried out (Kivlahan, Walker, Donovan, & Mischke, 1985; Support Services International, 1996b). Efforts to conduct evaluation outcome studies were often hampered by shifting administrative control of these programs, resulting in varying program regulations and expectations, and in a consequent lack of continuity in treatment objectives. From the late 1960s until 1971, reservation-based alcohol services and prevention were the responsibility of the Office of Economic Opportunity. Between 1971 and 1978, the oversight of such programs was the duty of the National Institute on Alcohol Abuse and Alcoholism; in 1978, this duty was finally assigned to the Indian Health Service. Between 1978 and 1988, the Indian Health Service embarked on a major effort to expand services—particularly for adolescents, community prevention, aftercare, family treatment, and urban Indian programs (Burns, 1995). These alcohol rehabilitation programs were based on the medical model and focused on abstinence; they combined a Twelve-Step approach with some alcohol education components, health care provision, and very limited assistance with aftercare needs (e.g., housing and educational/vocational training). Successful sobriety maintenance included individuals' involvement in treatment programs as both patients and later as peer counselors, membership in a Native Spirituality or Christian church, or in Alcoholics Anonymous (AA), and reintensification of a traditional belief system (Weisner, Weibel-Orlando, & Long, 1984).

May (1986) reported that success rates of 20–40% (based on such criteria as 12–18 months of sobriety and sustained employment or lack of arrest) were found as a result of treatment within some programs—a level comparable to treatment success rates in the majority culture. McDonald, Morton, and Stewart (1993) reported that problems for treatment facilities included understaffing, underfunding, and long waiting lists.

Until the last few years, factors contributing to treatment success have been largely unknown because of the scarcity of treatment outcome studies. A recent study conducted by Support Services International (1996b) suggests that for treatment success, younger Native people require family involvement, availability of trained counselors capable of processing post-traumatic events of violence and abuse, and long-term aftercare within a stable living environment. This study has also recommended the development of gender-specific groups for young Native women; these groups should address health, the traditional and evolving role of women, family expectations and personal needs, parenting skills, and financial stabilization (education and vocational training). Child care is perceived as an important need, if not a basic requirement, for treatment success. A survey conducted by Hussong et al. (1994) reported that Native women with a median age of 30 were interested in outpatient treatment programs that would provide stability, particularly social support and access to social services. This survey also suggested that such programs be exclusively Native and provide transportation and child care. Other research by Support Services International (1996a) has suggested that young men, as well as young women, require gender-specific groups; the men's groups should focus upon roles and expectations of men, communication skills, psychoeducation, and conflict resolution skills regarding the dynamics of family violence.

THE NEED FOR ALTERNATIVE
TREATMENT APPROACHES

Within the diversity of tribes, the common factor for Native people is their affiliation with their extended families and, depending upon the tribe, with clans or societies. Unfortunately, this basic characteristic of tribal life has seldom been investigated as a significant factor affecting Natives' use of alcohol or other substances. This neglect may be related to the adoption of non-Native theoretical models within prevention and treatment programs, which minimize the importance of the family within the process of behavioral change. Whereas individually based non-Native clinical models advocate separation of the client from the pathological family and the development of healthy individuality, a traditional Native perspective focuses on an increased awareness of family and community values, and on subordination and assimilation of the individual into the larger extended family and tribal community (LaFromboise, Trimble, & Mohatt, 1993).

Tribal communities are made up of large extended families, with substance abusers being individual members of these smaller units of the tribe. For recovery to be effective, a tribal individual needs the support of family members (who can include biological or nonbiological siblings, uncles, aunts, and cousins) in order to gain assistance and access to resources, and recognition for attempts to implement behavioral change and spiritual reconnection. "Family networks composed of linked households are the central unit through which employment advice, transportation, financial assistance, food, equipment, and information are exchanged" (Miller & Pylypa, 1995, p. 17).

Thomas (1981) notes that relationships between individuals in these small social systems are personal, systematic, fixed by birth and descent, structured, agreed upon, and predictable. A Native person is trained in family relationships and traditions; social position is determined by family connections (Swinomish Tribal Mental Health Project, 1991). Within the tribe, extended families compete for available resources. The importance of the Native person's extended family cannot be overestimated. The primary support system for a substance user lies within the family. When activated to assist an individual, family members can help with the acquisition of housing, financial support, and lend emotional support.

Some families with chronic, intergenerational problems (e.g., spouses of different tribes, different religions, or ethnicities; family members who have transgressed tribal rules/expectations and values) experience varying degrees of support from their family members. These families often require more intervention by social service units of the tribe or by urban agencies because of violations of both tribal boundaries and ethical norms. Weisner et al. (1984) found that heavy drinkers, particularly men, who came from heavy-drinking families were perceived as chronic and dysfunctional by the Native community and lacked family resources.

Historically, behavioral change has primarily been perceived within Native alcohol treatment programs as two-dimensional: Before treatment an individual abused alcohol, and after treatment he or she was abstinent. A middle ground—that is, moderate use of alcohol—was not conceptualized as a viable alternative for those with pronounced and debilitating alcohol use problems. This dichotomous characterization contrasts with the expectations and freedom of behavior allowed nonproblem drinkers. For those Native people who can manage their drinking (evidenced through moderate frequency, duration, and amount, coupled with maintenance of functionality and responsibility), moderate and socially-controlled patterns of alcohol use are accepted. These somewhat conflicting social rules can prove extremely challenging for the heavy drinker, who must thoroughly restructure his or her drinking habits (preferably in the form of complete abstention) in the midst of social norms that support moderate drinking for socially-controlled drinkers, while imposing total temperance on those perceived as "problem" drinkers. In addition to reconciling these varying latitudes of acceptance, a heavy drinker must also either overcome or integrate the emotional repercussions of labeling.

Aftercare treatment has involved reinforcement of abstinence and has depended upon a combination of outpatient treatment with long-term involvement in AA or similar support groups, wherein individuals are dealt with in a reinforcing and empathetic manner from a standpoint that addictive/excessive use of substances is beyond their control. Today, most substance abuse services are focused on a Twelve-Step model of complete abstinence from alcohol or other drugs. Although assessment of success has been primarily qualitative in method (Lowery, 1994), AA has proven to be an effective treatment for a few addicted individuals; as many as 10% of people seeking help are able to maintain long-term abstinence with this method of treatment (Mail & Johnson, 1993; Weibel-Orlando, 1989). Unfortunately, abstinence-based services exclude 90% of the substance-using population, primarily because of the strict requirement that users declare utter lack of control over their substance use and demonstrate a concerted effort to embrace abstinence-based principles of living. Not only does this style of treatment disenfranchise a substantial number of people in need, but many aftercare or treatment programs also appear to provide limited assistance with the acquisition of basic skills for daily living—such as locating and pursuing vocational options, developing an understanding of credit and bank accounts, and devising a process for rebuilding and maintaining adequate family relationships (Weibel-Orlando et al., 1984).

THE ROLE OF HARM REDUCTION IN THE NATIVE COMMUNITY

"Harm Reduction" Defined

"Harm reduction" is defined in the first section of this book (see also Marlatt & Tapert, 1993). Briefly, harm reduction is designed to minimize the harmful consequences and reduce the risks of alcohol and other drug use (as well as of high-risk sexual behaviors). Harm reduction strategies are community-based and are employed from the bottom up rather than the top down. The issues and problems associated with substance use are viewed as public health concerns rather than as moral or criminal in nature. The most controversial aspect of harm reduction is the fact that abstinence, or even a willingness to attempt abstinence, is not a requirement for participation in harm-reduction-based programs. Although *abstinence continues to be the ideal goal,* any steps toward reducing use and/or harmful consequences related to use are acceptable and supported. This remains the most difficult component of this model for many people to accept, and Native communities can have particular difficulty because of their history of tragic consequences related to alcohol abuse (and, to a lesser extent, the abuse of other drugs). However, because commitment to abstinence is not a requirement, the usual high-threshold barrier to entering treatment does not exist. This means that access to and, ideally, utilization of treatment and prevention options can be greatly increased.

As discussed in previous sections of this chapter, conventional treatment and prevention programs in Native communities have been, at best, only moderately effective. Harm reduction strategies may encourage more Native individuals, families, and communities to participate in treatment and prevention programs. This increased participation is a primary goal of harm reduction and provides a compelling argument for the implementation of these strategies in Indian country.

For Native communities, the harm reduction model offers an additional advantage in efforts to reduce substance use problems and their sequelae. In parallel with the Native focus on community- and family-driven priorities, harm reduction connotes a focus upon ascertaining a community's needs and desires prior to determining a plan of action for substance use reduction. One of the core principles of harm reduction that aligns well with traditional Native values is the pragmatic emphasis upon community outreach as the primary intervention context. This community focus suggests that the substance user is an inseparable part of his or her environment, and that in order to make a genuine change in substance use behavior, he or she must find ways of appropriately coping and functioning in the presence of permanent environmental conditions and behavioral cues. Harm reduction resists the dichotomous approach to substance use reduction; instead, it proposes an array of options, with principal emphasis on the substance user's perception of his or her use patterns and on self-initiated behavior change strategies.

Personal goals and methods for achieving those goals are part and parcel of the harm reduction model. This approach bodes well with the fact that substance users are generally resistant to strict, imposed rules for behavior, and instead prefer to decide for themselves how and what to change about their substance use practices. Many substance users find harm reduction congruent with their initial ambivalence about change and tendency to shy away from available treatment resources. Instead of forcing a user to conform to a conventional abstinence-centered philosophy, harm reduction allows the user to progress at his or her own pace, while offering resources in a manner that implies true choice in the absence of judgment.

The harm reduction philosophy espouses three central beliefs. First, addiction or other excessive behavior occurs along a continuum of risk, ranging from minimal to extreme. Second, changing excessive behavior is a stepwise process, with complete abstinence being the final step. Any movement in the direction of reduced harm is viewed as positive. And, third, sobriety or complete abstinence is simply not for everybody. The final principle permits substance users to be given unconditional support and characterized as "normal"; it allows them to choose moderate levels of substance consumption freely, as a possible and admirable alternative to complete abstinence.

As stated by the executive director of the Harm Reduction Coalition (Clear, 1997), harm reduction recognizes harm to be multidimensional, affecting the self, loved ones, and the community. In its work, harm reduction seeks to address both the range and the depth of harm through a combination of practical, direct services and longer-term humanitarian goals. The method for achieving substance use reduction is individually tailored to meet the needs and personal goals of the substance user; goal attainment is supported and assisted by family and community members and by health care providers who subscribe to the harm reduction philosophy.

The somewhat loosely prescriptive process for harm reduction is to provide individuals with continued education, information, and emotional support, thereby enabling them to make educated decisions regarding lifestyle choices and habits within the realistic scope of their own lives. Harm reduction supports individuals in being competent and responsible in their entire lives, including (but not limited to) their substance use and subsequent sexual behavior. Support is offered through nonpunitive responses; mutual support and accountability exist between the individuals and the communities in which they live. This approach suggests that through self-empowered and self-imposed goal setting, the locus of change is shifted to the individual. An individual typically responds to this strategy with an optimistic attitude, which allows for more positive and sustained change.

A Theoretical Model for Native Harm Reduction Programs

The advantages of harm reduction include both its community-driven, grassroots-level methodology (an appealing and commendable characteristic) and its practical, common-sense principles, which can be interwoven with public health models subscribing to the notion that behavior change occurs in gradual, measurable steps. A proper matching of harm reduction methodology with public health theory and intervention development strategies has the potential to result in a substance use reduction program that is respectful of and appealing to a Native community—an element that contributes to long-term program sustainability. Fortunately, the linkage between harm reduction and public health has already been recognized by Native treatment providers, as well as by Indian Health Service administrators. The theoretical model supported by the Indian Health Service (1996a) and harm reduction experts alike as a guide for the development of harm/risk reduction programs is the transtheoretical model (TTM) of behavior change.

Developed by Prochaska and DiClemente (1986), the TTM views reduction in alcohol or other substance use as a step-by-step process that requires rethinking the context in which the substance is utilized. By reconstructing the situations that activate and reinforce drinking, for example, an alcohol user can identify psychological triggers, peer pressure, stressful circumstances that evoke the need for alcohol use, and patterns of coping behaviors that lead to further drinking. The TTM has been shown to effectively predict alteration in substance use behaviors, demonstrating marked versatility and robustness (Prochaska & DiClemente, 1992).

The "steps of change" or "stages of change" represent ordered categories along a continuum of motivational readiness to change a particular behavior. Transitions between the stages of change are influenced by a set of independent variables known as the "processes of change." The model also incorporates a series of intervening or outcome variables. These include "decisional balance" (the balance between the pros and cons of change), "self-efficacy" (confidence in one's ability to change across situational contexts), situational temptations to engage in the behavior, and behaviors that are specific to a given situation.

The model is defined by a five-stage process of behavior change: (1) "precontemplation," (2) "contemplation," (3) "preparation," (4) "action," and (5) "maintenance." Precontemplation is the stage at which there is no intention to change behavior in the foreseeable future. Many individuals in this stage are unaware or underaware of the consequences of their behavior. Contemplation is the stage in which people are aware that a problem exists and are seriously thinking about overcoming it, but have not yet make a commitment to take action. Contemplators are much more open to feedback and information about their problem and how to change it than precontemplators are. Preparation is a stage that combines intention and behavioral criteria. Individuals in this stage are intending to take action in the next month or have unsuccessfully taken action in the past year.

Action is the stage in which individuals modify their behavior, experiences, or environment in order to overcome a problem behavior. Action involves the most overt behavioral changes and requires considerable commitment of time and energy. With most problem areas, the action stage has been defined as lasting up to 6 months (Prochaska, Redding, Harlowe, Rossi, & Velicer, 1994). Maintenance is the stage in which people work to prevent relapse and consolidate the gains attained during action. Sustaining behavior change is difficult, especially when the environment is filled with cues that can trigger a problematic behavior. Relapse is the norm for most behavior change attempts, although relapse is less likely to occur in maintenance than it is in the action stage. People can remain in the maintenance stage for 3–5 years and yet still experience temptations to relapse (Prochaska et al., 1994).

A visual metaphor for a person's progression along the stages of change is a child's "Slinky" toy, a lengthy, spiral, spring-like object. It is well accepted and borne out in practice (Marks, 1996) that people will often revert to an earlier stage, which is then repeated. Relapse is seen as leading back to either the contemplation stage, from which the individual may again attempt to change, or to the precontemplation stage, during which the individual succeeds (at least temporarily) in avoiding thinking about the behavior as a problem.

Another fundamental component of the TTM is the process dimension of change; this element provides an understanding of how shifts in behavior occur. Change processes are both covert and overt activities and experiences that individuals engage in when they attempt to modify problem behaviors. Each process is a broad category encompassing multiple techniques, methods, and interventions traditionally associated with disparate theoretical orientations. The TTM involves 10 processes of change, which receive differential application during the five stages of change (Prochaska et al., 1994). These 10 processes are consciousness raising, counterconditioning, dramatic relief, environmental reevaluation, helping relationships, reinforcement management, self-liberation, self-reevaluation, social liberation, and stimulus control. People use different processes of change during various stages. Earlier stages of change are considered experiential and include cognitive and affective processes, such as the impact of triggers upon behavioral change, as well as the effect of mood upon decision making. The action stage is the point of transition, where the processes of change shift from cognitive to behavioral. In the contemplation stage, for example, the processes include information seeking and evaluation of one's behavior. In the action and maintenance stages, processes include changing the environment to build supports for new behaviors, to minimize risk-associated stimuli, and to develop new responses to these stimuli (Marks, 1996; Prochaska et al., 1994).

Finally, the TTM of behavior change accounts for slips or relapse in substance use behavior. When viewed through a tribal perspective, behavioral stages and processes become a circular process, with the inevitability of alterations and slips.

Bringing It All Together: Making Harm Reduction Work in Native Communities

As just noted, Native people view behavioral change as a circular process wherein relapse is possible. This recognition of relapse as a potential reality has resulted in preparation on the part of Native communities for substance use to recur. To attend to this natural and repeated phenomenon, more stringent expectations are placed on those who appear to refrain successfully from substance use, primarily to ensure their sincerity and continued commitment to remain substance-free; essentially, the level of these expectations corresponds to the qualities and capacities typical of someone in the maintenance stage of behavior change. Given these intense and monitored expectations, an individual is watched closely and with a fair amount of skepticism, as relapse is thought to be a threatening possibility.

Within this context, harm reduction provides a much-needed supportive environment for the substance user, who has a personal investment in changing behavior and meeting the expectations of his or her cultural community. Applying harm reduction in the Native community requires an understanding of a community member's dual priorities: gaining personal mastery over substance use problems, and regaining the respect and trust of other community members. In work within a harm reduction methodology, it is vitally important that the perceived norms and role expectations voiced by the Native community be made a part of an individual's long-term plan for substance use reduction. This element may not always be clearly articulated by the substance user, but will invariably be alluded to in the course of conversation centering upon reasons for substance use, outcome expectancies, and reflections upon how the larger community views substance use. Convergent with the notion that the individual can never be completely taken out of the environment, addressing cultural expectations and tribal values is necessary for smooth transitions between stages of change, regardless of which stage has been reached, which processes are involved, or what level of moderation is realistically attainable.

The model of the behavior change continuum is consistent with many tribes' conceptualization of the true nature of the process of substance use reduction. However, the more tolerant harm reduction model deviates from traditional Native views in reference to the expectation of total elimination of the substance. Although abstinence is the ultimate goal of harm reduction efforts in general, it is not a goal that is imposed upon an individual who voices a preference for moderation. In contrast, harm reduction efforts in the Native community would need to describe complete abstinence more explicitly and concretely as a goal worth striving for, given community values and familial expectations for "problem" drinkers (as described earlier in this chapter). This is not to say that abstinence must be advocated as it currently is in conventional, medical models, but instead that abstinence should be made an alternative that is in agreement with the Native individual's cultural environment.

The emphasis on integrating Native belief systems and cultural norms into substance use recovery programs is not new. Thirty years ago, Leon (1968) argued that only the development by Indian (Native) people of a treatment program, coupled with a new identity, would offer a workable solution to the problem of Indian (Native) alcoholism. The current Indian Health Service practice of offering contracts for alcohol programs is consistent with Leon's assertion, since it appears to offer an even greater degree of local control than was previously conceived of (Hall, 1986). The use of traditional, cultural practices and medicines in treatment has been investigated by a number of researchers (Fleming, 1994; Jilek, 1978, 1981; Shore, 1972; Waldram, 1990; Weibel-Orlando, 1984). Researchers and treatment providers express the opinion that local Native community control, cultural sensitivity in the form of incorporating traditions that are relevant and meaningful to a specific tribal group, and the consistent use of traditional practices in treatment are positive steps (Lowery, 1994; McDonald et al., 1993; Weibel-Orlando, 1987).

Finally, the Native community has a multitude of currently practiced traditional customs that function to elicit candid responses in a supportive manner; these customs are based in Native value systems that appreciate and nurture the well-being of the individual for the betterment of the whole community. One such practice that aligns well with harm reduction, in that it provides an opportunity for open discussion of community members' feelings and reflections on a given issue, is the Talking Circle (Stone, 1982). The Talking Circle, commonly facilitated by a selected, well-respected community member, creates a setting wherein each member of the Circle can be heard and not criticized. It is a venue for self-expression and for learning about the feelings and opinions of other community members; it is about personal respect for others' words and physical space, and it is intended to provide an environment for open group process.

Generally beginning with the facilitator, each Circle participant offers comments pertaining to a previously agreed-upon topic for discussion. The person speaking holds a feather or other sacred object to signify himself or herself as the message carrier; each speaker expresses heartfelt, honest opinions, and is always careful not to chastise the words, opinions, or stories of any other speaker. In a Talking Circle, each member can speak only for himself or herself, and must take personal responsibility and ownership of stated remarks. Unstated ethics suggest that statements should not be made directly to other members of the Talking Circle; this is not the place for working out quarrels. Silence while the speaker is talking is a sign of respect, and when the speaker finishes and the feather is passed to the next speaker, silence persists from all other members until it becomes their turn to speak (Squeoch, 1995).

The Talking Circle provides a wonderful occasion for eliciting community feedback on conceptualizations of how alcohol has affected Native people in general and the local community specifically. The same venue can be utilized as a focus group for devising solutions to alcohol problems; for discerning mechanisms for reconciling differences between role expectations and individuals' actual capacity to meet those expectations; for ascertaining specific elements that must be present in local alcohol reduction programs; for deciding upon a treatment staff structure (perhaps even for identifying particular people to fill new or vacant positions); for healing through prayer and the sharing of medicines; and for discussing new ways of understanding alcohol as a substance that can be managed in moderation.

CONCLUSION

In order to make and, even more importantly, to maintain behavioral change, the Native substance abuser requires a harm reduction model of care that assumes gradual elimination of chemical use, with expansion of life skills, acquisition of a mature, responsible lifestyle, and reconnection with family and community. For optimum treatment effectiveness, utilization of family resources is the preferred method of stabilization for the substance abuser. In the event that the family is unable to provide adequate support (e.g., in a case of dysfunction or abandonment), utilization of the available social service programs and case management services is the next best option; social service providers may function as surrogate family members, representing external emotional and practical reinforcement. These surrogate family/social service programs require an understanding of Native family and community dynamics, along with an ability to customize treatment plans that are amenable to both the individual's needs and the requirements operating within existing network structures generally found in extended families. The ideal prototypical treatment plan involves the family in group process activities, such as Talking Circles, sweat lodges, and larger community events wherein traditional Native values are supported and revered.

To be successful, the services provided by either the family or the social service agency will require an investment in long-term stabilization, with an emphasis on a harm reduction approach of stepwise substance use reduction, gradual elimination of substance-use-related problems, basic life skills training, and reintroduction to community standards and expectations. It is possible to follow a new path when it is placed within the known territory of extended family characteristics. The harm reduction approach provides a method by which Native substance abusers can pursue recovery within treatment programs capable of working with the necessary components of lifestyle dynamics that allow for gradual change and recognition of the processes of change.

REFERENCES

Bach, P. J., & Bornstein, P. H. (1981). A social learning rationale and suggestions for behavioral treatment with American Indian alcohol abusers. *Addictive Behaviors, 6,* 75–81.

Bachman, J. G., Wallace, J. M., Jr., O'Malley, P. M., Johnston, L. D., Kurth, C. L., & Neighbors, H. W. (1991). Racial/ethnic differences in smoking, drinking, and illicit drug use among American high school seniors, 1976–1989. *American Journal of Public Health, 81,* 372–377.

Beauvais, F. (1992). An integrated model for prevention and treatment of drug abuse among American Indian youth. *Journal of Addictive Diseases, 11*(3), 68–80.

Beauvais, F. (1996). Trends in drug use among American Indian students and dropouts, 1975 to 1994. *American Journal of Public Health, 86*(11), 1594–1598.

Beauvais, F., & LaBoueff, S. (1985). Drug and alcohol abuse intervention in American Indian communities. *International Journal of the Addictions, 20,* 139–171.

Beiser, M. (1984). Flower of the two soils: Emotional health and academic performance of Native North American Indian children. *Journal of Preventive Psychiatry, 2,* 365–369.

Bennion, L. J., & Li, T. K. (1976). Alcohol metabolism in American Indians and whites: Lack of racial differences in metabolic rate and liver alcohol dehydrogenase. *New England Journal of Medicine, 294,* 9–13.

Bouey, P. (1997). Chemical dependency and it's specific effects on a person living with HIV/AIDS. *In the Wind, 8*(4), 3.

Burns, T. R. (1995). How does Indian Health Service relate administratively to the high alcoholism mortality rate? *American Indian and Alaska Native Mental Health Research, 6*(3), 31–45.

Chavez, G. F., Cordero, J. F., & Becerra, J. E. (1989). Leading major congenital malformations among minority groups in the U. S., 1981–1986. *Journal of the American Medical Association, 261*(2), 205–209.

Clear, A. (1997, Spring). Welcoming address: First National Harm Reduction Conference. *Harm Reduction Communication,* No. 4, pp. 1–13.

Cockerham, W. C. (1977). Patterns of alcohol and multiple drug use among rural white and American Indian adolescents. *International Journal of the Addictions, 12,* 271–285.

Daisy, F., & Marlatt, G. A. (1998). *Drinking pattern, ethnic identity, and alcohol outcome expectancy: Comparison between Asian, African American, American Indian, and Caucasian.* Manuscript in preparation, University of Washington.

Escalante, F. (1980). Group pressure and excessive drinking among Indians. In J. O. Waddel (Ed.), *Drinking behavior among southwest Indians* (pp. 183–204). Tucson: University of Arizona Press.

Fenna, D., Mix, L., Schaefer, D., & Gilbert, J. A. L. (1971). Ethanol metabolism in various racial groups. *Canadian Medical Association Journal, 105,* 472–475.

Ferguson, F. N. (1976). Stake theory as an explanatory device in Navajo alcoholism treatment response. *Human Organization, 35,* 65–78.

Fleming, C. M. (1994). The Blue Bay healing center: Community development and healing as prevention. *American Indian and Alaska Native Mental Health Research, 4,* 134–165.

Forslund, M. A. (1978). Functions of drinking for Native American and white youth. *Journal of Youth and Adolescence, 7,* 327–332.

Gregory, D. (1992). Much remains to be done. *American Indian and Alaska Native Mental Health Research, 4*(3), 89–94.

Gurnee, G. G., Virgil, D. E., Krill-Smith, S., & Crowley, T. J. (1990). Substance abuse among American Indians in an urban treatment program. *American Indian and Alaska Native Mental Health Research, 3*(3), 17–26.

Hall, R. L. (1986). Alcohol treatment in American Indian populations: An indigenous treatment modality compared with traditional approaches. *Annals of the New York Academy of Sciences, 472,* 168–178.

Han, P. K., Hagel, J., Welty, T. K., Ross, R., Leonardson, G., & Keckler, A. (1992). Cultural factors associated with health risk behavior among Cheyenne River Sioux. *American Indian and Alaska Native Mental Health Research, 5*(3), 15–29.

Hughes, S. P., & Dodder, R. A. (1984). Alcohol consumption patterns among American Indian and white college students. *Journal of Studies on Alcohol, 45,* 433–439.

Hussong, R. G., Bird, K., & Murphy, C. V. (1994). Substance use among American Indian women of childbearing age. *Indian Health Service Primary Care Provider,* 196–199.

Indian Health Service. (1995). *Trends in Indian health—1995.* Washington, DC: U.S. Government Printing Office.

Indian Health Service. (1996a). *Aberdeen area adolescent alcohol and other drug abuse prevention system.* Aberdeen, SD: Indian Health Service, Division of Field Health, Aberdeen Office.

Indian Health Service. (1996b). *Indian Health Service fact sheet* [On-line]. Available: http://www.ihs.gov/9Vision/ThisFacts.html.

Institute of Medicine (IOM). (1990). *Broadening the base of treatment for alcohol problems.* Washington, DC: National Academy Press.

Jaimes, M. A. (1992). American Indian women: At the center of indigenous resistance in contemporary North America. In M. A. Jaimes (Ed.), *The state of Native America: Genocide, colonization, and resistance* (pp. 311–344). Boston: South End Press.

Jilek, W. G. (1978). Native renaissance: The survival and revival of indigenous therapeutic ceremonials among North American Indians. *Transcultural Psychiatric Research Review, 15,* 117–147.

Jilek, W. G. (1981). Anomic depression, alcoholism and a culture-congenial Indian response. *Journal of Studies on Alcohol,* (Suppl. 9), 159–170.

Kivlahan, D. R., Walker, R. D., Donovan, D. M., & Mischke, H. D. (1985). Detoxification recidivism among urban American Indian alcoholics. *American Journal of Psychiatry, 142*(12), 1467–1470.

Kuklinski, D. M., & Buchanan, C. B. (1997). Assault injuries on the Hualapai

Indian reservation: A descriptive study. *Indian Health Service Primary Care Provider,* 22(4), 60–64.

LaFromboise, T. D., & Rowe, W. (1983). Skills training for bicultural competence: Rationale and application. *Journal of Counseling Psychology,* 30(4), 589–595.

LaFromboise, T. D., Trimble, J. E., & Mohatt, G. V. (1993). Counseling intervention and American Indian tradition: An integrative approach. In D. R. Atkinson, G. Morten, & D. W. Sue (Eds.), *Counseling American minorities* (pp. 145–170). Dubuque, IA: William C. Brown.

Leland, J. (1981). The context of Native American drinking: What we know so far. In T. C. Harford & L. S. Gaines (Eds.), *Social drinking contexts* (NIAAA Research Monograph No. 7, pp. 173–205). Rockville, MD: U.S. Department of Health and Human Services.

Leon, R. L. (1968). Some implications for a preventative program for American Indians. *American Journal of Psychiatry,* 125.

Leung, P. K., Kinzie, J. D., Boehnlein, J. K., & Shore, J. H. (1993). A prospective study of the natural course of alcoholism in a Native American village. *Journal of Studies on Alcohol,* 54, 733–738.

Levy, J., & Kunitz, S. (1974). *Indian drinking: Navajo practices and Anglo-American theories.* New York: Wiley-Interscience.

Lowery, C. T. (1994). *Life histories: Addiction and recovery of six Native American women.* Unpublished doctoral dissertation, University of Washington.

Mail, P. D. (1985). Closing the circle: A prevention model for Indian communities with alcohol problems. *Indian Health Service Primary Care Provider,* 10, 2–5.

Mail, P. D., & Johnson, S. (1993). Boozing, sniffing, and toking: An overview of the past, present, and future of substance use by American Indians. *American Indian and Alaska Native Mental Health Research,* 5(2), 1–33.

Marks, R. (1996). Right behavior. *AIDS Information Newsletter,* 8(2), 16.

Marlatt, G. A., & Tapert, S. F. (1993). Harm reduction: Reducing the risks of addictive behaviors. In J. S. Baer, G. A. Marlatt, & R. McMahon (Eds.), *Addictive behaviors across the lifespan* (pp. 243–273). Newbury Park, CA: Sage.

Martin, H. W. (1974). Correlates of adjustment among American Indians in an urban environment. *Human Organization,* 23(4), 290–295.

May, P. A. (1986). Alcohol and drug misuse prevention programs for American Indians: Needs and opportunities. *Journal of Studies on Alcohol,* 47(3), 187–195.

May, P. A. (1992). Alcohol policy considerations for Indian reservations and bordertown communities. *American Indian and Alaska Native Mental Health Research,* 4(3), 5–59.

May, P. A., & Hymbaugh, K. J. (1989). A macro-level fetal alcohol syndrome prevention program for Native Americans and Alaska Natives: Description and evaluation. *Journal of Studies on Alcohol,* 50(6), 508–518.

May, P. A., & Moran, J. R. (1995). Prevention of alcohol misuse: A review of health promotion efforts among American Indians. *American Journal of Health Promotion,* 9(4), 288–299.

McDonald, J. D., Morton, R., & Stewart, C. (1993). Clinical concerns with American Indian patients. *Innovations in Clinical Practice: A Source Book,* 12, 437–454.

Medicine, B. (1982). New roads to coping: Siouan sobriety. In S. M. Manson (Ed.),

New directions in prevention among American Indian and Alaskan Native communities (pp. 189–213). Portland: Oregon Health Sciences University.

Miller, B. G., & Pylypa, J. (1995). The dilemma of mental health paraprofessionals at home. *American Indian and Alaska Native Mental Health Research, 6*(2), 13–33.

Meketon, M. J. (1983). Indian mental health: An orientation. *American Journal of Orthopsychiatry, 53*(1), 110–115.

Mohatt, G., & Blue, A. W. (1982). Primary prevention as it relates to traditionality and empirical measures of social deviance. In S. M. Manson (Ed.), *New directions in prevention among American Indian and Alaskan Native communities* (pp. 91–116). Portland: Oregon Health Sciences University.

Moncher, M. S., Holden, G. W., & Trimble, J. E. (1990). Substance abuse among Native-American youth. *Journal of Consulting and Clinical Psychology, 58*(4), 408–415.

Napoleon, H. (1991). Yuuyaraq: The way of being human. In E. Madsen (Ed.), *Yuuyaraq: The way of being human.* Fairbanks: Center for Cross-Cultural Studies, University of Alaska.

National Native American Aids Prevention Center. (1996). Substance abuse and HIV/AIDS: Intravenous drug use. *In the Wind, 7*(2), 1–2.

Neligh, G. (1990). Mental health problems affecting Indian people. In G. Neligh (Ed.), *Mental health programs for American Indians: Their logic, structure and function* (pp. 25–85). Denver: University of Colorado Health Sciences Center.

Norman, M. C. (1992). Alcoholic beverage control policy: Implementation on a northern plains Indian reservation. *American Indian and Alaska Native Mental Health Research, 4*(3), 120–125.

Oetting, E. R., Beauvais, F., & Edwards, R. (1988). Alcohol and Indian youth: Social and psychological correlates and prevention. *Journal of Drug Issues, 18,* 87–101.

Price, J. A. (1972). The migration: An adaptation of American Indians to Los Angeles. In H. M. Bahr (Ed.), *Native Americans today: Sociological perspectives.* New York: Harper & Row.

Prochaska, J. O., & DiClemente, C. C. (1986). The transtheoretical approach. In J. C. Norcross (Ed.), *Handbook of eclectic psychotherapy* (pp. 163–200). New York: Brunner/Mazel.

Prochaska, J. O., & DiClemente, C. C. (1992). Stages of change in the modification of problem behaviors. In M. Hersen, R. M. Eisler, & P. M. Miller (Eds.), *Progress in behavioral modification* (pp. 184–214). Sycamore, IL: Sycamore Press.

Prochaska, J. O., Redding, C., Harlowe, L., Rossi, J., & Velicer, W. (1994). Transtheoretical model of change and HIV prevention: A review. *Health Education Quarterly, 21*(4), 471–486.

Reed, T., Kalant, H., Gibbins, R., Kapur, B., & Rankin, J. (1976). Alcohol and acetaldehyde metabolism in Caucasians, Chinese and Amerinds. *Canadian Medical Association Journal, 115,* 851–855.

Rowell, R. M. (1990). Native American stereotypes and HIV/AIDS: Our continuing struggle for survival. *SIECUS Report, 9*–15.

Rowell, R. M., & Bouey, P. D. (1997). Update on HIV/AIDS among American Indians and Alaska Natives. *Indian Health Service Primary Care Provider, 22*(4), 49–53.

Schaefer, J. M. (1981). Firewater myths revisited: Review of findings and some new directions. *Journal of Studies on Alcohol, 9,* 99–117.

Shore, J. H. (1972). Three alcohol programs for American Indians. *American Journal of Psychiatry, 128,* 1450–1454.

Shore, J. H., Manson, S. M., Bloom, J. D., Keepers, G., & Neligh, G. (1987). A pilot study of depression among American Indian patients with Research Diagnostic Criteria. *American Indian and Alaska Native Mental Health Research, 1*(2), 4–15.

Squeoch, M. D. (1995). *Talking Circle: Conducting the Talking Circle.* Toppenish, WA: Yakima Indian Nation.

Stone, S. (1982). Cultural program for alcoholism. In J. S. Putnam & T. C. Hansen (Eds.), *Indian and Alaska Native mental health seminars* (pp. 411–432). Seattle, WA: Indian Health Board.

Support Services International. (1996a). *Final report: A case study of family violence in four Native American communities.* Silver Spring, MD: Indian Health Service.

Support Services International. (1996b, December). *Evaluation of the Indian Health Service adolescent regional treatment centers.* Silver Spring, MD: Indian Health Service.

Swinomish Tribal Mental Health Project. (1991). *A Gathering of wisdoms—Tribal mental health: A cultural perspective.* Mount Vernon, WA: Veda Vangarde.

Thomas, R. T. (1981). The history of North American Indian alcohol use as a community-based phenomenon. *Journal of Studies on Alcohol,* (Suppl. 9), 29–39.

Trimble, J. E. (1984). Drug abuse prevention research needs among American Indians and Alaskan Natives. *White Cloud Journal, 3,* 22–34.

U.S. Bureau of the Census. (1992). *1990 census of population: General population characteristics—United States.* Washington, DC: U.S. Government Printing Office.

Waldram, J. B. (1990). The persistence of traditional medicine in urban areas: The case of Canada's Indians. *American Indian and Alaska Native Mental Health Research, 4*(1), 9–29.

Weibel-Orlando, J. (1984). Indian alcoholism treatment programs as flawed rites of passage. *Medical Anthropology Quarterly, 15*(3), 62–67.

Weibel-Orlando, J. (1986–1987, Winter). Drinking patterns of urban and rural American Indians. *Alcohol Health and Research World,* pp. 8–12, 54.

Weibel-Orlando, J. (1987). Culture-specific treatment modalities: Assessing client-to-treatment fit in Indian alcoholism programs. In W. M. Cox (Ed.), *Treatment and prevention of alcohol problems: A resource manual* (pp. 261–283). New York: Academic Press.

Weibel-Orlando, J. (1989). Treatment and prevention of Native American alcoholism. In T. Walts & R. Wright (Eds.), *Alcoholism in minority populations* (pp. 121–139). Springfield, IL: Charles C Thomas.

Weibel-Orlando, J., Weisner, T. S., & Long, J. (1984). Urban and rural Indian drinking patterns: Implications for intervention policy development. *Substance and Alcohol Actions/Misuse, 5,* 45–57.

Weisner, T. S., Weibel-Orlando, J. C., & Long, J. (1984). "Serious drinking," "White man's drinking" and "teetotaling": Drinking levels and styles in an urban American Indian population. *Journal of Studies on Alcohol, 45,* 237–250.

PART FOUR

CAN HARM REDUCTION PLAY A ROLE IN U.S. DRUG POLICY?

CHAPTER TEN

Harm Reduction
and Public Policy

KENNETH R. WEINGARDT
G. ALAN MARLATT

Since the turn of the century, drug control policy in the United States has been characterized primarily by prohibition; the possession, use, and distribution of most psychoactive substances are expressly forbidden by authority of law. Beginning in 1909 with the passage of the Smoking Opium Exclusion Act, legislation passed by the federal government has served to criminalize almost all pharmacological agents that might be used to alter consciousness. The Controlled Substances Act of 1970 (as amended in 1984, 1986, and 1988) is the controlling national drug legislation of today, and applies to all psychoactives considered dangerous by the government.

The Controlled Substances Act divides drugs into five categories or schedules. Schedule I drugs are thought to have the highest potential for abuse and no accepted medical use, and are thus the most strictly controlled. Examples of Schedule I drugs include heroin, LSD, marijuana, and various "designer drugs" (chemicals such as MDMA designed to mimic the pharmacological effects of controlled drugs; see Chapter 6). Schedule II drugs, including morphine and cocaine, are thought to have limited accepted medical uses, but also have a high potential for abuse. Drugs placed on Schedules III, IV, and V (e.g., barbiturates, benzodiazepines) have accepted medical uses and are thought to have progressively lower abuse potential (the higher the number, the lower the potential for abuse) (Hart, 1994).

Over the past decade, governmental attempts to enforce the prohibition of these controlled substances have dramatically intensified. The

Federal Anti-Drug Abuse Act of 1988 established as a policy goal of the U.S. government the "creation of a drug-free America," and was seen by many as the formal declaration of the "war on drugs." The Anti-Drug Abuse Act of 1988 established an Office of National Drug Control Policy (ONDCP) to set priorities and objectives for national drug control, to promulgate a National Drug Control Strategy on an annual basis, and to oversee this strategy's implementation (see ONDCP, 1997).

The ONDCP has come to codify desirable outcomes as "goals" in the annual National Drug Control Strategy. During the Bush administration, the sole objective of drug policy was to reduce the overall level of drug use, as measured by reductions in nationwide survey-based measures. Consequently, 5 out of the 9 goals in the National Drug Control Strategy under President Bush were simply to achieve reductions in use as measured by the National Household Survey on Drug Abuse. The primary mechanism used to achieve these goals was a dual emphasis on interdiction and domestic law enforcement (Nadelman, 1989; Reuter & Caulkins, 1995).

Beginning in 1994, the Clinton administration made significant steps toward a more balanced National Drug Control Strategy by moving the focus away from casual and intermittent drug use, and calling for a reduction in law enforcement's share of total expenditures, while increasing the proportion of federal funding targeted for treatment. The goals of the most recent (1997) National Drug Control Strategy reflect, in principle, this more balanced approach. The five goals for the 1997 strategy were as follows:

> 1) Educate and enable America's youth to reject illegal drugs as well as alcohol and tobacco, 2) Increase the safety of America's citizens by substantially reducing drug-related crime and violence, 3) Reduce health and social costs to the public of illegal drug use, 4) Shield America's air, land and sea frontiers from the drug threat, and 5) Break foreign and domestic drug sources of supply. (ONDCP, 1997)

Although these goals certainly appear to reflect a multifaceted, balanced drug control strategy, examination of fiscal year (FY) 1997 budgetary appropriations for each of these goals provides a different picture. Appropriations for goals intended to reduce the supply of available drugs by strengthening domestic law enforcement efforts (Goal 2), interdicting drugs at our borders (Goal 4), and disrupting and dismantling major national and international drug producers and traffickers (Goal 5) accounted for 68% of the $15.2 billion spent on drug control by the federal government in FY 1997. Only 33% of the budget went to efforts aimed at reducing demand for drugs (e.g., prevention and treatment) (National Criminal Justice Reference Service [NCJRS], 1998). Despite considerable rhetoric to the contrary, the relative level of investment in demand reduction programs evident in current federal drug control spending is virtually identical to the proportion invested in prevention and treatment throughout the 1980s—approximately 30% (Jarvik, 1990). Although annual National Drug Control Strategies under the Clinton administration have repeatedly called for a significant expansion in treatment and a reduction in law enforcement's overall share of total federal expenditures (Reuter & Caulkins, 1995), budget figures clearly indicate that the necessary funds have not been reallocated to implement this shift in policy.

THE 1997 NATIONAL DRUG CONTROL STRATEGY: EVALUATING THE EFFECTIVENESS OF CURRENT DRUG CONTROL POLICY

In this section, we outline the stated goals of the 1997 National Drug Control Strategy and examine a wide variety of data in an effort to determine how effective existing policy initiatives have been at achieving these goals.

Goal 1. Educate and enable America's youth to reject illegal drugs as well as alcohol and tobacco. In an effort to estimate the prevalence of drug use among U.S. citizens 12 years of age or older, the National Institute of Drug Abuse (NIDA) has conducted the National Household Survey every 2 or 3 years since 1972. The results of the survey conducted in 1995 indicate that more than a third of all Americans aged 12 and over admitted to having tried an illicit drug, and an estimated 12.8 million Americans (about 6% of the population) admitted to having used illegal drugs within the past 30 days. Although the magnitude of this figure may seem shocking, it actually represents a decrease in reported drug use relative to previous National Household Survey data. When viewed longitudinally, the data for adults reveals a gradually declining trend in use of all types of drugs since the early 1980s (Newcomb, 1992; Substance Abuse and Mental Health Services Administration [SAMHSA], 1996).

Recent trends in drug use among America's youth, however, are quite different. The National Senior Survey, administered annually by the Monitoring the Future Study at the University of Michigan, has polled high school seniors about their alcohol, drug, and tobacco use annually since 1975. In 1996, the Monitoring the Future Study reported that the use of illicit drugs among eighth-graders had risen 150% over the past 5 years, and that almost one in four high school seniors had used marijuana within the past 30 days (Johnston, 1996). Overall, the National Household Survey data indicate that in 1995, 10.9% of youth aged 12–17 had used illicit drugs within the 30 days preceding the survey, up from only 5.3% in 1992 (SAMHSA, 1996).

In sum, then, it appears that recent prevention efforts have met with little success. The widespread media attention focused on the recent rise in youth drug use prompted President Clinton to propose a 22% annual increase in his FY 1998 budget allocation for prevention efforts (NCJRS, 1998). Though this is certainly a step in the right direction, it remains to be seen whether the $1.8 billion proposed to be allocated for youth prevention will be used to develop innovative, empirically validated programs that acknowledge the realities of experimental drug use among adolescents, or whether any additional funding will be invested in existing zero-tolerance, abstinence-oriented programs such as Drug Abuse Resistance Education (D.A.R.E.).

D.A.R.E. was developed in 1983 by the Los Angeles Police Department and the Los Angeles school district; it consists of a series of weekly lessons taught to fifth- and sixth-graders by uniformed police officers, who lecture and assign homework on the dangers of alcohol, drugs, and gangs. In the 1980s, D.A.R.E. quickly became the nation's standard antidrug curriculum. The company that develops and sells the D.A.R.E. curriculum boasts that police officers working with D.A.R.E. now lecture in 70% of school districts nationwide.

Although there is considerable controversy surrounding the conclusions that can be drawn from studies that have evaluated the effectiveness of the D.A.R.E. program, it is a well-documented fact that teen drug use has skyrocketed in recent years, despite the widespread popularity of D.A.R.E. and the ever-increasing financial investment that has been made in it. In the most rigorous and comprehensive evaluation of the D.A.R.E. program conducted to date, Ennett, Tobler, Ringwalt, and Fleming (1994) pointed out what is perhaps one of the most troublesome implications of D.A.R.E.: "[It] could be taking the place of other, more beneficial drug education programs that kids could be receiving."

Goal 2. Increase the safety of America's citizens by substantially reducing drug-related crime and violence. The primary vehicle through which a substantial reduction in drug-related crime and violence is to be achieved is the strengthening of domestic law enforcement efforts. In 1997 alone, the federal government spent $8.1 billion—or 53% of its total budget for drug control—on domestic law enforcement efforts (NCJRS, 1998). This emphasis on the penal or criminal justice approach has been a consistent part of federal drug control policies ever since the "war on drugs" was formally declared in 1988.

Much of the justification for the current criminal justice approach to drug control comes from the well-documented connection between drugs and violent crime. The apparent rationale behind drug control policies emphasizing law enforcement and criminal justice interventions is that drugs cause crime, and that declaring a "war on drugs" will put a stop to drug-related crime. In discussing the relationship of drug policy to violent crime, however, it is of paramount importance to distinguish between violence caused by actual drug use or substance abuse (i.e., "drug-induced" violence, or violence caused by the actual physical and/or mental alterations brought on by use of illicit drugs) and violence that is a by-product of the high stakes involved in the illicit drug trade (i.e. "drug-prohibition-related" violence, or violence resulting from participation in the violent but lucrative drug trade under circumstances of drug prohibition) (New York County Lawyers Association [NYCLA], 1996).

Recently, the Department of Justice (Roth, 1994) conducted a comprehensive search of all of the existing evidence on the relationship between drugs and violence, and issued a report of the findings. Some key findings relevant to this discussion are as follows:

1) Of all psychoactive substances, alcohol is the only one whose consumption has been shown to commonly increase aggression . . .
2) Illegal drugs and violence are linked primarily through drug marketing: disputes among rival distributors, arguments and robberies involving buyers and sellers, property crimes committed to raise drug money, and more speculatively, social and economic interactions between illegal drug markets and surrounding communities. (Roth, 1994, pp. 1–2)

In 1993 NYCLA formed a Drug Policy Task Force whose purpose was to develop and urge implementation of rational and workable alternatives to current drug policy. This task force consisted of a "blue-ribbon" panel of prominent and respected individuals drawn from legal, medical, and academic circles, as well as from each branch of government—legislative, executive, and judicial, including four members of the New York State Supreme Court. The panel engaged in extensive study, public hearings, discussion, and analysis of various issues within the scope of the drug policy debate. In its 1996 report, the NYCLA task force reached conclusions virtually identical to those reached in the Department of Justice report quoted above:

There is no doubt that some forms of drug use may result in undesirable, unacceptable and anti-social behavior. However, it appears that the overwhelming causes of violent crimes, which often find categorization under the heading of "drug related" are caused by various factors unrelated to actual pharmacological effects of controlled substance upon human behavior. Rather, much of the violent crime can be said to be "drug prohibition-related," insofar as it results from the high costs, and huge profits and great stakes involved in the world of drug commerce as it is carried on in the cities, states, and nations throughout the world. (NYCLA, 1996)

As one commentator remarked, "People aren't killing each other because they are high on drugs, any more than Al Capone ordered the execution of rival bootleggers because he was drunk" (Siegel, 1994, quoted in NYCLA, 1996, p. 14). Ethan Nadelman, a vocal opponent of current drug policy, would agree: "If we were to criminalize alcohol again, we would have the same alcohol-associated violence we had during prohibition. . . . In fact, the criminalization of drugs is the chief source of drug-related violence, and it breeds all sorts of other problems" (1992, p. 210).

In summary, some consensus seems to have emerged that the U.S. government's emphasis on the criminal justice approach to controlling illegal drugs not only has failed to resolve the problems of violent crime, but has exacerbated them. But some readers might object: "What about the government figures indicating that the incidence of violent crime in America has evidenced a sharp decline in recent years? Doesn't that mean that the 'war on drugs' is finally working?" Not necessarily. Even if such figures accurately reflect a substantial decrease in "prohibition-related" crime, it is important to remember that any reductions achieved under current policies have come at a tremendous social cost. The social costs of prohibitionist drug control policies, as well as current policies designed to reduce the social and health costs of illegal drug use itself, are explored next.

Goal 3. Reduce health and social costs to the public of illegal drug use. On its face, the third goal represents the most significant departure from the policies of the Bush administration, which focused entirely on achieving reductions in drug use through reducing supply. Much to the credit of the Clinton administration, the inclusion of a goal to reduce the "health and social costs" of drug use, instead of focusing exclusively on the reduction of drug use itself, is certainly a step toward addressing the realities of the social problems associated with substance abuse. As mentioned previously, however, budget allocations for this goal lag far behind the proportion of funds allocated for the more traditional goals of drug control policy, including domestic law enforcement, international efforts, and interdiction efforts. Only $3.4 billion out of the total $15.2 billion budget for drug control spending in FY 1997 (22%) was allocated for this goal (NCJRS, 1998).

Furthermore, an initial reading of this goal suggests that it might embrace non-abstinence-based interventions designed to reduce the physical and societal harm experienced by active drug users (e.g., needle exchange, substance substitution, outreach efforts); however, examination of the specific objectives tied to this goal indicate that harm reduction interventions are not among the initiatives supported. The vast majority (over 90%) of funds allocated for this goal in FY 1997 were tied to funding existing abstinence-oriented treatment, to training and credentialing of professionals who deliver such treatment, and to treatment research. The remaining funds allocated for this goal were earmarked primarily for promoting the national adoption of drug-free workplace programs that emphasize drug testing, and for expanding community-based antidrug coalitions (e.g., in schools, businesses, law enforcement agencies, social service organizations, religious organizations, etc.) (NCJRS, 1998). In sum, although this policy goal may superficially seem like a refreshing change of course for drug control policy, a closer inspection reveals that it is philosophically consistent with the traditional zero-tolerance approach that stigmatizes, marginalizes, and often outright criminalizes drug users.

Just as the continued emphasis on prohibitionist, criminal justice approaches toward drug-related crime seem to have exacerbated rather than alleviated the level of violence in our communities, so does current drug policy exacerbate the very social and health problems that it was ostensibly designed to reduce. A case in point is the ever-increasing number of individuals who are incarcerated because of violations of drug laws (McMillon, 1993). A report released on January 8, 1998 by the National Center on Addiction and Substance Abuse at Columbia University determined that the number of inmates and prisoners in the nation had more than tripled since 1980, and that illegal drugs and alcohol had helped lead to the imprisonment of four out of five inmates (Wren, 1998). In absolute numbers, each week since 1979, more than 900 new prisoners have been incarcerated (Holmes, 1994). According to the Bureau of Justice Statistics, as of mid-1997, 1 of every 155 U.S. residents was behind bars (Reuters, 1998). The costs of constructing the many new prisons required to house this population, to expand existing ones, and to provide shelter, food, clothing, and medical care for those already incarcerated was more than $30 billion in 1994, up from $4 billion in 1975 (Holmes, 1994).

The absolute economic costs of incarcerating those who violate drug laws are staggering. However, these figures do not speak to the equally troublesome yet less quantifiable social costs that our criminal justice approach to drug policy has wrought. As the NYCLA Task Force points out,

> Imprisoning individuals for drug use causes further detriment to those individuals and their families, destroying family cohesion and undermining rehabilitation efforts. . . . Studies have shown that children whose primary caretakers have spent significant amounts of time in prison are more likely to manifest symptoms of anxiety, depression, behavioral difficulties and juvenile delinquency, which may often be followed by adult criminal activity. (NYCLA, 1996, p. 9)

As for the incarcerated individuals themselves, the 1998 Columbia University study found that only 17% of those who needed drug treatment actually received it while in prison. Joseph Califano, Jr., the chairman of the center that sponsored the report, said that releasing inmates without treating their addictions was "tantamount to visiting criminals on society" (quoted in Wren, 1998, p. A14). Even if untreated drug users are able to stay out of jail, their criminal record decreases the likelihood of successful employment and complete rehabilitation; this in turn has an adverse impact on the financial, emotional, and social stability of their households, as well as of the larger community. Furthermore, incarcerated offenders bring their experience of violent prison culture back home upon release. Many inner-city neighborhoods have already been turned into literal war zones because of the illicit drug trade (NYCLA, 1996).

Another social cost of prohibitionist drug policies in the United States has been the erosion of civil liberties tolerated in the name of the "war on drugs." This erosion has become so extreme that some commentators have gone so far as to claim:

> The Bill of Rights is in danger of becoming meaningless in cases involving drugs. Tenants charged with no crime are evicted from homes where police believe drugs are being sold. Public housing projects are sealed for house to house inspections. The Supreme Court has permitted warrantless searches of automobiles, the use of anonymous tips and drug courier profiles as the basis for police searches, and the seizure of lawyer's fees in drug cases. (Grinspoon & Bakalar, 1994, p. 357)

As the NYCLA task force pointed out, "what might be called the 'drug exception' to the Constitution threatens the civil liberties of every citizen since precedents set in the context of a drug case are later cited to justify limitations of civil rights in other contexts" (p. 18). With the increasing prevalence of drug testing, citizens' rights to privacy have been further eroded in the name of the "drug war." In addition, concerns about "due process" and morality have arisen through increased use of civil forfeiture laws, which deprive innocent families of substantial assets (and sometimes their homes) because of the actions of a single member of the household.

Rhetoric aside, it seems that current federal drug control policy has failed to make significant headway toward reducing the social costs of drug abuse. In fact, many individuals in the judiciary, the medical establishment, and the legal profession have concluded, as they have done in regard to "drug-related crime," that current drug policy has incurred a far higher social cost than the social costs associated with illegal drug use itself. What then of public health effects? Has the 1997 National Drug Control Strategy goal to reduce the health costs of illegal drug use been successful?

Objective 2 associated with Goal 3 in the 1997 strategy is to "reduce drug-related health problems, with an emphasis on infectious diseases" (ONDCP, 1997). Although this is certainly a laudable objective, the 1997 strategy fails to articulate any concrete mechanisms by which this reduction is to be achieved. Meanwhile, the overwhelming emphasis on law enforcement in the current strategy has had a multitude of untoward effects on public health. Because drug use is treated as a criminal offense in this country, fears of arrest, stigmatization, and even removal of children from their homes prevent substance users from availing themselves of the counseling and health care resources available.

Due to the illegal status of many dangerous drugs, the quality and purity of drugs available on the street are completely unregulated. This results in the production and consumption of adulterated drugs, which in turn results in more disease and death from drug use than would be the case if production and distribution were regulated—for example, by the Food and Drug Administration (Association of the Bar of the City of New York, 1994; Nadelman, 1998). In sum,

> It appears that present drug control laws themselves have directly led to an increase in the health risks associated with drug use and substance abuse. In addition to those dangers posed by lack of quality control and safety regulations governing illegal drugs, drug paraphernalia laws, together with a failure to promote needle exchange programs, have resulted in the preventable spread of AIDS and other similarly transmitted diseases to users, their partners and children. (NYCLA, 1996, p. 11)

Goal 4. Shield America's air, land, and sea frontiers from the drug threat; and Goal 5. Break foreign and domestic drug sources of supply. The final two goals constitute the primary emphasis of U.S. international drug control and interdiction efforts. They accounted for approximately $5 billion (33%) of total drug control spending in FY 1997, equivalent to the budget for all treatment and prevention efforts combined (NCJRS, 1998). In essence, these goals are aimed at stopping the movement of drugs from the sources of production to the United States, and at curbing production of drugs in foreign nations. To these ends, the federal government spends billions of dollars annually to help source and transit countries to eradicate crops and destroy major drug-trafficking organizations, as well as to conduct "flexible operations to detect, disrupt, deter and seize illegal drugs in transit to the United States and the U.S. borders" (ONDCP, 1997, Goal 4, Objective 1).

In February 1997, pursuant to a congressional request, the U.S. General Accounting Office (GAO) summarized the findings of its previous work on international drug control and interdiction efforts, focusing on "1) the effectiveness of U.S. efforts to combat drug production and the movement of drugs into the United States; 2) Obstacles to implementation of U.S. drug control efforts; and 3) suggestions to improve operational effectiveness" (U.S. GAO, 1997). In the process of preparing the summary report, investigators reviewed 59 prior GAO reports. They also

> . . . spoke with appropriate officials and reviewed planning documents, studies, cables, and correspondence at the Departments of Defense, State, and Justice— primarily the Drug Enforcement Agency; the U.S. Coast Guard, the U.S.

Customs Service; the U.S. Agency for International Development; the U.S. Interdiction Coordinator; and ONDCP in Washington D.C. (U.S. GAO, 1997)

The investigative team from the GAO'S Office of International Relations and Trade Issues also met with senior Bolivian, Peruvian, and United Nations law enforcement and drug control officials responsible for counternarcotics programs. In a surprisingly candid appraisal, the GAO investigators concluded:

> Despite long-standing efforts and expenditures of billions of dollars, illegal drugs still flood the United States. We have reported on obstacles faced by the United States and host countries in their efforts to reduce illegal drug supplies. Although these efforts have resulted in some successes, including the arrest of traffickers and the eradication, seizure, and disruption of the transport of illegal drugs, they have not materially reduced the availability of drugs. (U.S. GAO, 1997)

The report went on to identify a plethora of reasons for U.S. counternarcotics programs' lack of success: (1) drug traffickers have become sophisticated, multibillion-dollar industries that quickly adapt to U.S. drug control efforts; (2) efforts are constrained in source and transit countries by competing economic and political policies; and (3) drug traffickers are increasingly resourceful in corrupting source and transit countries' institutions. We would like to offer an additional, more parsimonious reason for the failure of U.S. efforts to reduce the supply of illegal drugs. Simply put, where there is demand, supply will follow. As William S. Burroughs (1959) observed in his novel "Naked Lunch,"

> The addict in the street who must have junk to live is the one irreplaceable factor in the junk equation. When there are no more addicts to buy junk there will be no junk traffic. As long as junk need exists, someone will service it. (p. xi)

SUPPLY REDUCTION, DEMAND REDUCTION, USE REDUCTION, AND HARM REDUCTION

Use Reduction: The Common Goal of Supply and Demand Reduction

Although the National Drug Control Strategy has evolved to become what appears to be a multicomponent, balanced strategy, its overwhelming emphasis has always been and continues to be reducing the *supply* of available drugs. In recent years, however, there has been growing acknowledgment that prevention and treatment efforts designed to reduce the *demand* for illegal drugs should constitute an integral component of drug control policy. Increasing investment in demand reduction efforts constitutes a welcome change for U.S. drug control policy. What many fail to recognize, however, is this

> ... despite their disagreements, demand-side and supply-side advocates share a common allegiance to what might be called the *use reduction* paradigm. This is the view that the highest, if not exclusive, goal of drug policy should be to reduce (and if possible, to eliminate) psychoactive drug use. (MacCoun, in press)

The stated goal of the 1988 Anti-Drug Abuse Act was, after all, the "creation of a drug-free America."

A troublesome conclusion that emerges from our critique of contemporary drug control strategy is that the desired reductions in the prevalence of use have simply not been achieved. In fact, the data suggest that drug use among teens has been steadily increasing in recent years. Even more disturbing is the fact that the strengthened law enforcement and interdiction efforts constituting the primary focus of the current strategy are themselves a source of many drug-related problems, such as drug-prohibition-related crime (Nadelmann, 1989).

Distinguishing Use Reduction from Harm Reduction

The use reduction paradigm as it is embodied in the 1997 National Drug Control Strategy consists of a host of policies and interventions whose collective aim is to achieve total prohibition of illicit drugs. Thus, current prohibition policy is driven by a set of assumptions in which behavior is forbidden and infractions are subject to punishment; the objective is total suppression (Glazer, 1974, cited in Erikson, 1990). Such an objective in turn requires the assumption that the criminal justice approach could conceivably result in the total suppression of drug use in U.S. society (i.e., the "creation of a drug-free America"). Other assumptions underlying the prohibitionist perspective are that drugs (and drug users) are essentially immoral; that psychoactive drugs are inherently dangerous; and that legal proscriptions on drug use are necessary to protect the well-being of users, the people around them, and society at large.

An alternative set of interventions, programs, and policies, collectively referred to as "harm reduction," has been advocated throughout this book. The harm reduction approach entails quite a different set of goals and assumptions. According to one commentator, these alternative approaches are, to varying degrees "based on the premise that the desire to alter consciousness is a normal human trait, a drive as deep as the need for food, shelter and love (Siegel, 1989; Weil, 1972)" (Aldrich, 1990, p. 547). Harm reduction advocates argue that this motivation to alter consciousness and subjective mood states has led people to use drugs for their psychoactive properties throughout recorded history. Despite the best efforts of those working in the criminal justice system, this inherent desire to alter consciousness also ensures that people will continue to use drugs in the future. Harm reduction proponents thus recognize the futility of trying to eliminate drug use entirely; they focus on identifying the best ways to minimize the harm that results from drug use, rather than on attempting to eliminate it altogether. Other assumptions underlying the harm reduction perspective are that certain psychoactive drugs are relatively safe; that decisions to use drugs are not inherently immoral; and that drug users are not malicious criminals, but individuals with maladaptive habits in need of treatment.

Public health professionals have taken the lead in promoting harm reduction as an alternative to traditional drug policy approaches in the United States. Des Jarlais (1995), in an editorial for the *American Journal of Public Health*, has described harm reduction as consisting of the following working list of basic components:

1. Nonmedical use of psychoactive drugs is inevitable in any society that has access to such drugs. Drug policies cannot be based on a utopian belief that nonmedical drug use will be eliminated.
2. Nonmedical drug use will inevitably produce important social and individual harm. Drug policies cannot be based on a utopian belief that all drug users will always use drugs safely.
3. Drug policies must be pragmatic. They must be assessed on their actual consequences, not on whether they symbolically send the right, the wrong, or mixed messages.
4. Drug users are an integral part of the larger community. Protecting the health of the community as a whole therefore requires protecting the health of drug users, and this requires integrating the drug users within the community rather than attempting to isolate them from it.
5. Drug use leads to individual and social harms through many different mechanisms, so a wide range of interventions is needed to address these harms. These interventions include providing health care (including drug abuse treatment) to drug users; reducing the number of persons who are likely to begin using some drugs; and particularly, enabling users to switch to safer forms of drug use. It is not always necessary to reduce nonmedical drug use in order to reduce harms. The harm reduction perspective thus would be particularly amenable to using research findings. . . . The harm reduction perspective emphasizes the need to base policy on research rather than on stereotypes of (legal and illegal) drug users. (Des Jarlais, 1995, pp. 10–11)

Of the wide variety of harm reduction interventions described throughout this volume, those that have received the highest level of support within recent National Drug Control Strategies are those interventions designed to reduce demand. This certainly makes sense, for strategies designed to reduce both supply and demand have as their primary objective achieving reductions in use, and use reduction remains the primary goal of U.S. drug control policy.

Demand Reduction as Harm Reduction

"The initial step [in the adoption of harm-reduction strategies] is to reduce reliance on criminal justice measures against users and develop proactive, creative health promotion and protection strategies to achieve demand reduction . . . [for] supply reduction will not work as long as demand is maintained" (Erikson, 1990, p. 567). Strategies designed to reduce demand can be thought of as the most effective subset of harm reduction strategies, for the least harm occurs when drugs are not used at all. For example, prevention efforts focused on discouraging drug use before it begins not only reduce but eliminate the harm that can result from such use. Similarly, users who successfully complete a treatment program through which they are able to achieve and maintain abstinence have thus eliminated their demand for drugs and the resultant harm to themselves and their communities.

Efforts to delay or eliminate the onset of drug use are referred to as "primary" or "universal" prevention; such efforts typically focus on education as a means of maintaining abstinence. When drug use or experimentation has already begun but has not yet engendered significant problems for the user, educational efforts designed to eliminate or minimize the harm resulting from such use are referred to as "secondary" or "selective" prevention. If primary and secondary prevention efforts fail, and an individual's substance use becomes problematic, they typically receive substance abuse treatment—which is sometimes referred to as "tertiary" or "indicated" prevention (Institute of Medicine, 1994).

Most primary and secondary prevention programs (including the D.A.R.E. program) have been derived from the social influences model. The social influences model posits that adolescent substance abuse is initiated and maintained because of social influences, both direct (parents, peers) and indirect (the mass media) (Marlatt, Baer, & Quigley, 1995). Social inoculation theory (see Donaldson, Graham, Piccinin, & Hansen, 1995) recognizes that adolescents' decisions about whether or not to use alcohol or other drugs depends upon their ability to resist these overwhelming social pressures. The goal of prevention programs developed under these models is to inoculate children against these untoward social influences.

Although advocates of the social influences and social inoculation models can certainly point to a few successes, such as the Minnesota Smoking Prevention Program (Luepker, Johnson, Murray, & Pechacek, 1983) and the Life Skills Training Program (Dusenbury, Botvin, & James-Ortiz, 1989), evaluations of the impact of resistance skills training programs such as D.A.R.E. have generally failed to show overall effects (e.g. Donaldson et al., 1995; Ennett et al., 1994). Future prevention programs must go beyond the confines of present theories by incorporating student input in program development.

The second modality of demand reduction that has been employed within the context of a larger policy of drug prohibition is substance abuse treatment. As the ONDCP (1997) points out, "effective treatment programs can help individuals end dependence on addictive drugs, thereby reducing consumption. In addition, such programs can reduce indirectly the consequences of addictive drug use on the rest of society" (p. 54). A widely cited study conducted by the California Department of Alcohol and Drug Problems (Gerstein et al., 1994) estimated that $209 million cost of providing treatment for 150,000 individuals in 1991–1992 generated an estimated $1.5 billion in savings—a 7:1 return on investment. The U.S. Government's 1996 Treatment Improvement Evaluation Study concurred with Gerstein et al.'s (1994) findings that treatment reduces drug use from 40 to 50 percent, that health improves after treatment, and that all types of treatment can be effective (Center for Substance Abuse Treatment, 1996).

It stands to reason, however, that treatment can only be effective for those drug users who are actually able to gain entrance to a treatment program. The ONDCP is cognizant of the barriers that present users from seeking treatment:

> The willingness of chronic drug users to undergo treatment is influenced by the availability of treatment programs, affordability of services, access to publicly-funded programs or medical coverage, personal motivation, family and employer support, and potential consequences of admitting a dependency problem. (ONDCP, 1997, p. 56)

Under current policies, these "potential consequences" include arrest, incarceration, seizure of assets and property, loss of one's job, or loss of child custody. Furthermore, "in many communities, the demand for help far exceeds treatment capacity. Being unable to enter treatment may discourage chronic users from maintaining a commitment to end chemical dependency" (ONDCP, 1997, p. 56).

The ONDCP identified lowering entry barriers to treatment programs as one of its 1997 initiatives to reduce health and social problems. The main focus of this initiative seems to be on increasing the number of available publicly funded treatment slots. Although this would certainly be welcome, supplying enough slots in traditional substance abuse treatment programs to meet demand is not enough. In the context of current public policy, even if free treatment on demand were available for every person who indicated that he or she wanted to stop using substances, many would stay away from treatment. Why? By the very nature of the fact that certain individuals have a "problem" with drugs, they are unable to maintain sobriety. Unfortunately, the U.S. treatment establishment perceives total abstinence as the only acceptable treatment outcome; consequently, treatment centers routinely discharge clients who can't stop using, as well as those who resume use after a period of abstinence.

Substance abuse treatment in the U.S. is high-threshold not only because there are not enough slots available. It is high-threshold because it generally requires complete abstinence; typically employs aggressive and confrontational tactics; and, perhaps most importantly, operates within an official federal policy that treats users as criminals who have much to lose by presenting themselves for treatment (see Marlatt, 1996). Despite the progress that has been made in recent years toward developing treatment interventions that reduce the psychological barriers to treatment entry (Miller & Heather, in press), substance abuse treatment in the United States continues to be high-threshold because the legal barriers caused by prohibitionist drug control policies remain in place.

In summary, prevention and treatment efforts designed to reduce demand for drugs are an important subset of harm reduction strategies. However, the harm reduction approach goes beyond efforts to decrease the prevalence of substance use by acknowledging the fact that some individuals will inevitably be unwilling or unable to reduce their levels of drug use. Under current U.S. policies, these individuals are marginalized and criminalized. If prevention and treatment strategies are unsuccessful for some subset of the population who cannot remain abstinent, then innovative harm reduction strategies, such as needle exchange, substance substitution, and changing the route of drug administration, can be employed to minimize the adverse effects of their use. Unfortunately, numerous obstacles must be overcome before harm reduction proponents will be able to bring about any fundamental change in U.S. drug control policy. Before we turn our attention to a discussion of current public debate surrounding the adoption of harm reduction strategies, however, a point of clarification is in order.

HARM REDUCTION IS NOT LEGALIZATION

As Nadelman (1998) points out,

> Most proponents of harm reduction do not favor legalization. They recognize that prohibition has failed to curtail drug abuse, that it is responsible for much of the crime, corruption, disease, and death associated with drugs, and that its costs mount every year. But they also see legalization as politically unwise and as risking increased drug use. (pp. 113–114)

Drug policy "alternatives are best understood not as polar opposites, but as a variety of points along a spectrum, with the most prohibitionist policies at one extreme, and the most libertarian ones at the other" (Nadelmann, 1992, p. 205). The harm reduction approach is compatible with a wide range of policy options that lie on the spectrum between total legalization and total prohibition. This spectrum is represented graphically as the continuum of policy options in Figure 10.1.

By this point, the reader should be familiar with the policy option at the extreme right of Figure 10.1. This policy of "total prohibition" is currently the law of the land in the United States. The policy option at the extreme left of the figure, labeled "total legalization," is the libertarian position that thoughts and conduct concerning the substances one chooses to ingest should be free from governmental control, interference, or restriction. Consequently, advocates of total legalization believe that all substances that are currently controlled by the government should be available on a completely unregulated free market.

Although supporters of prohibition policies sometimes act as if total legalization is the only alternative to prohibition, a good many policy options lie between these two extremes. In one class of policy options, drugs are legalized, but the government exercises varying degrees of control over the markets in which they are bought and sold. For example, in the "controlled availability" option (Chesher & Wodack, 1990), some or all controlled substances would be available through a government monopoly, outside of which criminal sanctions would be used to police drug sales. In this option, federal and state governments could regulate the sale and possession of illicit drugs in the same way they currently regulate alcohol and tobacco products.

Similarly, in the "medicalization" option, drugs would be made legal, but would only be available to drug-dependent users with a prescription from a medical practitioner. With medicalization, criminal justice sanctions would also be employed against those who buy or sell drugs outside official channels. The medicalization option was recently brought to the forefront of public consciousness when voters in the November 1996 elections passed initiatives making medicinal marijuana available in both California and Arizona. In California, Proposition 215 requires only an oral "doctor's recommendation" for marijuana use by patients with AIDS, cancer, glaucoma, or other illnesses (Pollan, 1997). In Arizona, Proposition 200 requires a written prescription from two licensed physicians for medicinal

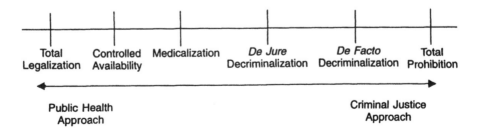

FIGURE 10.1. Spectrum of drug control policies.

marijuana, and limits its availability to persons afflicted with the most serious illnesses; this proposition also mandates treatment and probation instead of incarceration for most people convicted of drug use and possession (Ferguson, 1997). In a striking testament to the federal government's commitment to current policies of total prohibition and use reduction, both propositions were quickly subjected to legal challenges.

In another class of policy options, known as "decriminalization," the possession, use, and distribution of psychoactive substances would continue to be expressly forbidden by authority of law (i.e., drugs would remain illegal), but penalties for the violation of such laws would be reduced, eliminated, or selectively enforced "on condition that the quantity of the drug is below a defined level considered to be for personal use only" (Chesher & Wodack, 1990, p. 556). If the criminal penalties for drug law violations are officially reduced or eliminated via legislative action, the policy is referred to as "simple decriminalization" or "*de jure* decriminalization" (Bertrand, 1990). If criminal penalties remain on the books, but law enforcement agencies are allowed considerable discretion in deciding whether or not to enforce them (particularly the penalties applying to those substances deemed least addictive or offensive), the policy is referred to as "*de facto* decriminalization" (Bertrand, 1990). The Dutch have embraced this policy option and have used it in their attempt to "normalize" drug users without officially condoning their drug use. Hence "normalization" refers to a policy of *de facto* decriminalization.

To varying degrees, harm reduction interventions are compatible with every one of these policy options, including prohibition. For example, under a policy of medicalization, addicts would be able to reduce the risk of infection and overdose by having access to sterile injection equipment and drugs of known quality and purity. Furthermore, medicalization would bring addicts into contact with health and social resources that they might not otherwise avail themselves of. As reported in Chapter 2, the Swiss government conducted a 3-year nationwide trial of a medicalization scheme, wherein approximately 1,000 heroin addicts with at least two unsuccessful treatment attempts were given legal prescriptions to use heroin. In July 1997, the Swiss government reported that criminal offenses and the number of criminal offenders among study participants had dropped 60%, that participants' illegal heroin and cocaine use had declined dramatically, that their stable employment had increased from 14% to 32% and that their physical health had improved dramatically (Nadelmann, 1998, p. 120).

Official drug control policies of decriminalization, both *de facto* and *de jure,* are also quite compatible with the harm reduction approach. In Europe, harm reduction strategies such as needle exchange, condom distribution, street outreach, and the establishment of safe, sanitary "injection rooms" have been successfully pursued within the context of an official drug control policy of *de facto* decriminalization (see Nadelmann, 1998, and Chapter 2). Even in the context of the official U.S. policy of total prohibition, some harm reduction policies have taken root. For example, 115,000 Americans are currently enrolled in federally monitored methadone maintenance programs. Although these programs only have enough openings to treat 10–20% of heroin addicts, and many argue that methadone maintenance should be integrated with mainstream medicine (as it has been in Europe, Australia, New Zealand, and Canada; Nadelmann, 1998), the very existence of oral methadone treatment in the United States reminds us that harm reduction interventions and any official drug control policy are not necessarily mutually exclusive. However, it stands to reason that the farther one moves away from the "total prohibition" end of the spectrum, the easier it is to implement strategies that are designed to reduce drug-related harm.

Now that we have clarified the relationship between harm reduction interventions and official drug control strategies, we turn our attention to the factors that may be preventing U.S. policy makers from implementing innovative, empirically validated interventions that successfully reduce drug-related harm. As a vehicle for this discussion, we explore the specific policies and attitudes that have prevented the widespread adoption of needle exchange programs in the United States.

NEEDLE EXCHANGE PROGRAMS: A CASE STUDY IN RESISTANCE TO HARM REDUCTION POLICY

With remarkable consistency, the U.S. government has aggressively resisted harm reduction (Kirp & Bayer, 1993; Reuter & MacCoun, 1995). For example, there are probably more than one million injecting drug users in this country, and injection drug use accounts for about one third of all AIDS cases. A considerable body of evidence demonstrates that needle exchange programs can bring about significant reductions in HIV transmission (DesJarlais, Friedman, & Ward, 1993; Lurie & Reingold, 1993). Yet there are fewer than 100 needle exchange programs operating in the United States. (MacCoun, in press)

Why does the United States have so few needle exchange programs in operation? Despite endorsement of such programs by the National Academy of Sciences and the Centers for Disease Control, "both the White House and Congress block allocation of AIDS or drug-abuse prevention funds for needle exchange, and virtually all state governments retain drug paraphernalia laws, pharmacy regulations, and other restrictions on access to sterile syringes" (Nadelmann, 1998, pp. 115–116). The reasons for opposition to harm reduction policies in general, and needle exchange programs in particular, are many and varied (Reuter & MacCoun, 1995). In this section, we evaluate a number of factors that may account for the resistance to harm reduction initiatives such as needle exchange.

A "Trojan Horse" for Legalization

Opponents of the harm reduction approach often contend that harm reduction is a "trojan horse" for drug legalization. Two proponents of this view describe it as follows:

> Although reducing the harm caused by drug use is a universal goal of all drug policies, policy proposals called "harm reduction" proposals include a creative renaming of the dismantling of legal restrictions against the use and sale of drugs. The essential components of legalization policies are couched within this concept. Much of the driving force behind the harm reduction movement also centers on personal choice and "safe" habits for drug use.... What is needed today is not the dismantling of restrictive drug policies. Rather a strong national policy should seek to reduce the harm of drug use through harm prevention (for example, by creating drug-prevention programs) and harm elimination (by implementing broader interdiction and rehabilitation efforts). ... We do not need new experiments to tell us what we have already learned from legal alcohol and tobacco. Those experiments have already been done at the cost of great human suffering. (DuPont & Voth, 1995, p. 462)

These authors are mistaken in their assumption that harm reduction efforts are directed only at illicit drug use (Chapters 4 and 5 of this book describe harm reduction approaches to the use of two legal drugs, alcohol and tobacco) or only at substance use in general (Chapter 7 describes harm reduction programs applied to high-risk sexual behaviors and the prevention of HIV infection). They are also mistaken in equating harm reduction with drug legalization, since harm reduction initiatives have been successfully implemented under a wide range of existing drug control policies. They are most mistaken in their insistence that "we do not need new experiments to tell us what we have already learned" about the use of legal and illegal drugs. In the absence of such experimentation, critics are free to speculate on the harmful consequences of "relaxing" legal restrictions on drug use.

Fear of "Sending the Wrong Message"

Another argument, once voiced by former "drug czar" William Bennett and Governor Pete Wilson of California, is that needle exchange programs (as well as other harm reduction initiatives) somehow "send the wrong message"—in other words, that they encourage or increase illicit drug use or other illicit behaviors. The logic by which this process occurs "is rarely articulated in any detail, suggesting that for its proponents, the proposition is self-evident" (MacCoun, in press).

In a recent insightful article appearing on harm reduction, MacCoun (in press) explores the potential mechanisms by which the "wrong message" might be "sent." One potential mechanism is what he refers to as the

> *rhetorical mechanism*—the notion is that irrespective of their effectiveness in reducing harms, harm reduction programs literally communicate messages that encourage drug use.... Without intending to do so, harm reduction sends tacit messages that are construed as approval—or at least the absence of strong disapproval—of drug consumption. (MacCoun, in press)

MacCoun points out that whether or not such rhetorical effects occur is an empirical question, and that without evidence concerning the kinds of unintended inferences that users and nonusers draw from harm reduction messages, this hypothesis is purely speculative.

A second possible mechanism that MacCoun elaborates upon is the "compensatory behavior mechanism"—the hypothesis that "even if no one took harm reduction to imply government endorsement of drugs, harm reduction might still influence levels of drug use indirectly through its intended effect—that is, by reducing the riskiness of drug use." The argument here is that public response to needle exchange programs and other harm reduction initiatives might be similar to drivers' response to improvements in automobile safety and mandatory seat belt laws: They compensate by driving faster and more recklessly than they would have before (Chirinko & Harper, 1993). In other words, a reduction in the risk of injection might lead drug users to take fewer precautions than before, raising the probability of their unsafe conduct to a higher level. "In both domains, some of the safety gains brought about by a reduction in the probability of harm given unsafe conduct have been offset by increases in the probability of that conduct" (MacCoun, in press). The available data, however, do not support the hypothesis of completely off-setting effects (Hughes, 1995; Stetzer & Hofman, 1996).

In sum, there is no empirical support for either a rhetorical or a compensatory behavior mechanism that could provide justification for policy makers' fear that needle exchange programs or other harm reduction interventions "send the wrong message" and thus result in increased drug use and drug-related harm. Perhaps more importantly, there *does* exist an impressive body of literature suggesting that needle exchanges do not increase illicit drug use (Lurie & Reingold, 1993; Watters, Estilo, Clark, & Lorvick, 1994; see also Chapter 7).

However, as MacCoun (in press) is quick to point out, "the empirical success record for needle exchange does not constitute blanket support for the harm reduction movement. Each intervention must be assessed empirically on its own terms."

Politics and Public Opinion

Supply reduction strategies resulting in the seizure of a boatload of cocaine, or a decrease in "drug-related" crime due to strengthened domestic law enforcement, are immediate and easily publicizable substantiations of a politician's promise to "get tough on drugs." The payoff from demand reduction strategies, such as increasing in the number of available treatment slots or improving the effectiveness of prevention programs, is generally more long-term and less glamorous.

As those familiar with politics will readily attest, public opinion is a fickle creature that does not always follow the dictates of logic and reason. This is certainly true in the case of public opinion concerning drug control policy. Research on human decision making suggests a number of ways in which such public opinion could be influenced by factors other than objective data. For example, researchers investigating judgment and decision making have found that people often "judge the probability of an uncertain event by the degree to which it is similar in essential properties to its parent population" (Kahneman & Tversky, 1972, p. 431). In the drug policy arena, the operation of this "representativeness heuristic" may help the public and their elected representatives

> justify harsh policies on the basis of a mental model that fails to differentiate drug use from abuse. Their mental image of a drug user is that of a formerly productive citizen inevitably driven to illness, financial ruin and criminality. Each new instance that fits the model reinforces the stereotype and the general conclusion, irrespective of the actual proportion of users that end up in this sorry state. (Beyerstein & Hadaway, 1990, p. 691)

Another psychological factor that may adversely influence public opinion about drug policy is the "availability heuristic." This heuristic is a mental rule of thumb according to which people's estimates of the probability of an event's occurrence are influenced by the ease with which examples come to mind (Tversky & Kahneman, 1974). "Thus, voters are more likely to become agitated about the dangers of relatively rare events such as drug overdoses, but more complacent about the far greater toll exacted by preventable illnesses or traffic fatalities" (Beyerstein & Hadaway, 1990, p. 692). The reason is that instances of the former readily spring to mind as a result of media exposure, while instances of the latter do not.

Conservativism and Morality

Many reasons for opposition to harm reduction policies are based on what MacCoun refers to as "consequentialist" grounds. "They are characterized primarily by the belief that harm reduction will be counterproductive, either by failing to reduce average harm, or by increasing drug use enough to increase total harm" (MacCoun, in press). Other grounds for opposing needle exchange or other harm reduction initiatives are what MacCoun calls "symbolic." The moral and political climate in the United States for at least the past decade could fairly be described as conservative. Along with conservative attitudes comes a general antagonism toward users of "hard drugs," partly stemming from the strong association between drugs and crime. Furthermore, many conservatives view addiction is a voluntary state, and consequently feel that drug users do not deserve help because they "did it to themselves." Finally, conservative Americans cling tightly to the notion that drug abuse is a "bad act"—a transgression against social rules that is deserving of punishment. Consequently, they are led to prefer a criminal justice rather than a public health approach to drug control policy.

CONCLUSIONS

In this concluding chapter, we have stated our criticisms of the current U.S. drug policy. To state such views in public (or in a publication) is in itself likely to provoke opposition from government officials who endorse and promote the "party line" of zero tolerance. Sometimes this lack of tolerance for opposing views can lead to censorship.

To take a personal example, one of us (G. Alan Marlatt) and some colleagues were asked to prepare a paper on the topic of keeping the drug-dependent individual in treatment. The paper was initially presented at a research conference sponsored by NIDA in May 1994, and was to be published in a research monograph entitled *Beyond the Therapeutic Alliance: Keeping the Drug-Dependent Individual in Treatment* (Onken, Blaine, & Boren, 1997). Our chapter for this monograph was entitled *Help-Seeking by Substance Abusers: The Role of Harm Reduction and Behavioral–Economic Approaches to Facilitate Treatment Entry and Retention* (Marlatt, Tucker, Donovan, & Vuchinich, 1997). In it, we reviewed the literature on correlates of help seeking for drug treatment and made several recommendations to facilitate treatment entry and retention. Harm reduction was recommended as a promising approach that may lower barriers to treatment, thus encouraging more people to seek help for their drug and alcohol problems. We completed the manuscript and submitted it for publication to NIDA in 1996.

After our chapter in the monograph was approved by the editors at NIDA, we assumed that it would appear in print as we wrote it. We were wrong. We received word that publication of the entire monograph was being held up because of some "official concern" with the conclusions presented in the final two paragraphs of the chapter. We attempted to modify the final paragraph and to "tone down" our criticisms of contemporary drug policy so that the publication of the monograph would not be delayed further. We sent in an edited ending, as requested, and awaited the publication of the final monograph (Onken, Blaine, & Boren, 1997).

When we received the final published version of our chapter in the monograph (Marlatt et al., 1997), we were surprised and dismayed to learn that the concluding paragraph of our manuscript had been cut entirely from the final published version. We had received no official word that our work had been censored prior to its publication. We were not given a choice as to whether we still wanted the chapter published. Those who have read the published chapter have told us that it ends "suddenly" and seems to come to no particular conclusion. To rectify this unfortunate situation, we would like to close this chapter (and this book) by presenting readers with the missing final paragraph. The conclusions drawn are relevant to both the original chapter and the material we have presented throughout the present book:

The various U.S. communities that are concerned with the drug problem are at a crossroads. Do we attempt to move forward in our efforts to understand and reduce the drug problem by learning from the scientific evidence on interventions, help-seeking and recovery patterns for substance disorders, and by drawing from the European harm reduction experiments those aspects of their programs that are likely to work well in the U.S.? Or, do we continue expanding the already costly "war on drugs" and neglecting intervention efforts, even in the face of the AIDS epidemic, which is now spreading into the heterosexual (including pediatric) community, primarily through sexual contact with I.V. drug users? Some may not see the choice as being quite so clear cut, and perhaps they are right. However, the stakes are too high not to engage in the debate.

REFERENCES

Aldrich, M. R. (1990). Legalize the lesser to minimize the greater: Modern applications of ancient wisdom. *Journal of Drug Issues, 20*(4), 543–553.

Association of the Bar of the City of New York. (1994). A wiser course: Ending drug prohibition. *The Record, 49*(5), 523.

Bertrand, M. A. (1990). Beyond antiprohibitionism. *Journal of Drug Issues, 20*(4), 533–542.

Beyerstein, B. L., & Hadaway, P. F. (1990). On avoiding folly. *Journal of Drug Issues, 20*(4), 689–700.

Burroughs, W. S. (1959). *Naked lunch.* New York: Grove Press.

Center for Substance Abuse Treatment. (1996, September). *The National Treatment Improvement Evaluation Study, preliminary report: The persistent effects of substance abuse treatment—One year later.* Rockville, MD: U.S. Department of Health and Human Services.

Chesher, G., & Wodack, A. (1990). Evolving a new policy for illicit drugs. *Journal of Drug Issues, 20*(4), 555–561.

Chirinko, R. S., & Harper, E. P. (1993). Buckle up or slow down?: New estimates of offsetting behavior and their implications for automobile safety regulation. *Journal of Policy Analysis and Management, 123,* 270–296.

Des Jarlais, D. C. (1995). Harm reduction: A framework for incorporating science into drug policy [Editorial]. *American Journal of Public Health, 85*(1), 10–11.

Des Jarlais, D. C., Friedman, S. R., & Ward, T. P. (1993). Harm reduction: A public health response to the AIDS epidemic among injecting drug users. *Annual Review of Public Health, 14*, 413–450.

Donaldson, S. I., Graham, J. W., Piccinin, A. M., & Hansen, W. B. (1995). Resistance-skills training and onset of alcohol use: Evidence for beneficial and potentially harmful effects in public schools and in private Catholic schools. *Health Psychology, 14*(4), 291–300.

DuPont, R. L., & Voth, E. A. (1995). Drug legalization, harm reduction, and drug policy. *Annals of Internal Medicine, 123*, 461–469.

Dusenbury, L., Botvin, G. J., & James-Ortiz, S. (1989). The primary prevention of adolescent substance abuse through the promotion of personal and social competence. *Prevention in Human Services, 7*(1), 201–224.

Ennett, S. T., Tobler, N. S., Ringwalt, C. L., & Fleming, R. L. (1994). How effective is D.A.R.E.?: A meta-analysis of Project D.A.R.E. outcome evaluations. *American Journal of Public Health, 84*, 1394–1401.

Erikson, P. G. (1990). A public health approach to demand reduction. *Journal of Drug Issues, 20*(4), 563–575.

Ferguson, S. (1997, January 6). The battle for medical marijuana. *Nation*, pp. 14–17.

Gerstein, D. R., Johnson, R. A., Harwood, H. J., Fountain, D., Suter N., & Malloy, K. (1994). *Evaluating recovery services: The California Drug and Alcohol Treatment Assessment (CALDATA)*. Sacramento: California Department of Alcohol and Drug Programs.

Grinspoon, L., & Bakalar, J. B. (1994). The war on drugs: A peace proposal. *New England Journal of Medicine, 330*(5), 357–360.

Hart, R. (1994). U. S. drug laws: An introduction. *New England Journal of Medicine, 330*(5), 356–357.

Holmes, S. A. (1994, November 6). The boom in jails is locking up lots of loot. *The New York Times*, p. E3.

Hughes, J. R. (1995). Applying harm reduction to smoking. *Tobacco Control, 4*, S33–S38.

Institute of Medicine. (1994). *Reducing risks for mental disorders: Frontiers for preventive intervention research*. Washington, DC: National Academy Press.

Jarvik, M. E. (1990). The drug dilemma: Manipulating the demand. *Science, 250*, 387–392.

Johnston, L. (1996). *Monitoring the Future Study—1996* [Press release]. Ann Arbor: University of Michigan.

Kahneman, D., & Tversky, A. (1972). Subjective probability: A judgment of representativeness. *Cognitive Psychology, 3*, 430–454.

Kirp, D. L., & Bayer, R. (1993). The politics. In J. Stryker & M. D. Smith (Eds.), *Dimensions of HIV prevention: Needle exchange* (pp. 77–98). Menlo Park, CA: Henry J. Kaiser Foundation.

Luepker, R. V., Johnson, C. A., Murray, D. M., & Pechacek, T. F. (1983). The prevention of cigarette smoking: Three year follow-up of an educational program for youth. *Journal of Behavioral Medicine, 6*(1), 53–62.

Lurie, P., & Reingold, A. L. (Eds.). (1993). *The public health impact of needle exchange programs in the United States and abroad*. Berkeley: School of Public Health, University of California at Berkeley/San Francisco; Institute for Health Policy Studies, University of California at San Francisco.

MacCoun, R. J. (in press). Toward a psychology of harm reduction. *American Psychologist.*

Marlatt, G. A. (1996). Harm reduction: Come as you are. *Addictive Behaviors, 21*(6), 777–788.

Marlatt, G. A., Baer, J. S., & Quigley, L. A. (1995). Self-efficacy and addictive behaviors. In A. Bandura (Ed.), *Self-efficacy in changing societies* (pp. 289–315). New York: Cambridge University Press.

Marlatt, G. A., Tucker, J. A., Donovan, D. M., & Vuchinich, R. E. (1997). Help-seeking by substance abusers: The role of harm reduction and behavioral-economic approaches to facilitate treatment entry and retention. In L. S. Onken, J. D. Blaine, & J. J. Boren (Eds.), *Beyond the therapeutic alliance: Keeping the drug-dependent individual in treatment* (NIDA Research Monograph No. 165, pp. 44–84). Rockville, MD: U.S. Department of Health and Human Services.

McMillon, R. (1993). Hard time: Mandatory minimum sentencing comes under congressional scrutiny. *American Bar Association Journal, 79,* 100.

Miller, W. R., & Heather, N. (in press). *Treating addictive behaviors.* New York: Plenum Press.

Nadelmann, E. A. (1989). Drug prohibition in the United States: Costs, consequences, and alternatives. *Science, 245,* 939–946.

Nadelmann, E. A. (1992). America's drug problem: A case for decriminalization. *Dissent, 39*(2), 205–212.

Nadelmann, E. A. (1998). Commonsense drug policy. *Foreign Affairs, 77*(1), 111–126.

National Criminal Justice Reference Service (NCJRS). (1998). *Federal drug control spending by goal and function, FY 1996–1998* [On-line]. Available: http://www.ncjrs.org [January 25, 1998].

Newcomb, M. D. (1992). Substance abuse and control in the united states: Ethical and legal issues. *Social Science and Medicine, 35*(3–4), 471–479.

New York County Lawyers Association (NYCLA). (1996). *Report and recommendations of the Drug Policy Task Force.* New York: Author.

Office of National Drug Control Policy (ONDCP). (1997). *National drug control strategy for 1997* [On-line]. Available: http://www.ncjrs.org [January 25, 1998].

Onken, L. S., Blaine, J. D., & Boren, J. J. (Eds.). (1997). *Beyond the therapeutic alliance: Keeping the drug-dependent individual in treatment* (NIDA Research Monograph No. 165). Rockville, MD: U.S. Department of Health and Human Services.

Pollan, M. (1997, July 20). Living with medical marijuana (California Proposition 215). *New York Times Magazine,* p. 22.

Reuter, P., & Caulkins, J. P. (1995). Redefining the goals of national drug policy: Recommendations from a working group. *American Journal of Public Health, 85*(8), 1059–1063.

Reuter, P., & MacCoun, R. (1995). Drawing lessons from the absence of harm reduction in American drug policy. *Tobacco Control, 4,* S28–S32.

Reuters. (1998, January 19). 100,000 additional inmates in U.S. jails: The prison population rises to 1.7 million. *The Seattle Times,* p. A4.

Roth, J. A. (1994). *Psychoactive substances and violence* (Research in Brief Series). Washington, DC: U.S. Department of Justice.

Stetzer, A., & Hofman, D. A. (1996). Risk compensation: Implications for safety interventions. *Organizational Behavior and Human Decision Processes, 66,* 73–88.

Substance Abuse and Mental Health Services Administration (SAMHSA). (1996). *Preliminary estimates from the 1995 National Household Survey on Drug Abuse.* Rockville, MD: U.S. Department of Health and Human Services.

Tversky, A., & Kahneman, D. (1974). Judgment under uncertainty: Heuristics and biases. *Science, 185,* 1124–1131.

U.S. General Accounting Office (GAO). (1997, February 27). *Drug control: Long-standing problems hinder U.S. international efforts* (Report No. GAO/NSIAD-97-75). Gaithersburg, MD: Author.

Watters, J. K., Estilo, M. J., Clark, G. L., & Lorvick, J. (1994). Syringe and needle exchange as HIV/AIDS prevention for injection drug users. *Journal of the American Medical Association, 271,* 115–120.

Weil, A. (1972). *The natural mind: An investigation of drugs and the higher consciousness.* Boston: Houghton-Mifflin.

Wren, C. S. (1998, January 9). Alcohol or drugs tied to 80% of inmates. *The New York Times,* p. A14.

Index

'i' indicates an illustration; 'n' indicates a note; 't' indicates a table

Lightning Source UK Ltd.
Milton Keynes UK
17 March 2010

151514UK00001B/28/P